HELPING THE NONCOMPLIANT CHILD

Helping the Noncompliant Child

SECOND EDITION

Family-Based Treatment for Oppositional Behavior

ROBERT J. McMAHON
REX L. FOREHAND

Foreword by Sharon L. Foster

THE GUILFORD PRESS
New York   London

© 2003 The Guilford Press
A Division of Guilford Publications, Inc.
72 Spring Street, New York, NY 10012
www.guilford.com

Paperback edition 2005

Printed in the United States of America

This book is printed on acid-free paper.

Last digit is print number: 9   8   7   6   5   4

Library of Congress Cataloging-in-Publication Data

McMahon, Robert J. (Robert Joseph), 1953–
  Helping the noncompliant child : family-based treatment for oppositional behavior / by
Robert J. McMahon, Rex L. Forehand.—2nd ed.
     p. cm.
Includes bibliographical references and index.
   ISBN 1-57230-612-2 (hc)   ISBN 1-59385-241-X (pbk)
   1. Family psychotherapy.   2. Child rearing.   3. Conduct disorders in children.
I. Forehand, Rex L. (Rex Lloyd), 1945–   II. Title.
   RC488.5.M398 2003
   649'.64—dc21
                                                                2003001947

To our partners, Joanne and Lell;
our children, Patrick, Colleen, Laura, and Greg;
our mothers, Mary Wells McMahon
and Sara H. Forehand;
and to our fathers, Robert J. McMahon, Jr.,
and Rex L. Forehand, who passed away during the
preparation of this book

About the Authors

Robert J. McMahon, PhD, is Professor of Psychology at the University of Washington in Seattle. He is also a member of the Conduct Problems Prevention Research Group and Principal Investigator at the Seattle site of the Fast Track Project, an NIMH-funded multisite, longitudinal investigation of the prevention of early-starting conduct problems in high-risk children. Dr. McMahon has coedited a number of books, including *The Effects of Parental Dysfunction on Children* (2002, Kluwer Academic/Plenum Press) and *Preventing Childhood Disorders, Substance Abuse, and Delinquency* (1996, Sage) (both with Ray DeV. Peters), and serves on the editorial boards of several journals.

Rex L. Forehand, PhD, is Professor of Psychology at the University of Vermont and Regents Professor Emeritus at the University of Georgia. He is also Principal Investigator of a CDC-funded parenting project. Dr. Forehand is coauthor of *Parenting the Strong-Willed Child* (2002, McGraw-Hill) and *Making Divorce Easier on Your Child: 50 Effective Ways to Help Children Adjust* (2002, McGraw-Hill) (both with Nicholas Long). He is a member of 10 editorial boards.

Foreword

Many copies of *Helping the Noncompliant Child* have had favored places on my bookshelf since the first edition was published in 1981. My copies disappeared with regularity as graduate student supervisees treating noncompliant children asked, "What should I do?" I discussed the case with them, then handed them my copy of *Helping the Noncompliant Child* and said, "Come back when you've read this." They came back with a more sophisticated understanding of noncompliance and its assessment and treatment. Unfortunately, they rarely returned my copies of the book.

Times have changed in the 20-plus years since the first edition appeared, in part because of the efforts and successes of scientists like Bob McMahon and Rex Forehand. Parent training is now widely used both in treatment and in prevention settings. Parent training has become part of many interventions aimed at populations that span the age spectrum from preschool to adolescence. Many of the scientifically based practices described in this volume, too, have come into widespread use as part of contemporary childrearing in the United States. For example, many parents found "time out" to be an unusual discipline strategy in the early days of parent training. Now it is not uncommon to hear a parent in a public place caution a young child on the verge of misbehaving with the words, "Do you want a time out?"

The science of treatment and prevention that underscores this volume has changed as well. We understand the evolution of conduct problems more fully than we did when this book was first crafted. A growing number of increasingly sophisticated clinical trials have evaluated interventions to reduce and prevent child behavior problems such as noncompliance and aggression. Treatment and prevention scientists are more ambitious in their goals, seeking to disseminate evidence-based interventions in an effort to take the most efficacious and effective interventions into public health arenas. They are also more humble, recognizing that even the best of our interventions do not reach or help every troubled child and family.

The second edition of *Helping the Noncompliant Child* reflects the growing sophistication of the field. McMahon and Forehand have completely revised and updated the volume to reflect the research they and others have conducted over the last two decades. Much of this research underscores the importance of intervening with young children and noncompliance as a way of preventing more serious, entrenched problems as the child ages and the child's difficulties compound. Portions of the book also draw from the authors' extensive experience implementing the approach with families in clinic and school settings.

The book retains the strengths of the original—it is clear, specific, and contains the materials a clinician needs to implement the approach. It is also a model of the scientist-practictioner approach at its best, showing the cumulation of systematic knowledge over many years of research, translated into methods clinicians can use to intervene with young children and their caregivers and to assess whether their efforts are successful. Many of the specific implementation suggestions derive from an impressive body of research that systematically evaluated not only the outcomes of the program, but also some of the specific parameters that could be incorporated to make the approach more efficacious and acceptable. Although many variations of parent training exist, few are as well researched and replicated as this one.

Like the children McMahon and Forehand treated in the early days of parent training, *Helping the Noncompliant Child* has matured. The roots of the approach, firmly grounded in science, provided the nutrition for evolution and growth. Changes from the earlier volume reflect the growing integration of behavioral interventions with children, with a focus on the broader context in which parents and children operate. The volume extends intervention to consider the couple's relationship, the child's behavior in the school, and parent adjustment, when necessary for the success of parent training. McMahon and Forehand also consider applications of the approach to children with difficulties in addition to noncompliance, such as attentional problems, medical problems, and developmental disabilities. At the same time, the authors never lose sight of the fact that the goal of parent training with young children is to improve the child's compliance with directives—not to create a docile child, but rather to give the child a good start on a developmental trajectory that will lead to better relationships with family members, teachers, and peers, and will reduce the likelihood of future problems as the child matures.

How long a "shelf life" will this version of *Helping the Noncompliant Child* have on my bookshelf? Not long, I suspect. After all, some things do not change. Graduate students still need to know how to treat noncompliant children by using the best available strategies. People still forget to return the books they find most useful. And top notch scientist-practitioners like McMahon and Forehand continue to refine their work to bring the best of available science and practice to the treatment community—and ultimately to children and families.

SHARON L. FOSTER, PHD
Alliant International University

Preface

The purpose of this book is to provide a detailed description of the Helping the Non-compliant Child (HNC) program, which is designed to teach parents to improve their young children's noncompliance and related oppositional behavior. The program is formulated on social learning principles and is designed primarily for the parents of 3- to 8-year-old children. We have been extensively involved in the development, implementation, and evaluation of this parent training program over the past 30 years. The impetus for the first edition of HNC in 1981 was the large number of "how to do it" inquiries from other mental health professionals that came about as the applicability and success of HNC became known. That volume, which was one of the first behaviorally oriented parent training manuals, has been well received.

So, why a second edition? In the 20-plus years since publication of the first edition of HNC, several events have occurred that necessitated revision of this book. First, we now have a much better picture (albeit still somewhat incomplete and evolving) of the developmental pathways by which young children go on to develop serious conduct problems in later childhood and adolescence. It has become clear that early child noncompliance is a "keystone" behavior in the early starter pathway of conduct problems. Similarly, the importance of family processes and parenting practices throughout this period, but especially during the preschool and early school-age periods, has been increasingly well documented. Second, our experiences, and those of others, in implementing the HNC program have led us to refine and extend our intervention and assessment procedures. Those improvements are reflected in this volume. Third, although the basic empirical evaluations of HNC were described in the first edition, there have been a number of important additions to the research support for HNC that we felt were important to include. Fourth, although HNC was originally developed as a *treatment* for child noncompliance, it has become increasingly clear to us and others that interventions such as HNC can also play an important role in the *prevention* of more serious conduct problems that develop later in childhood and adolescence. Finally, as before, we hope that dissemination of our current work will lead to the replication and extension of our procedures by others.

This book is intended for professionals and paraprofessionals who are involved in counseling parents of young children who present with problems of noncompliance or other oppositional conduct problems, whether in traditional treatment settings or in a preventive context. There are several prerequisites that are essential for effectively using this book. Foremost is a basic knowledge of social learning principles, child development, and an awareness of typical problems experienced by young children. In addition, experience in behavioral counseling is also desirable. We should also point out that there is some question as to whether simply reading a training manual of this type is sufficient for utilizing its contents effectively in the clinical setting. In training graduate students and mental health professionals, we use written and videotaped materials, in conjunction with modeling, role playing, and guided practice of the therapist skills. Discussion and verbal feedback are also extensively employed. Finally, as noted above, we consider our work in parent training to be an ongoing process. Many of the refinements and adaptations to the HNC program that have been incorporated into this second edition are evidence of that process. We hope that such refinements will continue as a result of our own endeavors as well as those of other clinical researchers.

This edition consists of 10 chapters and 4 appendices. The first chapter provides a context for the HNC parent training program by describing the "normal" development of compliance and noncompliance, and then focusing on the role of noncompliance in the development of early-starting conduct problems. In Chapter 2, we provide an overview of parent training as an intervention approach for treating child conduct problems, with particular attention paid to the model of parent training developed by Dr. Constance Hanf and the various parent training programs derived from it (including the one described in this book). Chapter 3 provides an overview of the HNC program. The fourth chapter describes the assessment methods and procedures that we employ. Emphasis is placed on the use of multiple measures (including direct observation of parent–child interaction) to formulate a treatment plan and to evaluate the success of treatment. Chapters 5–7 provide detailed instructions on the implementation of the HNC program. Chapter 5 focuses on how to provide feedback to parents concerning the assessment findings and how to describe the HNC program to them. We also provide a session-by-session example of the program in outline form. The sixth chapter focuses on the Phase I (Differential Attention) skills of attends, rewards, and ignoring. In Chapter 7, we present the Phase II (Compliance Training) skills concerned with the clear instructions sequence and standing rules. Applications of the parenting skills to siblings and to situations outside the home are also presented in this chapter. In Chapter 8, we describe four sets of adjunctive interventions that we have developed to enhance the effectiveness and generalization of our treatment effects. Chapter 9, which was written by our colleague Karen Wells, describes how the HNC program can be adapted for special populations, including children with attention-deficit/hyperactivity disorder, children who are abused and neglected, children with developmental disabilities, children with enuresis or encopresis, and children in medical and inpatient psychiatric settings. In Chapter 10, we present a comprehensive review of research with the HNC parent training program. The chapter concludes with an overview of some of our current efforts in the area of prevention. Appendices include a greatly expanded set of parent handouts and record sheets, some of the assessment measures that we employ, and one of the adjunctive interventions.

As in all endeavors of this nature, there are many individuals who have played critical roles in our thinking and practice. Constance Hanf was the initial guiding light for HNC, and for many other parent training programs derived from her pioneering work. The seminal work of Jerry Patterson, John Reid, and their colleagues at the Oregon Social Learning Center has played, and continues to play, a critical role in our understanding of the primary role of the family in the development of conduct problems. We have also benefited from the writings of, and our discussions with, Russ Barkley, Chuck Cunningham, Mark Dadds, Tom Dishion, Jean Dumas, Sheila Eyberg, Sharon Foster, Hy Hops, Alan Hudson, Judy Hutchings, Kate Kavanagh, Eric Mash, Carol Metzler, Laurie Miller Brotman, Ron Prinz, Matt Sanders, Stephen Scott, Danny Shaw, Jim Snyder, Bob Wahler, Hill Walker, and Carolyn Webster-Stratton. Thanks also to the "regulars" at the Social Learning and the Family Preconference at AABT and to colleagues in the Conduct Problems Prevention Research Group (Karen Bierman, John Coie, Ken Dodge, Michael Foster, Mark Greenberg, John Lochman, and Ellen Pinderhughes).

In the more than 20 years since we wrote the first edition of *Helping the Noncompliant Child*, we have had the good fortune to work with wonderful colleagues who have contributed directly to the evolution of the HNC parent training program. Three of those individuals have been particularly influential: Mark Roberts, Karen Wells, and Nicholas Long. In addition, we have had the opportunity to work with dedicated students and postdoctoral fellows over the years at the University of Georgia, the University of British Columbia, and the University of Washington. They include Lisa Armistead, Beverly Atkeson, Cynthia Baum, Steve Beck, Cathy Bond, Jeri Breiner, Susan Cross Calvert, Glen Davies, Ron Fauber, Gene Flessati, Bill Furey, Ken Green, Doug Griest, Steve Hobbs, Lew Humphreys, Kim Johnson, Betty King, Karla Klein, Beth Kotchick, Julie Kotler, Bob Leahy, Karen Lehman, Patricia Long, Jimmy Middlebrook, Bryan Neighbors, Steve Peed, Patricia Resick, Dana Rhule, Katie Robbins, Tim Rogers, Ric Steele, Amanda Thomas, Georgia Tiedemann, and Michelle Wierson. We would also like to express our appreciation to our colleagues "in the trenches" who have provided important assistance and ideas over the years, especially Tom DuHamel, Lew Humphreys, Loyd Nicholson, and Nancy Slough. Sandy Gary, Julie Kotler, and Ann Shaffer provided invaluable "in-house" editorial support and feedback throughout. Thanks also to Sharon Foster and Nick Long for their thoughtful and constructive reviews of earlier versions of the manuscript.

We are extremely grateful to the many children and parents with whom we have worked with over the years. We hope that we have improved their lives by some small measure.

It is pro forma for authors to express their appreciation to publishing staff and family members for their long-suffering patience during the preparation of the book. In our case, this appreciation is genuine and deep-seated. At The Guilford Press, Editor-in-

Chief Seymour Weingarten has been a supporter and advocate of *Helping the Noncompliant Child* since the beginning, and his willingness to stay with us during the many fits and starts that have characterized the preparation of this second edition speaks to his endurance and, perhaps, to his potential for canonization. Although a relative newcomer to the project, Senior Editor Barbara Watkins provided incredibly helpful assistance and direction in shaping the final nature of the book. Senior Production Editor Laura Specht Patchkofsky was instrumental in the final production process. Thanks, too, to Executive Editor Kitty Moore, for her kind words and encouragement.

Closer to home, our families have supported our efforts and tolerated our absences through long nights, missed weekends, and preoccupied minds, with far fewer expressions of annoyance than we expected or deserved. Finally, special thanks goes to Reverend Thomas F. McMahon, CSV—academic role model and favorite uncle.

Contents

HELPING THE NONCOMPLIANT CHILD

CHAPTER 1

Child Compliance
and Noncompliance

In this chapter, we first define "compliance" and "noncompliance" as they are used in this book. The role of compliance and noncompliance in normal development is presented. We then focus on developmentally inappropriate aspects of these two behaviors. Relevant DSM-IV diagnostic categories are presented, followed by a description of the "early starter" pathway for the development of serious conduct problems.

"No!" Is there a word more familiar to parents of toddlers? Indeed, not only do all children learn to say "no" to their parents, doing so is considered a normal characteristic of the developing 2- to 3-year-old. Moreover, saying "no" may even be an expression of a toddler's emerging sense of identity, self-regulation, and independence (Greenspan, 1991). However, for some families, what begins as apparently age-appropriate behavior develops into a severe and unmanageable problem. In such cases, parents feel frustrated, helpless, and ineffective as their children become more and more defiant and oppositional. Such children refuse to follow directions and rules set by parents, teachers, and other adults. In short, these children are excessively *noncompliant*, consistently refusing to initiate or complete actions requested by other people.

The focus of this book is on the development of excessive noncompliance in young (3- to 8-year-old) children, the assessment of noncompliance (and related conduct problems) in children who are referred for treatment, and especially the description of effective family-based intervention procedures for dealing with these children.

DEFINITIONS OF COMPLIANCE
AND NONCOMPLIANCE

Defining what is meant by compliance and noncompliance is a difficult task. One operational definition of *compliance* is "appropriate following of an instruction to perform a specific response within a reasonable and/or designated time" (Schoen, 1983, p. 493).

1

Forehand (1977) noted the importance of distinguishing between the *initiation* of compliance within a reasonable time after a command given by an adult and the *completion* of the task specified in the command. With respect to the initiation of compliance, it is necessary to determine an appropriate time interval to allow the child to begin compliance. These intervals have typically ranged from 5 to 15 seconds, partly depending upon the age of the child. (As will be seen later, we employ a 5-second criterion for initiation of compliance.)

In the first edition of this book (Forehand & McMahon, 1981), we defined *noncompliance* as the refusal to initiate or complete a request made by another person. This typically occurs when one person (e.g., a parent or teacher) issues a command or instruction to another person (i.e., a child). However, it also involves failure to follow a previously stated rule that is currently in effect (e.g., "You may not hit your sister"). Whining, playing with matches, fighting, destroying property, "smart-talking," and many other child inappropriate behaviors can be viewed as noncompliance using such a conceptualization. In addition, many of these inappropriate behaviors are used frequently by children to either escape from or avoid having to follow through on a command or rule. Thus, we view noncompliance as a *keystone* behavior in the child's social development. We will have more to say about this later. It is important to note that compliance and noncompliance, by definition, are interactional processes that involve the person who gives the command or makes the rule (in this case, the parent or teacher) and the person to whom the command or rule is directed (the child). It is also the case that there are bidirectional effects: the child's characteristics and previous behavior concerning compliance and noncompliance affect the parent's behavior toward the child, as well as vice versa (Kuczynski & Hildebrandt, 1997; Maccoby & Martin, 1983; Patterson, 1997). This focus on the interactional aspects of compliance and noncompliance with parental behavior is key to the conceptualization of their role in children's social development, the assessment of the problem in clinic-referred families, and the design of effective interventions.

In developmental research with normal children, a number of distinctions have been made between various types of compliance and noncompliance. With respect to compliance, a primary distinction has been made between "situational" compliance, which is based on an expectation of punishment or reward, and "receptive" (Maccoby & Martin, 1983) or "committed" (Kochanska & Aksan, 1995) compliance, which occurs in the context of a general willingness to cooperate. Receptive/committed compliance is considered to be a more developmentally advanced form of compliance and is associated with internalization of parental rules (Kochanska, Coy, & Murray, 2001). Kochanska and colleagues (2001) found that situational compliance stabilized by age 2 but committed compliance increased until age 3 in a sample of children followed from ages 1 to 4. Thus, in terms of social development, normal children engage in progressively greater proportions of committed compliance as they move through the preschool period.

With respect to noncompliance, Kuczynski and Kochanski (1990; Kuczynski, Kochanski, Radke-Yarrow, & Girnius-Brown, 1987) described four types, which reflect varying degrees of developmental sophistication: (1) direct defiance, in which the noncompliance is accompanied by hostile, angry, or oppositional behavior; (2) passive noncompliance, in which the child ignores the parental command; (3) simple noncompliance, in which the child acknowledges the command but refuses to comply, although not in an angry, oppositional manner; and (4) negotiation, in which the child attempts to renegotiate the nature or conditions of the command. Direct defiance and passive noncompliance, which are seen as the least developmentally sophisticated strategies, are predictive of externalizing behavior problems at age 5. Negotiation is viewed as the most developmentally sophisticated strategy. However, it is important to note that, for some children, negotiation strategies may serve as a manipulative means for the child to escape from or avoid the parent's instruction (Walker & Walker, 1991).

THE SIGNIFICANCE OF COMPLIANCE AND NONCOMPLIANCE

So, why is it useful or important to help children develop appropriate levels of compliance and noncompliance? It is clear that child compliance and noncompliance are significant concerns for parents and teachers. Approximately 50% of parents of nonreferred 4- to 7-year-olds reported "disobedience at home" to be a problem (Achenbach & Edelbrock, 1981). Noncompliance is consistently rated as a primary reason for referral by parents who bring their children to outpatient mental health clinics for assistance. For example, 80–90% of parents of referred 4- to 7-year-old children reported noncompliance in the home to be a problem (Achenbach & Edelbrock, 1981). It is also the case that a parent's report of high levels of noncompliance at home (and to a lesser extent at school) is among the better discriminators of children's referral status (Achenbach & Edelbrock, 1981; Achenbach, Howell, Quay, & Conners, 1991; Dumas, 1996).

Similarly, teachers place a great deal of importance on compliance in the classroom setting. In several large surveys, Walker and colleagues (noted in Walker, 1995) found that "child complies with teacher commands" and "follows established classroom rules" were rated by teachers as the two most important behaviors for classroom adjustment out of 56 behaviors. In addition, the items "child behaves inappropriately in class when corrected (e.g., shouts back, defies the teacher, etc.)" and "child ignores teacher warnings or reprimands" were rated, respectively, as the third and tenth least acceptable behaviors out of 51 maladaptive behaviors.

Finally, noncompliance is a concern for parents of children with special needs of various types. For example, both parents (Tavormina, Henggeler, & Gayton, 1976) and teachers (Wehman & McLaughlin, 1979) of children with mental retardation rated noncompliance as the most significant problem that they faced in dealing with these children. In pediatric psychology outpatient services, noncompliance is the parent's top behavioral concern (e.g., Charlop, Parrish, Fenton, & Cataldo, 1987). Noncompliance also has been identified as a significant problem in subpopulations in the school setting, such as children with behavior disorders or developmental disabilities (see Walker & Walker, 1991).

What are "normal" rates of compliance and noncompliance? This is extremely difficult to answer because of the many variations in relevant parameters that occur across studies. These parameters include definition and measurement, the nature of the sample (normal, at-risk, clinic-referred), age of the child, nature of the task, and the experimental setting.

Having noted these difficulties in interpretation, there are data that provide some guidelines. For example, Whiting and Edwards (1988) reported the percentage of child compliance to parental commands in observational studies of 12 cultures. Compliance was 72% for 2- to 3-year-olds, 79% for 4- to 5-year-olds, and 82% for 6- to 8-year-olds. Girls were generally more compliant than boys. Brumfield and Roberts (1998) reported compliance rates of 32% for 2- and 3-year-old children and 78% for 4- and 5-year-old children in a standardized situation. There was no evidence of sex effects. In his review of normative studies, the second author of this volume (Forehand, 1977) reported 60–80% compliance rates to parental commands in "normal" preschool-age children. He suggested that compliance rates less than 60% were clinically significant; however, he also noted that there is a great deal of overlap between clinic and nonclinic groups. An observational study of children's compliance to teacher commands in kindergarten through grade 3 classrooms reported compliance rates ranging from 72% (for maladjusted children) to 90% (for well-adjusted children) (Strain, Lambert, Kerr, Stagg, & Lenkner, 1983). Similarly, Jacobs and colleagues (2000) reported that noncompliance occurred 17% of the time in which there was an opportunity to comply. The bottom line is that there is a limited amount of normative data on this important issue (Forehand, 1977; Houlihan, Sloane, Jones, & Patten, 1992).

THE DEVELOPMENT OF COMPLIANCE AND NONCOMPLIANCE IN NORMAL (NONREFERRED) CHILDREN

Significant advances have been made in the delineation of the development of compliance and noncompliance in nonreferred children since the first edition of this book was published. Research by Joan Grusec, Claire Kopp, Leon Kuczynski, Grazyna Kochanska, and their colleagues has been especially relevant. A book edited by Grusec and Kuczynski (1997) summarizes many areas of research that focus on the role of parenting in children's internalization of values.

The development of compliance has been viewed as important because of the critical role that it plays in many seminal areas of development, including autonomy, internalization of moral values (i.e., conscience), self-control, and socialization. The second and third years of life are particularly important for the emergence of these skills (e.g., Kochanska, Tjebkes, & Forman, 1998; Kopp, 1982). Children begin to develop the ability for self-regulation at this age. Part of this emergent skill is the cognitive capability to understand parental commands and the physical ability to carry them out (Schroeder & Gordon, 2002). Parental expectations with respect to socialization of the child increase, but so does the child's "negativism" (Wenar, 1982), which is a function of the child's increasing autonomy. As Kuczynski and Hildebrandt (1997) point out, "at a time that children are more and more *able* to comply, they become less and less *willing* to comply" (p. 241). However, as children progress through the preschool period, they gradually become more cooperative, with increasing skill in the use of negotiation strategies (e.g., Kuczynski & Kochanska, 1990). Thus, by the time that most children begin elementary school, they are well situated to handle the increasing social demands that will be placed on them as they enter school and are faced with an expanded social context of peers and other adults (i.e., teachers) with whom it is necessary to get along.

The work of developmental psychologists has been central in describing the development of compliance and noncompliance in nonreferred, "normal" children during the toddler and preschool periods. However, the theoretical and empirical contributions of child clinical and developmental psychopathology researchers such as Gerald Patterson, Robert Wahler, Susan Campbell, and Daniel Shaw suggest that the generalization of this developmental sequence to high-risk or clinic-referred children may be questionable. It is clearly the case that some children amplify and solidify their noncompliant behavior during the preschool period. Patterson (1982) described noncompliant children as displaying "arrested socialization," and it has been suggested that perhaps these children are expressing more developmentally immature forms of noncompliance (Kuczynski & Hildebrandt, 1997). How does this happen, and why? We now turn to an examination of compliance and noncompliance in the context of "deviant" development.

COMPLIANCE AND NONCOMPLIANCE AS "DEVIANT" DEVELOPMENT

The Role of Noncompliance in the Development of Conduct Problems

Noncompliance appears to be a keystone behavior in the development of conduct problems. As we will demonstrate, noncompliance appears early in the progression of conduct problems, plays a critical role in the development of both overt and covert conduct problem behaviors, and continues to be manifested in subsequent developmental periods (e.g., Chamberlain & Patterson, 1995; Edelbrock, 1985), playing a role in these children's subsequent academic and peer relationship problems. Excessive noncompliance is integral to the development of the coercive cycle (Patterson, Reid, & Dishion, 1992) in the "early starter" pathway of conduct problems, which we will describe later in the chapter. Low levels of compliance are also associated with referral for services in children with conduct problems (e.g., Dumas, 1996). Furthermore, intervention research has shown that when clinicians target child noncompliance, other conduct problem behaviors also improve as well (Parrish, Cataldo, Kolko, Neef, & Egel, 1986; Russo, Cataldo, & Cushing, 1981; Wells, Forehand, & Griest, 1980).

Diagnostic Categories

Noncompliance may be manifested in a variety of child behavior disorders. Relevant categories from the current edition of the *Diagnostic and Statistical Manual of Mental Disorders* (4th ed.—Text Revision) (DSM-IV-TR; American Psychiatric Association,

2000) are listed in Table 1.1. The two diagnostic categories that are most relevant to child noncompliance—oppositional defiant disorder (ODD) and conduct disorder (CD)—are described in the attention-deficit and disruptive behavior disorders section of the DSM-IV-TR. The behaviors comprising these two diagnostic categories are often referred to as "conduct problems."

The essential feature of ODD is a "recurrent pattern of negativistic, defiant, disobedient, and hostile behavior toward authority figures" (p. 100). The pattern of behavior must have a duration of at least 6 months, and at least four of the eight behaviors listed in Table 1.2 must be present. The behaviors must have a higher frequency than would be observed in other children of a comparable age and developmental level. Furthermore, the behaviors must lead to significant impairment in social or academic functioning.

The essential feature of CD is a "repetitive and persistent pattern of behavior in which the basic rights of others or major age-appropriate societal norms or rules are violated" (p. 93). At least 3 of the 15 behaviors listed in Table 1.3 must have been present in the past 12 months, with at least 1 of the behaviors present in the past 6 months. The behaviors are categorized into four groups: (1) aggression toward people and animals, (2) destruction of property, (3) deceitfulness or theft, and (4) serious violations of rules. One of the two subtypes of CD described in the DSM-IV is relevant to this discussion. The childhood-onset type is defined by the onset of at least 1 of the 15 behaviors prior to 10 years of age. (The adolescent-onset type, by definition, will not be a focus in this book.) The severity of CD (mild, moderate, severe) may be noted, based on the number of behaviors and their relative seriousness. Although ODD includes behaviors, such as noncompliance, that are also included in CD, it does not involve the more serious behaviors that represent violation of either the basic rights of others or age-appropriate so-

TABLE 1.1. DSM-IV Child Behavior Disorders and Related Conditions Associated with Child Noncompliance

Primary disorders	
Oppositional defiant disorder	Adjustment disorder with disturbance of conduct
Conduct disorder	Adjustment disorder with mixed disturbance of emotions and conduct
Attention-deficit/hyperactivity disorder	Disruptive behavior disorder not otherwise specified

Related conditions	
Child or adolescent antisocial behavior	Noncompliance with treatment
Parent–child relational problem	Problems related to abuse or neglect
Sibling relational problem	

Other disorders	
Mood disorders	Encopresis
Psychotic disorders	Mental retardation
Enuresis	Autistic disorder

TABLE 1.2. DSM-IV Symptoms of Oppositional Defiant Disorder

1. Loses temper
2. Argues with adults
3. Actively defies or refuses to comply with adults' requests or rules
4. Deliberately annoys people
5. Blames others for his or her mistakes or misbehavior
6. Touchy or easily annoyed by others
7. Angry and resentful
8. Spiteful or vindictive

Note. Adapted from American Psychiatric Association (2000). Copyright 2000 by the American Psychiatric Association. Adapted by permission.

TABLE 1.3. DSM-IV Symptoms of Conduct Disorder

<u>Aggression toward people and animals</u>

1. Bullies, threatens, or intimidates others frequently
2. Initiates physical fights frequently
3. Used a weapon that can cause serious physical harm to others (e.g., a bat, brick, broken bottle, knife, gun)
4. Physically cruel to people
5. Physically cruel to animals
6. Has stolen while confronting a victim (e.g., mugging, purse snatching, extortion, armed robbery)
7. Forced someone into sexual activity

<u>Destruction of property</u>

8. Deliberately engaged in fire setting with the intention of causing serious damage
9. Deliberately destroyed others' property (other than by fire setting)

<u>Deceitfulness or theft</u>

10. Has broken into someone else's house, building, or car
11. Lies to obtain goods or favors or to avoid obligations (i.e., "cons" others) frequently
12. Has stolen items of nontrivial value without confronting a victim (e.g., shoplifting, but without breaking and entering; forgery)

<u>Serious violations of rules</u>

13. Stays out at night despite parental prohibitions frequently, beginning before age 13 years
14. Has run away from home overnight at least twice while living in parental or parental surrogate home (or once without returning for a lengthy period)
15. Truant from school frequently, beginning before age 13 years

Note. Adapted from American Psychiatric Association (2000). Copyright 2000 by the American Psychiatric Association. Adapted by permission.

cietal norms or rules. Thus, if a child meets the diagnostic criteria for both disorders, only the diagnosis of CD is made.

Children with a variety of other DSM-IV diagnoses may present with problems of noncompliance, either as symptomatic of that particular diagnostic category or because of comorbid ODD or CD. Children with attention-deficit/hyperactivity disorder (ADHD) often present with problems of noncompliance (Barkley, 1998b). There are several possible reasons for this. Children with ADHD often do not seem to listen when spoken to directly, they may fail to initiate compliance, and they often fail to follow through on instructions or tasks. This type of noncompliance is not due to oppositional behavior per se, but rather the child's inattention problems. However, as noted later (see also Chapter 9), there is also a very high rate of comorbidity between ADHD and ODD or CD. Thus, children with ADHD may also be noncompliant as a function of their oppositional behavior.

If noncompliance is accompanied by conduct problem behaviors in which there is a "violation of the rights of others or of major age-appropriate societal norms and rules" (American Psychiatric Association, 2000), and is related to a specific psychosocial stressor that has occurred within the past 3 months, then a diagnosis using one of the adjustment disorder categories (e.g., with disturbance of conduct or with mixed disturbance of emotions and conduct) would be appropriate. Problems with noncompliance may be severe enough to warrant intervention, even if the child does not meet the diagnostic criteria for one of the disorders just discussed. The diagnosis of disruptive behavior disorder not otherwise specified may be used in situations in which the child presents with a number of oppositional or conduct problem behaviors, but which do not meet the frequency criteria specified in the DSM-IV for ODD or CD. This may often be the case when the child is 3–4 years of age.

There are several conditions listed in the DSM-IV that are not considered to be "mental disorders" that may be relevant for children who are presenting with noncompliance as a primary problem. (It should be noted that third-party payers typically do not cover these "V code" diagnoses.) These include child or adolescent antisocial behavior, parent–child relational problem, sibling relational problem, noncompliance with treatment, and problems related to abuse or neglect. A diagnosis of child or adolescent antisocial behavior might be employed in situations in which the child has engaged in more isolated acts of antisocial behavior, rather than the pattern of such activities specified for CD. A parent–child relational problem diagnosis might be used in situations in which the focus of the intervention is on parent–child interaction (as is the case in parent training). A diagnosis of sibling relational problem could be considered if the focus of clinical attention involves coercive sibling interactions (e.g., excessive arguing, fighting). Noncompliance with treatment may be an appropriate diagnosis in situations in which the focus of the clinician's attention is on the child's failure to adhere to a medical regimen, such as daily urine testing for a child with diabetes or regular use of an inhaler by a child with asthma (Huszti & Olson, 1999; Manne, 1998). This particular form of noncompliance is quite important, as it can have direct implications for the child's physical well-being (see Chapter 9).

Child compliance and noncompliance are salient for children in abusive and neglecting families. On the one hand, physically abused toddlers (1–2½ years old) have been shown to demonstrate a pattern of "compulsive compliance" in which they quickly comply to maternal directives and inhibit negative behavior, at a time when normal children are demonstrating increased noncompliance as part of the development of autonomy (Crittenden & DiLalla, 1988). While this response style is adaptive in the sense that it functions to reduce abuse, it has negative implications for these children's subsequent development of internal control of their own behavior. On the other hand, preschool and early school-aged children who have been physically abused and/or neglected are less compliant to maternal commands than are nonabused children (e.g., Egeland, Sroufe, & Erickson, 1983; Schindler & Arkowitz, 1986). A recent study found that physically abused, but not neglected, children (aged 3 and 4 years) demonstrated less committed compliance and more situational compliance than nonabused children (Koenig, Cicchetti, & Rogosch, 2000).

Finally, noncompliance and other oppositional behaviors may also be associated with mood disorders (e.g., juvenile-onset bipolar disorder), psychotic disorders, enuresis, encopresis, and developmental disabilities such as mental retardation and autistic disorder (American Psychiatric Association, 2000). While noncompliance is not a central feature of these disorders, it may be serious enough to become a focus of intervention.

Nondeviant Noncompliance

There are situations in which it may *not* be appropriate to intervene with child "noncompliance." One example is when the noncompliance is due to impaired language comprehension, such as in the case of deafness or a language disability (i.e., the child is not able to hear or process directives, so appears noncompliant). However, even in such cases, adaptations can be made to the parent training program to take into account the impaired language comprehension and to address noncompliance that is not a direct result of the disability (e.g., Forehand, Cheney, & Yoder, 1974; see also Chapter 9). Another example is noncompliance that, following a thorough assessment (see Chapter 4), is deemed to be developmentally appropriate.

The intervention program described in this book is intended for use with the range of children who present with the various diagnostic labels described above. The basic parent training program is designed for young children between the ages of 3 and 8 who present with noncompliance and other conduct problems. Adaptations to the basic parent training program for use with specific populations, such as children with ADHD, children who have been abused or neglected, children with developmental disabilities, children with enuresis or encopresis, children on inpatient psychiatric units, and children who must adhere to a medical regimen, are described in Chapter 9.

The Early Starter Pathway for the Development of Conduct Problems

Longitudinal studies have shown that there are multiple pathways that lead to the display of conduct problem behavior in childhood, adolescence, and adulthood. The most thoroughly delineated pathway, and the one that seems to have the most negative long-term prognosis, has been variously referred to as the "early starter" (Patterson, Capaldi, & Bank, 1991), "childhood-onset" (Hinshaw, Lahey, & Hart, 1993), or "life-course-persistent" (Moffitt, 1993) pathway. We will use the "early starter" label in this book. (The childhood-onset type of CD would seem to be a likely diagnostic outcome of this pathway.)

The early starter pathway is characterized by the onset of conduct problems in the preschool and early school-age years, and by a high degree of continuity throughout childhood and into adolescence and adulthood. As we noted in the preceding section, noncompliance is a keystone behavior in the development of conduct problems. It is thought that these children progress from relatively less serious (e.g., noncompliance, temper tantrums) to more serious (e.g., aggression, stealing, substance abuse) forms of conduct problem behavior over time; that overt behaviors (e.g., defiance, fighting) appear earlier than covert behaviors that occur behind the backs of adult caregivers (e.g., lying, stealing), and that later conduct problem behaviors expand the child's behavioral repertoire rather than replace earlier behaviors (e.g., Edelbrock, 1985; Patterson & Yoerger, 2002). Furthermore, settings in which the conduct problem behaviors occur broaden over time, from the home to other settings such as the school and the larger community. The risk for continuing on this developmental pathway through the elementary school years and into adolescence may be as high as 50% for children who display conduct problem behaviors at ages 3 and 4 (Campbell, 1995). As illustrated in Figure 1.1, although there is a high degree of continuity across the developmental period, the specific behaviors that are manifested will change as a function of the child's developmental stage and of particular opportunities presented in the child's environment (Moffitt, 1993).

As we will present in detail later, characteristics of the child (e.g., temperament) and coercive patterns of family interaction in the preschool years can lead to the development of high levels of child noncompliance. On school entry, the child's coercive style of interaction with parents and siblings (see below) is likely to extend to interactions with teachers and peers, resulting in frequent disciplinary confrontations with school personnel, rejection by peers, and continued coercive interchanges with parents (some of which now center around school-related behavioral and academic problems) (e.g., Patterson et al., 1992; Ramsey, Patterson, & Walker, 1990). By age 10 or 11, this recurrent constellation of negative events places the child at increased risk for association with deviant peer groups in middle school and high school. Both peer rejection (e.g., Coie, Lochman, Terry, & Hyman, 1992) and subsequent involvement with antisocial peers (e.g., Dishion, Patterson, Stoolmiller, & Skinner, 1991) are important ways in which the peer group serves to maintain and escalate conduct problem behavior during middle and late childhood and early adolescence. The child's conduct problem behaviors often become more serious, more frequent, and more covert (e.g., stealing) during this period. Figure 1.2 summarizes this developmental trajectory.

Children with conduct problems (in particular, boys) are also at increased risk for depression by the time they reach adolescence (see Ollendick & King, 1994). Capaldi (1991, 1992) found co-occurrence of conduct problems and depressive symptoms in an at-risk community sample of early adolescent boys in sixth grade. Over the next 2 years,

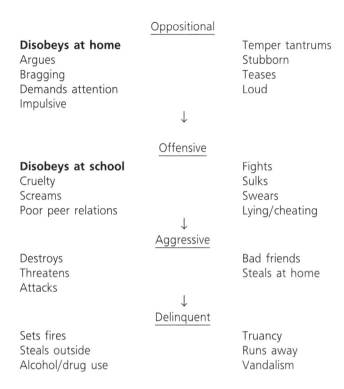

FIGURE 1.1. Developmental progression of conduct problem behaviors. Children in this nonreferred sample ranged from 4 to 16 years of age. From Edelbrock (1985). Reprinted by permission of the author.

the boys with conduct problems and depressive symptoms displayed higher levels of suicidal ideation than boys with only conduct problems or only depressive symptoms. They also displayed poor academic achievement and a high arrest rate (65%) by eighth grade. The boys with conduct problems who were depressed also appeared to initiate substance use at an earlier age than boys with only conduct problems.

Adolescents who have progressed along the early starter pathway are at significant risk for continuing to engage in more serious forms of conduct problem behavior throughout adolescence and into adulthood. As adults, they are at high risk for a subsequent diagnosis of antisocial personality disorder (APD); they are also at increased risk for other psychiatric diagnoses and a variety of negative life outcomes (e.g., lower occupational adjustment and educational attainment, poorer physical health) (e.g., Farrington, 2003; Kratzer & Hodgins, 1997; Moffitt, 1993).

Child and Family Risk Factors for Early Starting Conduct Problems

There is a growing body of evidence concerning the many individual and familial factors that may increase the likelihood of a child entering and progressing along the early

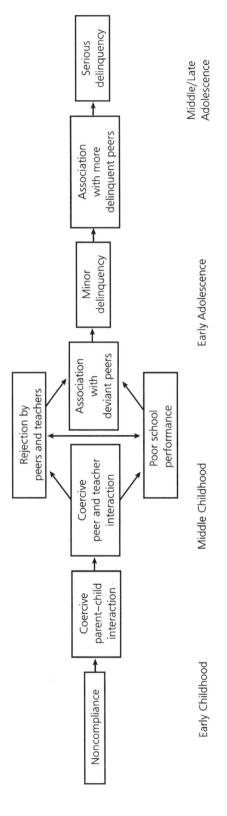

FIGURE 1.2. The early starter trajectory for the development of conduct problem behaviors. From Forehand and Wierson (1993). Copyright 1993 by the Association for Advancement of Behavior Therapy. Reprinted by permission.

starter pathway (for reviews, see Campbell, Shaw, & Gilliom, 2000; McMahon & Wells, 1998; Shaw, Bell, & Gilliom, 2000).

Child Risk Factors

A number of researchers have proposed that early hyperactivity is a significant (and perhaps necessary) risk factor for the early starter pathway (e.g., Loeber & Keenan, 1994; Moffitt, 1993). Certainly, there is ample evidence that children who display both conduct problems and hyperactivity (as in ADHD) display more serious and higher levels of conduct problems and that they have a poorer prognosis than do children with conduct problems or hyperactivity only (for reviews, see Abikoff & Klein, 1992; Hinshaw et al., 1993). Moffitt posits that subtle neuropsychological variations in the infant's central nervous system, which could be due to a variety of prenatal, perinatal, and/or postnatal difficulties (e.g., exposure to toxic agents, birth complications, heredity), increase the likelihood that the infant will be "temperamentally difficult," displaying characteristics such as irritability, hyperactivity, impulsivity, and the like.

The role of child temperament (usually viewed as involving relatively stable innate personality characteristics; Rothbart & Bates, 1998) has received increased attention from clinicians as a possible contributing factor to conduct problems (e.g., Forehand & Long, 2002; Greene & Doyle, 1999). Of particular interest is the temperamentally difficult child who, from very early in life, is intense, irregular, negative, and nonadaptable (Thomas, Chess, & Birch, 1968). Such a child is thought to be predisposed to the development of subsequent behavior problems, due to the increased likelihood of maladaptive interactions with family members. However, temperament has often been found to have a low to moderate relation to subsequent conduct problems in early and middle childhood, at best (e.g., Bates, Bayles, Bennett, Ridge, & Brown, 1991), and, in some cases, to have no relation (Aguilar, Sroufe, Egeland, & Carlson, 2000). Other investigators have shown that it is the combination of difficult temperament in infancy with other concurrently measured risk factors, such as maternal perception of difficulty, male gender, prematurity, and low socioeconomic status (SES) (Sanson, Oberklaid, Pedlow, & Prior, 1991), or inappropriate parenting (Bates et al., 1991), that best predicts subsequent conduct problems.

Another individual risk factor concerns the child's social-cognitive skills. Dodge and colleagues (Coie & Dodge, 1998; Crick & Dodge, 1994) have demonstrated that children with conduct problems display a variety of deficits in the processing of social information. For example, children with conduct problems have been shown to have deficits in encoding (e.g., lack of attention to relevant social cues, hypervigilant biases), to make more hostile attributional biases and errors in the interpretation of social cues, to have deficient quantity and quality of generated solutions to social situations, to evaluate aggressive solutions more positively, and to be more likely to decide to engage in aggressive behavior. These deficiencies and biases in social-cognitive skills have been shown to predict the subsequent development of conduct problems in kindergarten, and are associated with parental report of earlier harsh disciplinary practices (Weiss, Dodge, Bates, & Pettit, 1992).

Family Risk Factors

Child characteristics (e.g., difficult temperamental style and deficits in social information processing) may increase risk for both the development of an insecure attachment
to the parent (Greenberg, 1999) and a coercive style of interaction with family members
(Patterson et al., 1992; Snyder & Stoolmiller, 2002). These interaction patterns have
been implicated in the development of conduct problems. However, the relationship
between security of attachment in infancy and later conduct problems has been inconsistent. Attachment researchers (e.g., Greenberg, 1999; Lyons-Ruth, 1996) have noted
the necessity of adopting a transactional perspective in that attachment security is likely
mediated by other risk or protective factors (e.g., parenting practices, maternal depression, family adversity) over time.

The critical role of inadequate and punitive parenting practices in the development and maintenance of conduct problems has been well established. Types of parenting practices that have been closely associated with the development of child conduct
problems include inconsistent discipline, irritable explosive discipline, low supervision
and involvement, and inflexible, rigid discipline (Chamberlain, Reid, Ray, Capaldi, &
Fisher, 1997).

The potential role for so-called positive parenting practices as they relate to child
conduct problems has been less clear. Mother–child interactions of preschool-age children with conduct problems are characterized by lower levels of positive interaction
than those of a nondeviant control sample (Gardner, 1987); however, mothers of clinic-
referred children often do not differ in the frequency of specific positive behaviors (e.g.,
verbal rewards) directed toward their children (see Forehand, 1986, for a review).

The most comprehensive family-based formulation for the early starter pathway has
been the coercion model developed by Patterson and his colleagues (Patterson, 1982,
2002; Patterson et al., 1992). This model describes a process of "basic training" in conduct problem behavior occurring in the context of an escalating cycle of coercive parent–child interactions in the home that begins prior to school entry. According to this
model, rudimentary aversive behaviors, such as crying, may be instinctual in the new-
born infant. Such behaviors could be considered highly adaptive in the evolutionary
sense, in that they quickly shape the mother's behavior in ways necessary for the infant's
survival (e.g., feeding and temperature control). As most infants grow older, they substitute more appropriate verbal and social skills for their rudimentary coercive behaviors.
However, according to Patterson, a number of conditions increase the likelihood that
some children will continue to employ aversive control strategies. The proximal cause
for entry into the coercive cycle is thought to be ineffective parental management strategies, particularly in regard to child compliance to parental instructions during the preschool period. Child noncompliance is often coupled with negative, resistant behavior
that often results in parental withdrawal or failure to follow through with the command.

Negative reinforcement plays a particularly important role in the escalation and
maintenance of coercive behaviors, in that the coercive behavior on the part of one
family member (parent or child) is reinforced when it results in the removal of an
aversive event being applied to another family member. The upper section of Figure 1.3

illustrates how parent and child might be negatively reinforced for engaging in coercive behavior. In this example, the child's coercive behaviors are negatively reinforced when the parent withdraws the aversive stimulus (command). If the child stops whining, the parent's withdrawal of the command has also been reinforced by the identical process. In the lower section of Figure 1.3, the coercive interchange escalates. In this example, the parent's escalating coercive behavior is reinforced by the child's eventual compliance. The parent learns that the child will stop whining and eventually comply if the parent becomes louder and more negative.

As this "training" process continues over long periods, the rate and intensity of these coercive behaviors (including noncompliance) increase significantly, as family members' aggressive behaviors are reinforced. Furthermore, the child also observes his or her parents engaging in coercive responses. This provides the opportunity for modeling of aggression to occur (Patterson, 1982).

Coercive interactions with siblings also play an important role in the development of conduct problems (Garcia, Shaw, Winslow, & Yaggi, 2000; Snyder & Stoolmiller, 2002). Siblings of children with conduct problems often engage in comparable levels of coercive behavior, and coercive parent–child interactions interact with sibling coercion and conflict to predict subsequent child conduct problems.

The findings from several longitudinal studies with samples of preschool and early school-age children are consistent with the coercion model (e.g., Aguilar et al., 2000; Bates et al., 1991; Campbell, 1995; Campbell et al., 2000; Shaw et al., 2000). For example, the series of studies conducted by Campbell and her colleagues has shown that high levels of externalizing behavior problems during the preschool period, in conjunction with high levels of negative maternal control in observed parent–child interactions and

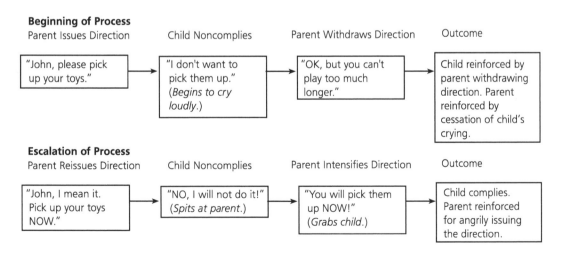

FIGURE 1.3. The coercive process between a parent and child. From Forehand and Long (2002). Copyright 2002 by McGraw-Hill. Reprinted by permission.

maternal personal and/or familial distress, predict subsequent externalizing problems several years later.

Although social learning theorists have focused on coercive processes within the family as the primary determinant of child *noncompliance* and other conduct problem behavior, a case can be increasingly made for the complementary contribution of parental responsivity to enhancing child *compliance*. Parental responsivity is a broad construct that includes dimensions such as warmth, sensitivity, involvement, positive reciprocity, and mutual compliance (Kochanska & Thompson, 1997; Maccoby & Martin, 1983). Such parental responsivity to the child appears to increase the likelihood of the child's readiness to comply. As such, it appears to function more as a parenting "style," rather than a parenting "practice" (Darling & Steinberg, 1993), by providing a broad context for more specific parent–child interactions. A number of investigations with non-referred (e.g., Parpal & Maccoby, 1985; Wahler, Herring, & Edwards, 2001), high-risk (e.g., Shaw, Keenan, & Vondra, 1994), and clinic-referred (e.g., Gardner, 1987; Wahler & Bellamy, 1997) children suggests that general parental responsivity to the child provides a context that is conducive to child cooperative behavior.

In addition to differences noted in parenting behaviors, the parents of children with conduct problems have more maladaptive social cognitions, including unrealistic expectations regarding their children's behavior, than do other parents. For example, these parents are more likely to misperceive child behaviors as negative (e.g., Holleran, Littman, Freund, & Schmaling, 1982; Wahler & Sansbury, 1990), to have fewer positive and more negative family-referent cognitions (Sanders & Dadds, 1992), and to perceive child conduct problem behaviors as intentional and to attribute them to stable and global causes (Baden & Howe, 1992). As a result, parents perceive their children as problematic. Furthermore, these negative perceptions of the child are associated with higher levels of maternal anger and overreactivity in child discipline (Slep & O'Leary, 1998). In addition, many parents, particularly those with limited experience with children, may not be acquainted with developmental norms and, thus, perceive age-appropriate behavior as being inappropriate. As a result, parents may have expectations that are unrealistically high for the child. For example, a parent might expect a child to be completely toilet trained before 2 years of age, or to be able to dress himself or herself without assistance before 3 years of age. Unrealistic parent expectations of child behavior may also exist because parents are experiencing depressive symptoms (e.g., Forehand & Brody, 1985). As a result of the depressive symptomatology, parents may have minimal tolerance for "normal" child behavior and, thus, unrealistically perceive the child as deviant (Forehand, McCombs, & Brody, 1987).

The parents of children with conduct problems are also at risk for increased levels of personal (e.g., depression, antisocial behavior, substance abuse, stress), interparental (e.g., marital conflict), and extrafamilial (i.e., insularity) distress. It is clear that parental depressive symptoms relate negatively to child adjustment (for reviews, see Cummings & Davies, 1994; Goodman & Gotlib, 1999). For the most part, maternal rather than paternal depressive symptoms have been the focus of attention. Relationships have been found between depressive symptoms and parenting practices, such as inept discipline, low responsiveness to children, and avoidance of conflict (Cummings & Davies, 1994;

Goodman & Gotlib, 1999), and, as noted above, negative perceptions of children and unrealistic expectations accompany parental depressive symptoms (e.g., Dumas & Serketich, 1994; Forehand et al., 1987). It also appears that maternal depressive symptoms may relate to the referral of children for noncompliance. Some children are referred by parents for noncompliance and other conduct problems when their behavior does not differ from that of nonclinic children (Rickard, Forehand, Wells, Griest, & McMahon, 1981). Mothers of clinic-referred, but nondeviant, children reported more depressive symptoms than did mothers whose children were clinic-referred and deviant.

Parental antisocial behavior has received increasing attention as both a direct and an indirect influence on the development and maintenance of conduct problems (see Frick & Loney, 2002). Parental APD (in combination with children's lower verbal intelligence) predicts the persistence of conduct problems over a 4-year period (Lahey et al., 1995). Parental antisocial behavior may also play an important role in parenting practices (e.g., Capaldi, DeGarmo, Patterson, & Forgatch, 2002; Frick et al., 1992; Patterson et al., 1992). For example, in a sample of boys at high risk for conduct problems, Patterson and colleagues (1992) reported that both paternal and maternal antisocial behavior was negatively correlated with parenting practices; furthermore, parental antisocial behavior mediated the effect of social disadvantage and divorce/remarriage transitions in predicting parental practices. Thus, parental antisocial behaviors may directly impact child behavior, indirectly impact child behavior through parenting, and play a role in the relationship between other family and extrafamilial variables and parenting.

Parental alcohol consumption and alcoholism are associated with child conduct problems (Pelham & Lang, 1993; West & Prinz, 1987). Furthermore, alcohol consumption by parents can influence parental perceptions of children's behavior and has a negative impact on parenting behaviors displayed toward children (e.g., inadequate monitoring, inconsistent and harsh discipline, indulgence, less problem solving) (El-Sheikh & Flanagan, 2001; Lang, Pelham, Atkeson, & Murphy, 1999; Pelham & Lang, 1993; Whipple, Fitzgerald, & Zucker, 1995). Pelham and Lang suggest that such characteristics may mediate the link between parental alcohol consumption and child noncompliance. They also point out that, not only can alcohol consumption have deleterious effects on parenting, but children's inappropriate behavior can lead to increases in parent alcohol consumption, thus perpetuating the cycle.

Parents of children with conduct problems also appear to experience higher frequencies of stressful events, both minor ones (e.g., daily hassles) and those of a more significant nature (e.g., unemployment, major transitions) (Capaldi et al., 2002; Webster-Stratton, 1990b). The effects of stress on child conduct problems may be mediated through maladaptive parental social cognitions (e.g., Johnston, 1996a; Wahler & Dumas, 1989) and parenting practices such as disrupted parental discipline (e.g., Forgatch, Patterson, & Skinner, 1988; Snyder, 1991), although the role of parenting behavior in mediating the association between parenting stress and child adjustment has not yet been rigorously tested (Deater-Deckard, 1998).

Conflict between parents that occurs in front of children or that involves children is a primary component of marital difficulties that lead to child conduct problems (e.g.,

Emery, 1999; Forehand, 1993; Long & Forehand, 2002b). Also, marital conflict appears to be more strongly associated with child conduct problems in samples of clinic-referred children than in samples of nonreferred children (O'Leary & Emery, 1984). It has been proposed that conflict between parents may operate through several different mechanisms to negatively impact children's behavior, including the disruption of parenting skills (Emery, 1999; Fincham, Grych, & Osborne, 1994), direct modeling of aggressive and coercive behavior, and the cumulative stressful effects of such conflict (Rutter, 1994). With respect to the latter, marital conflict may lead to maternal depressive symptoms and inconsistent parenting, which in combination may disrupt adaptive child behavior. Another possible mechanism has been proposed by Frick (1994); namely, that both child conduct problems and parental marital distress and conflict may be the result of parental antisocial behavior.

The impact of parental divorce on child functioning has been a hotly debated topic in recent years. Early work by Hetherington and her colleagues (e.g., Hetherington, Cox, & Cox, 1982) with preschool children indicated that divorce disrupted parenting and, particularly for boys, was associated with conduct problem behavior, including noncompliance. Reviews of more recent investigations have led to a more tempered conclusion: parental divorce has a *small* but statistically significant negative impact on children's behavior (e.g., Amato & Keith, 1991; Emery, 1999; Long & Forehand, 2002b). Thus, the magnitude of the difference between conduct problem behavior of children from divorced and nondivorced homes is smaller than initially thought. This results, in part, from the identification of a number of mechanisms that determine the magnitude of the effect of parental divorce on children. That is, it is not parental divorce per se that is necessarily detrimental for children, but rather factors that often are a part of the divorce process, such as interparental conflict and disruption of disciplinary practices (Emery & Forehand, 1994; Long & Forehand, 2002b). When divorcing parents engage in high levels of conflict, their parenting practices can be disrupted and their children may display various types of conduct problems (e.g., Emery, 1999; Fauber, Forehand, Thomas, & Wierson, 1990).

Relative to children living with both biological parents, children living in stepfamilies also are at a somewhat increased risk for conduct problems. Several explanations, including reduced involvement by parents and inadequate parenting, have been offered for children's difficulties in stepfamilies (e.g., Coleman, Ganong, & Fine, 2000; Demo & Cox, 2000; Lawton & Sanders, 1994).

Sources of stress on parents may not be limited to those occurring within or between parents. Wahler (1980; Wahler & Dumas, 1984) has identified parents whom he has labeled as "insular." These are individuals who have a high frequency of negative interactions and a low frequency of positive and supportive interactions with people from outside the immediate family (e.g., extended family, helping agencies). These individuals tend to be isolated from family, friends, neighbors, and the community. Insular parents perceive their children's behavior as more deviant than it is, engage in more ineffective discipline than noninsular parents, and have children who display oppositional behavior such as noncompliance (e.g., Dumas, 1984a, 1984b). Furthermore, when parent training is utilized, child behavior may improve, but maintenance of change does not occur in families where parents have high levels of insularity (Dumas & Wahler, 1983; Wahler & Afton, 1980).

Co-Occurrence of Risk Factors

Various child and family risk factors often co-occur, further increasing the likelihood of disrupted parenting practices and child conduct problems (Campbell et al., 2000; Sanders & Markie-Dadds, 1992). For example, a single mother who has just lost her job, is moderately depressed, and who perceives herself as socially isolated is likely at significant risk for being less able to engage in effective parenting practices, and her child is more likely to demonstrate conduct problems. As we emphasize throughout this volume, we consider parent training to be the core intervention for improving parenting and child conduct problem behaviors. However, assessment of broader family risk factors (see Chapter 4) is important, and, when appropriate, they may need to be incorporated into the intervention (see Chapter 5).

FINAL THOUGHTS

The focus on compliance and noncompliance in this book is important for a number of reasons. First, the development of compliance to parental instructions is an accomplishment that has important implications for the child's autonomy, self-regulation, internalization of moral values, and general socialization. Second, noncompliance is a major concern for parents and teachers of both normally developing children in the general population and children with special needs. Third, noncompliance is a major reason for the referral of young children for mental health services, it is a primary characteristic of ODD and CD, and it is associated with a variety of other child diagnoses and conditions. Finally, current theory and research indicate that noncompliance is a keystone behavior in the development of early starting conduct problems.

In the remainder of this volume, we focus on assessment and intervention strategies for 3- to 8-year-old children who are referred because of concerns regarding excessive noncompliance.

CHAPTER 2

Parent Training

In this chapter, we define parent training, provide a historical perspective of the stages of development of the parent training model, and list those parenting skills that are characteristic of this model and which appear across different types of parent training interventions. We then present an overview of the model of parent training developed by Constance Hanf and a comparison of the similarities and differences of the various parent training programs derived from it (including our own).

Parent training can be defined as an approach to treating child behavior problems by using

> procedures by which parents are trained to alter their child's behavior in the home. The parents meet with a therapist or trainer who teaches them to use specific procedures to alter interactions with their child, to promote prosocial behavior, and to decrease deviant behavior. (Kazdin, 1995, p. 82)

Parent training has received substantial attention during the past 30 years and has been applied to a broad array of child problems (see volumes by Briesmeister & Schaefer, 1998; Dangel & Polster, 1984; Schaefer & Briesmeister, 1989). These include ADHD, anxiety disorders, enuresis, sleep problems, feeding difficulties, and as an intervention for child abusing and neglectful parents. Parent training has also been employed with children with developmental disabilities (e.g., mental retardation, autism) and their families. However, parent training has been primarily employed in the treatment of preadolescent (i.e., preschool- to school-age) children's overt conduct problem behaviors such as temper tantrums, aggression, and excessive noncompliance, and it is in this area that parent training has the greatest empirical support. (As noted in Chapter 1, these children typically meet DSM-IV-TR (American Psychiatric Association, 2000) criteria for ODD or CD, although these behaviors may be manifested as part of, or in conjunction with, a variety of other diagnoses.) In recent reviews of various intervention approaches for child conduct problems, parent training has consistently emerged as the most successful intervention to date with these youngsters (e.g., Kazdin, 1995; McMahon & Wells, 1998).

THE DEVELOPMENT OF PARENT TRAINING

The concise definition of parent training presented at the beginning of this chapter fails to capture the historical antecedents of parent training or the sense of its active, ongoing development into a true "behavioral family therapy" (Griest & Wells, 1983; Wells, 1985). Since the earliest attempts to teach parents to alter their children's conduct problem behaviors (Williams, 1959), parent training has gone through three distinct stages of development (McMahon, 1991).

The first stage, which occurred during the 1960s and early 1970s, was concerned with developing a "parent training" model of intervention (O'Dell, 1974) and determining whether it was a viable approach to dealing with a wide variety of child behavior problems. Based on Tharp and Wetzel's (1969) triadic model, the parent training model employed a therapist (consultant) who worked directly with the parent (mediator) to alleviate the child's (target) conduct problem behavior. The underlying assumption of this model was that some sort of parenting skills deficit had been at least partly responsible for the development and/or maintenance of the conduct problem behaviors. The parent training model came about because of the confluence of several events (Kazdin, 1985): (1) the development of behavior modification techniques, especially reinforcement and punishment procedures based on operant conditioning, (2) the trend toward using paraprofessionals (including parents) to deliver mental health services, and (3) an awareness that utilizing parents as therapists could enhance the effectiveness of child therapy.

The parent training model presented several advantages over more traditional approaches to child therapy in which the therapist worked one-on-one with the child in hour-long weekly sessions (Berkowitz & Graziano, 1972). First, the importance of familial and broader contextual factors in the development and maintenance of conduct problem behavior suggested that clinically significant changes are unlikely when the child is treated "out of context." Second, even if the child's behavior improves in the treatment setting, the improvement will most likely dissipate when the child returns to the natural environment that produced the problems in the first place. Finally, parents have the greatest amount of contact with the child and the greatest control over the child's environment. By virtue of their parenthood, they also have the major moral, ethical, and legal responsibility to care for the child.

Although much of the research during this first stage of the development of parent training was limited to descriptive case studies or single-case designs with data collected in the clinic or laboratory (and less frequently in the home), the available evidence strongly supported the short-term efficacy of this approach in terms of immediate posttreatment improvements in both parent and child behavior. For example, children at posttreatment were less physically and verbally aggressive, more compliant, and less destructive, while their parents were less directive, controlling, and critical, and more positive toward their children (see O'Dell, 1974, for a review of these early studies). In the past 30 years, hundreds of studies focusing on parent training with children with conduct problems have appeared. Reviews of these investigations (e.g., McMahon, 1999; Miller & Prinz, 1990; O'Dell, 1974; Serketich & Dumas, 1996) indicate that teaching parents to change their children's behavior can be a highly effective intervention procedure.

Although the short-term efficacy of parent training in producing changes in both parent and child behaviors had been demonstrated repeatedly, the generalization of those effects had been less consistently documented. This concern about generalization of treatment effects led to the second stage in the development of parent training, which occurred from the mid-1970s to the mid-1980s. Forehand and Atkeson (1977) discussed four major types of generalization relevant to parent training interventions with children. *Setting generalization* refers to the transfer of intervention effects to settings in which intervention did not take place (e.g., from the clinic to the home or school), whereas *temporal generalization* pertains to the maintenance of intervention effects following termination. *Sibling generalization* concerns the transfer of the newly acquired parenting skills to untreated siblings in the family and the siblings' responding in the desired manner. *Behavioral generalization* refers to whether targeted changes in specific conduct problem behaviors are accompanied by improvements in other nontargeted behaviors.

Generalization is important for the success of a parent training approach from at least two perspectives (Forehand & Atkeson, 1977). In terms of treatment, generalization saves therapist time, since the therapist need not treat recurrences of previously treated problems, problem behaviors in new settings, all of the child's problem behaviors, or the behavior problems of the child's siblings. In terms of prevention, generalization minimizes repeated professional intervention and should result in a diminution of future behavior problems of the child (and siblings) (see Chapter 10). Assessing generalization also allows therapists to monitor the potential occurrence of any negative side effects of parent training.

Pertinent to the generalization of effects is the *social validity* or clinical significance of the effects of the intervention, which refers to whether therapeutic changes are "clinically or socially important" for the client (Kazdin, 1977, p. 429). Parent training interventions for the treatment of children with conduct problems have demonstrated their generalizability and social validity to varying degrees—some quite impressively, others to a moderate degree, and others not at all. As noted by several reviewers (e.g., Griest & Wells, 1983; Miller & Prinz, 1990; Serketich & Dumas, 1996), parent training is not uniformly successful, positive effects that are achieved are not always maintained, and some families are resistant to this therapeutic effort.

This emphasis on the generalization and social validity of treatment effects and the increased awareness of the multiple causal and maintaining factors of conduct problems led to the third and current stage of development of parent training. Since the mid-1980s, clinical researchers have focused on ways to enhance the effectiveness of parent training, not only with respect to short-term efficacy but especially with regard to generalization. Two factors have been key to this shift in focus: (1) an increased awareness of the role of developmental factors in developing behaviorally oriented interventions (Eyberg, Schuhmann, & Rey, 1998; Forehand & Wierson, 1993), and (2) the broadening of the conceptual basis of parent training to what is referred to as "behavioral family therapy" (Griest & Wells, 1983; Wells, 1985). Enhancements and expansions of the parent training model have included strengthening basic parenting skills; adding new parenting skills; focusing on parental personal and interparental adjustment factors, expectations, and social stressors; and incorporating multisystem approaches that focus on the child (peer and school domains) and broader ecological issues (Miller & Prinz, 1990). Although still developing (Miller & Prinz, 1990; Taylor & Biglan, 1998), the behavioral family therapy model has acknowledged and incorporated into intervention the variety of child, parent, and contextual variables that have been implicated empirically in the development and maintenance of conduct problems (see Chapter 1). Reviews of the effectiveness of recent iterations of parent training, which reflect the emphases noted above, find increasing evidence of generalization (e.g., Estrada & Pinsof, 1995; McMahon, 1999).

COMMON CATALOG OF PARENTING SKILLS

There are dozens of parent training interventions for preadolescent children with conduct problems. These interventions share some commonalities (Dumas, 1989; Kazdin, 1995; Miller & Prinz, 1990), including the following: (1) intervention is conducted primarily with the parents, with relatively less therapist–child contact; (2) therapists refocus parents' attention from a preoccupation with conduct problem behavior to an emphasis on prosocial goals; (3) the content of these programs typically includes instruction in the social learning principles underlying the parenting techniques; training in defining, monitoring, and tracking child behavior; training in positive reinforcement procedures, including praise and other forms of positive parent attention and token or point systems; training in extinction and mild punishment procedures such as ignoring, response cost, and time out (TO) in lieu of physical punishment; training in giving clear instructions or commands; and training in problem solving; and (4) therapists use didactic instruction, modeling, role playing, behavioral rehearsal, and structured homework exercises to promote effective parenting.

LIMITATIONS OF PARENT TRAINING

As already noted, parent training is not effective with all families. For example, Patterson (1974) reported that 22% of the treated families in his sample did not show improvement with parent training. Webster-Stratton, Hollinsworth, and Kolpacoff (1989) reported that approximately one-third of their sample did not have reliable and sustained improvement at a 1-year follow-up. Similarly, in our work, an examination of individual participants' data clearly indicates that some parents and children do not change on some of our outcome measures. Furthermore, as with other types of treatment for children, dropouts occur in parent training (Forehand, Middlebrook, Rogers, & Steffe, 1983). In a review of 22 parent training studies, Forehand and colleagues (1983) reported that the overall dropout rate was 28%. More recent studies report similar rates (e.g., Sanders, Markie-Dadds, Tully, & Bor, 2000).

Certain child and family characteristics may also limit the effectiveness of parent training (see McMahon, 1999, for a review). The child characteristic that has been shown to be most consistently associated with parent training outcome has been the severity of the child's conduct problem behavior: the more severe the child's behavior, the less positive the outcome. Child gender does not appear to be differentially associated with outcome. There are contradictory findings with respect to child age, with some, but not all, studies finding older children to be less responsive to parent training interventions (e.g., McMahon, 1999). We have found no differential treatment effect for our parent training program within the 3- to 8-year age range (McMahon, Forehand, & Tiedemann, 1985).

The relative effectiveness of parent training interventions with families of different ethnicities and from different cultural backgrounds has been largely unexplored (Forehand & Kotchick, 1996; Kotchick, Shaffer, Dorsey, & Forehand, in press). This is unfortunate, as ethnicity and culture do play critical roles in shaping childrearing attitudes and practices (Kotchick & Forehand, 2002) and to ignore these may alienate families seeking treatment. One study, using a parent training intervention similar to ours (i.e., Parent–Child Interaction Therapy—see below), found no differences between African American and European American families on pretreatment variables (e.g., child behavior problems, parent stress), number of treatment sessions completed, or point of dropout) (Capage, Bennett, & McNeil, 2001). Further research is needed in this area.

With respect to family characteristics, coercive and inconsistent parenting behaviors, maternal depressive symptoms, low marital satisfaction, negative life events, low SES, and maternal insularity have been associated with less positive outcomes (see Kotchick et al., in press). Parental perceptions of the child's adjustment prior to treatment and single-parent status have not been consistently associated with outcome.

THE HANF MODEL OF PARENT TRAINING

The parent training program described in this book, as well as a number of others described below, has its origins in the pioneering work of Constance Hanf (1969, 1970; Hanf & Kling, 1973), formerly a professor at the Oregon Health Sciences University. Although Dr. Hanf's work was not published or widely disseminated, she had a tremendous influence on the field through her supervision and training of clinical psychology interns and postdoctoral fellows. In addition to developing a program that taught parents a set of skills through a structured learning process, she strongly espoused the importance of (1) specifying difficulties in parent–child interactions in behavioral, observable, measurable terms, and (2) evaluating the outcome of the program through systematic data collection. As will be evident throughout this book and in the work of others (see below), Dr. Hanf's influence has been far-reaching.

Common Features of the Various Hanf-Based Programs

There are currently four primary variations of Hanf's original parent training program that are in wide use: (1) the version described in this volume ("Helping the Noncompliant Child," HNC), (2) Barkley's (1997) "Defiant Children" (DC), (3) Eyberg's (e.g., Eyberg & Boggs, 1998) "Parent–Child Interaction Therapy" (PCIT), and (4) Webster-

Stratton's (2000) "The Incredible Years: Early Childhood BASIC Parent Training Program" (BASIC).

In general, these programs focus on treating noncompliance and other oppositional behavior in preadolescent children, especially those of preschool and early school age. They vary in the primary mode of administration. HNC and PCIT are typically administered via individual contact with a therapist or trainer. BASIC is designed primarily to work with parents in a group setting. Group administration of DC is recommended, although it can be delivered to individual families. Characteristic of all Hanf-based parent training programs, therapists make extensive use of modeling and parent role play during sessions (in addition to didactic instruction and discussion) to teach parents, at a minimum, the skills of attends, rewards, ignoring, clear instructions, and TO. All of these programs also make extensive use of home practice assignments and exercises. Similar to Hanf, two of the programs (HNC, PCIT) describe behavioral performance criteria that the parent must meet for each parenting skill.

Manuals are available for each of the Hanf-based programs. All of the programs except PCIT have additional commercially available training materials, such as videotapes for training therapists and parallel books for the parents.

Three of the four Hanf-based programs (HNC, BASIC, PCIT) have significant empirical support as a result of extensive evaluation, and several external evaluations of child mental health or parenting programs have resulted in these programs being identified as effective interventions. (DC has not been empirically validated to the same extent as the other Hanf-based programs.)

In a recent review of "best practices" lists (Metzler, Eddy, & Taylor, 2002), HNC, BASIC, and PCIT were included as 3 of the top 21 evidence-based family-focused programs. HNC has been included on lists focusing on the treatment of conduct problems (Brestan & Eyberg, 1998) and intrafamilial child abuse (Saunders, Berliner, & Hanson, 2001), and the prevention of substance abuse and delinquency (Alvarado, Kendall, Beesley, & Lee-Cavaness, 2000; Webster-Stratton & Taylor, 2001) and "mental disorders" (Greenberg, Domitrovich, & Bumbarger, 2001). For example, the Strengthening America's Families Project (sponsored by the Office of Juvenile Justice and Delinquency Prevention and the Center for Substance Abuse Prevention) identified HNC as one of seven Exemplary I Programs (out of more than 500 programs examined) (Alvarado et al., 2000).

Comparison of the Various Hanf-Based Programs

Although these programs share a number of common features, they also vary in a number of ways. Following are brief descriptions of each of these Hanf-based parent training programs. Readers interested in more detailed information concerning these programs should refer to the primary sources cited below.

Barkley's "Defiant Children"

Russell Barkley worked with Dr. Hanf during his predoctoral internship at the Oregon Health Sciences University in 1976–1977. Because of his primary interest in children with

ADHD, Barkley first adapted the parent training program for this population (e.g., Barkley, 1981). The current adaptation for the parents of children with ADHD is described in Chapter 9. In 1987, Barkley published a manual describing his adaptation of the Hanf program for oppositional and noncompliant children (*Defiant Children: A Clinician's Manual for Parent Training*). A second edition of the manual was published in 1997 (Barkley, 1997). Although Barkley's adaptation can be administered in either a single-family or group format, he recommends group administration. Barkley has incorporated a number of additional components into his parent training program, including a token reinforcement system and an optional home-based reinforcement system for school problems. Because of these components, Barkley has indicated that this program is appropriate for children up to the age of 12. He specifically provides for booster sessions following termination of the parent training program. In contrast to most of the other Hanf-based programs, Barkley does not discuss the use of behavioral performance criteria for parents, nor does he include training in establishing household rules. His group format is more didactic and discussion-oriented than other Hanf-based programs; for example, he puts somewhat less emphasis on parent role play than do the other Hanf-based programs.

Eyberg's "Parent–Child Interaction Therapy"

Sheila Eyberg was affiliated with the Oregon Health Sciences University from 1971 to 1984 as an intern, postdoctoral fellow, and faculty member. During that time, she was exposed to Hanf's parent training work. As noted above, PCIT has remained quite close to Hanf's original program. More than the other Hanf variations, PCIT has emphasized the role of traditional play therapy techniques as part of the Child Directed Interaction (what we call Phase I) segment of the parent training program (Eyberg & Boggs, 1998). Children attend some, but not all, of the parent training sessions. Parents (without the child) attend a single "teaching" session at the beginning of each of the two phases of the parent training program. Parents receive didactic instruction, modeling, coaching, and role playing in all of the parenting skills to be covered in that phase. (In contrast, other Hanf-based programs tend to teach the skills sequentially within phase.) In subsequent coaching sessions within each phase, the therapist provides ongoing feedback to the parent as he or she practices the relevant skills with the child. PCIT specifically provides for four booster sessions over the course of the year following the conclusion of the parent training program (Rayfield, Monaco, & Eyberg, 1999). PCIT is the only Hanf-based program to continue to include spanking as one of several potential backups for the child's refusal to stay in TO. Hembree-Kigin and McNeil (1995) have published a clinician's manual (*Parent–Child Interaction Therapy*).

Webster-Stratton's "The Incredible Years: Early Childhood BASIC Parent Training Program"

The videotape modeling/group discussion program developed by Webster-Stratton (2000) differs the most from Hanf's original parent training program and from the other Hanf-based programs, as well. What is unique about this particular intervention is its use of a standard package of 10 videotape programs of modeled parenting skills shown by a therapist to groups of parents. Approximately 200 vignettes (each of which lasts approximately 2 minutes) include examples of parents interacting with their children in both appropriate and inappropriate ways. After each vignette, the therapist leads a discussion of the relevant interactions and solicits parents' responses to the vignettes. Session content is approximately 25% videotape modeling, 15% teaching, and 60% group discussion, problem solving, and support (Webster-Stratton & Herbert, 1994). Because children do not attend the group sessions, there are no behavioral performance criteria for parents. Parents are given homework exercises to practice various parenting skills with their children. The BASIC program teaches a somewhat broader array of skills than do the other Hanf-based programs, including the use of natural and logical consequences, "when-then" rules, and response cost. In addition, there are separate curricula available for parents of older (5–12 years) children, for educational support of the child during elementary school, for children's social skills training, for parental interpersonal skills, and for teacher training (Webster-Stratton, 2000).

Helping the Noncompliant Child

The program described in this volume was initially adapted by the second author (RLF) at the University of Georgia following completion of his clinical psychology internship with Dr. Hanf in 1970–1971. This adaptation is, along with PCIT, the closest to Hanf's original program. It differs from Hanf's program and from the other Hanf variations by having the child present throughout all of the treatment sessions and by its strong emphasis on teaching the child about the parenting skills through didactic instruction, modeling, and role playing. Similar to many of the Hanf-based programs, it includes instruction in establishing and following up on rules and the application of the parenting skills to situations that arise outside the home. We published the first edition of this volume (*Helping the Noncompliant Child: A Clinician's Manual for Parent Training*) in 1981. A detailed description of the HNC parent training program is provided in the chapters that follow. Several empirically based adjuncts have been developed to enhance generalization (see Chapter 8).

CHAPTER 3

Overview of the "Helping the Noncompliant Child" (HNC) Parent Training Program

In this chapter, we first present some of the necessary requirements for effective parent training, including characteristics of the training setting, who should attend sessions, the parenting skills that are taught, and the methods for teaching those skills. We then present overviews of the parent training program, the use of behavioral criteria to determine success in learning each parenting skill and the structure of sessions, and note the availability of additional training materials for the parent training program. Finally, we describe ethical considerations in the use of parent training to treat child noncompliance, engagement of families in the intervention, and therapist characteristics.

As noted in Chapter 1, we hypothesize that the child's noncompliant, inappropriate behavior is shaped and maintained through maladaptive patterns of family interaction, which reinforce coercive behaviors. As a logical outgrowth of this formulation, our intervention strategy involves teaching parents to change their behavior toward their child so as to incorporate more appropriate styles of family interaction. In the initial part of this chapter, we delineate some of the basic requirements for our parenting program to be effective.

THE TRAINING SETTING

Parent training can occur either in the home or in a clinic setting. There are advantages and disadvantages to each approach. Intervention in the home prevents the need for generalization from the clinic to the home to occur. However, home-based intervention requires substantially more time and expense on the part of the therapist (e.g., travel time and gas expenses). It is also the case that third-party payers typically will not pay for services provided outside of a clinic. As noted earlier, our program is based on a clinic training model, as this appears to be more efficient and therefore most likely to be employed by most mental health professionals. We have also spent substantial time and effort in our research endeavors to examine and facilitate generalization from the clinic to the natural environment (see Chapter 10).

Intervention is initiated and carried out with individual families rather than in groups in a clinic playroom similar to the one used for clinic observations. However, our parent training program has been adapted for use in a group format by several clinical researchers (e.g., Baum, Reyna McGlone, & Ollendick, 1986; Breiner & Forehand, 1982; Long & Forehand, 2000b; McMahon, Slough, & the Conduct Problems Prevention Research Group, 1996; Pisterman et al., 1989).

There are a few fundamental considerations in setting up the clinic playroom in which the parent training program will be conducted. The room should have a chair for each person (i.e., the therapist, parent[s], and child), various sets of age-appropriate toys, and an additional chair that serves as the TO chair. Because children with conduct problems often engage in destructive behavior, we recommend that the furniture be basic, functional, and durable, and that the room be furnished as minimally as possible. If possible, the light switch should either be out of the child's reach or taped or locked in the "on" position.

Toys should be conducive to joint play and facilitative of imaginative play (Cavell, 2000). Examples of such toys are building materials (e.g., Legos, building blocks, Lincoln Logs), crayons or markers with paper and coloring books, a dollhouse with furniture and people, cars and trucks, and farm or zoo animals. Toys that should be avoided include board games, aggression-facilitating toys (e.g., guns), and messy toys (e.g., bubbles, paints) (Hembree-Kigin & McNeil, 1995).

The placement of furniture and toys is also important. Toys should be placed in that part of the room farthest from the door, with chairs for the therapist and parent(s) placed between the toys and the door (see Figure 3.1). This layout (1) provides separate areas for discussion among adults and for toy play and (2) prevents the child from having easy access to the playroom door should the child decide to leave during the session!

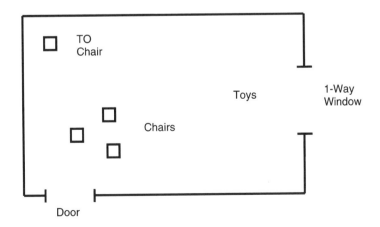

FIGURE 3.1. Example of playroom layout.

In an ideal situation, the playroom is equipped with a one-way window and a radio signaling device such as the "bug-in-the-ear" (a hearing-aid-like device converted to a radio receiver that the parent wears in his or her ear), giving the therapist the ability to unobtrusively talk to the parent from behind the window while the parent interacts with the child. However, these accoutrements are *not* necessary for the successful implementation of the program.

Sessions are optimally scheduled twice each week, with a session length of 75–90 minutes. We have found the more traditional format of weekly 50-minute sessions to be less successful. A 50-minute session usually does not permit adequate time for homework review, observation of parent–child interaction, and the extensive teaching and practice procedures employed in the program. In addition, weekly sessions increase the likelihood of an unacceptable level of performance decay. If parents are having difficulty implementing a procedure at home, they usually either stop using the skill or, worse, become proficient at using it incorrectly. By attending two sessions each week, parents receive a more constant level of feedback and training. When practical considerations (e.g., distance, insurance reimbursement, scheduling) prevent twice-weekly sessions, we strongly recommend that phone contact occur midway between the weekly sessions.

WHO SHOULD ATTEND SESSIONS

When two parents reside in the home, we encourage both to attend sessions. Two parents consistently implementing the program will be more effective than only one parent! In our clinical experience, both parents attend in about 50% of the cases. Not surprisingly, when only one parent is involved in treatment, it is usually the mother.

When only one parent attends sessions, we encourage that parent to share handouts with the second parent. The two parents also are encouraged to practice the skills together so that they both are using the skills.

In some cases, an extended family member (e.g., the child's grandmother) may be a coparent. In these cases, we encourage the involvement of that person. We have found particularly high levels of coparenting by extended family members in ethnic minority groups (e.g., African American) (Forehand & Kotchick, 1996; Kotchick et al., in press).

PARENTING SKILLS

Which skills can parents most effectively use to modify child noncompliance and other inappropriate behavior? As noted in Chapter 2, parent training interventions have tended to employ a number of similar teaching procedures and parenting skills (Dumas, 1989; Kazdin, 1995; Miller & Prinz, 1990). For young (3- to 8-year-old) children presenting with noncompliance, our research and clinical experience support the teaching of five core skills: giving attends, giving rewards, use of active ignoring, issuing clear instructions, and implementing time outs. These parenting techniques are described in detail in subsequent chapters, and Chapter 10 presents the data from studies examining these skills.

Our clinical experience has indicated that these skills should be taught in a specific order. In particular, the attending and rewarding skills from Phase I should be taught prior to teaching clear instructions and TO from Phase II. We strongly believe that these positive attention skills are critical to providing a more positive social context for the child and thus increase the likelihood of cooperative behavior (see Chapter 1). In addition, we have found that parents who are first taught a disciplinary procedure such as TO (which is a type of punishment) may terminate prematurely, as they often will have reduced their children's problem behaviors (albeit temporarily). Unfortunately, these parents have not learned any positive skills for interacting with their children or for maintaining their children's positive behavior. Therefore, for both ethical reasons and overall intervention effectiveness, we believe that, in nearly all cases, it is important to teach punishment procedures to parents later in the intervention process. However, it may sometimes be necessary to introduce nonphysical punishment procedures (e.g., TO) earlier in the program, when the child is extremely out of control (see Chapter 6, p. 128) or when working with physically abusive parents (see Chapter 9, pp. 190–192).

METHOD OF TEACHING

An extensive body of research indicates that modeling and role playing are the most effective teaching procedures in parent training (see O'Dell, 1985, for a review). These findings support our model for training parenting skills. Although we employ other teaching methods, such as instructing parents in what to do and giving them handouts describing the skill, we particularly emphasize modeling and role playing. In addition, parents are given homework assignments to employ the skill at home with their child. In this gradual shaping procedure, parents are told, are shown, practice, and generalize to the home each new skill. Parents also must meet specific performance criteria for a parenting skill before proceeding to the next skill (see below). This active approach to teaching parenting skills may be especially effective with disadvantaged parents (e.g., low SES, single parents) (Knapp & Deluty, 1989).

Similarly, our research (e.g., Davies, McMahon, Flessati, & Tiedemann, 1984) indicates the importance of actively including the child in the learning process. The child is present in the clinic playroom throughout the session; more importantly, the therapist and parent explain, model, and role play the parenting skills with the child before they are implemented "for real." This parent training program is one of the only ones of its type to involve the child as an active participant to this extent.

The sequence of instructional procedures that we follow for teaching the parenting skills is presented in Table 3.1.

An additional part of the teaching procedures consists of the therapist, in interactions with the parent, shaping how the parent should interact with his or her child. For example, in providing feedback to the parent during the instructional sequence just de-

TABLE 3.1. Sequence of Instructional Procedures for Teaching Each Parenting Skill

- Didactic instruction and discussion
- Therapist demonstrates skill through modeling and role playing
- Parent practices skill with therapist
- Child is taught skill
  - Therapist and parent explain and model skill for child
  - Child repeats skill verbally
  - Parent and child role play skill
- Parent practices skill with child (therapist provides ongoing cues and feedback)
- Parent practices skill with child (no ongoing therapist feedback)
- Parent is given handout describing the skill
- Homework assignment (parent records on data sheet)

scribed, the therapist can (1) provide positive reinforcement for appropriate parenting behavior ("Nice job of attending there!"), (2) provide corrective feedback ("Remember—no questions"), (3) prompt the parent as to what to say/do next ("Say, 'You're pushing the car up the tower' "), and (4) model a desired behavior ("You're pushing the car up the tower"). At other times, the therapist may ignore off-task comments by a parent. If such skills are good procedures to use with children, then they are also appropriate for the therapist to use with the parent!

OVERVIEW OF SKILLS TAUGHT IN THE PARENT TRAINING PROGRAM

The program consists of two phases: Differential Attention (Phase I) and Compliance Training (Phase II). In each phase a series of parenting skills is taught in a sequential manner. A synopsis of the skills that are taught in the parent training program is presented in Table 3.2.

During the Differential Attention phase of the intervention (Phase I), the parent learns to increase the frequency and range of social attention to the child and reduce the frequency of competing verbal behavior. A major goal is to break out of the coercive cycle of interaction by establishing a positive, mutually reinforcing relationship between the parent and child. In the context of the Child's Game, the parent is taught to increase the frequency and range of positive attention to the child; to eliminate verbal behaviors—commands, questions, and criticisms (Forehand & Scarboro, 1975; Johnson & Lobitz, 1974)—that are associated with inappropriate child behavior; and to ignore minor inappropriate behaviors. First, the parent is taught to attend to and describe the child's appropriate behavior. Moreover, the parent is required to eliminate all commands, questions, and criticisms directed to the child during the clinic training session. The second segment of Phase I consists of teaching the parent to use verbal (e.g., praise) and physical (e.g., hugs) attention contingent upon compliance and other appropriate behaviors (rewards). In particular, the parent is taught to use praise statements in which

TABLE 3.2. Outline of Skills Taught in the Parent Training Program

Phase I (Differential Attention)

Attends
- Attend to and describe child's appropriate behavior
- Verbally follow, do not direct, child's activity
- Do not ask questions, give commands, or teach

Rewards
- Give positive physical attention (e.g., hugs)
- Give nonspecific verbal praise
- Give verbal praise, labeling the desirable behavior

Ignoring
- No eye contact or nonverbal cues
- No verbal contact
- No physical contact

Phase II (Compliance Training)

Clear Instructions Sequence
- Clear Instructions
  - Reduce unclear instructions (such as chain, vague, question, etc.)
  - Employ clear instructions (get child's attention, state instruction clearly, wait 5 seconds)
- Consequences for Compliance and Noncompliance
  - Positive attention for compliance to the clear instruction (Path A) or to the warning (Path B)
  - Warning or Time-out sequence for noncompliance (Path C)

Standing Rules
- ("If . . . then" statement, continuously in effect, immediate time out)

Situations Outside the Home

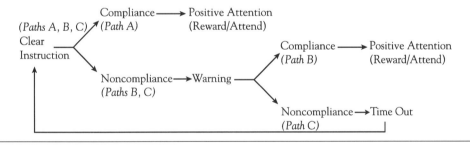

the child's desirable behavior is labeled (e.g., "You are a good boy for picking up the blocks"). Throughout Phase I, the therapist emphasizes the use of contingent attention to increase child behaviors that the parent considers desirable. The parent is also taught to actively ignore minor inappropriate behaviors. At home, the parent is required to structure daily 10- to 15-minute Child's Game sessions to practice the skills that were learned in the clinic. Near the end of Phase I, with the aid of the therapist, the parent formulates a list of child behaviors that he or she wishes to increase. The contingent use of attends and rewards to increase these behaviors is also discussed. The parent develops programs for use outside of the clinic to increase at least three child behaviors using the new skills.

In Phase II of the parent training program (Compliance Training), the primary parenting skills are taught in the context of the clear instructions sequence (see Table 3.2). The clear instructions sequence consists of three paths. The therapist first teaches the parent to use appropriate commands (clear instructions)[1] to increase the likelihood of child compliance. In the context of the Parent's Game, the therapist teaches the parent to give direct, concise instructions one at a time and to allow the child sufficient time to comply. If the child initiates compliance within 5 seconds of the clear instruction, the parent is taught to reward and attend to the child within 5 seconds of the compliance initiation (Path A). If the child does not initiate compliance, the parent learns to implement a brief TO procedure involving the following event sequence. The parent gives a warning that labels the TO consequence for continued noncompliance (e.g., "If you do not pick up the toys, you will have to sit in the chair"). If the child initiates compliance within 5 seconds, the therapist instructs the parent to provide positive attention (i.e., rewards and attends) for the child's compliance (Path B). If compliance does not occur within 5 seconds following the warning, the parent learns to implement a brief TO procedure that involves placing the child on a chair facing a wall (Path C). The child must remain in the chair for 3 minutes and be quiet and still for the last 15 seconds. Following TO, the parent returns the child to the uncompleted task and gives the clear instruction that originally elicited noncompliance. Compliance is followed by contingent attention from the parent. In practice with the child during the Parent's Game in the clinic, the parent is instructed to give a series of clear instructions and to provide appropriate consequences for compliance and noncompliance (i.e., the clear instructions sequence). In the home, the parent practices the use of clear instructions, positive consequences for compliance, and, finally, the use of the TO procedure for noncompliance.

When the parent is using the clear instructions sequence successfully in the home, the parent is taught to use standing rules as an occasional supplement to the clear instructions sequence. Standing rules are "if . . . then" statements ("If you hit your brother, then you must go to TO") that, once stated and explained to the child, are permanently in effect. Finally, the therapist instructs the parent in ways to implement the various Phase I and Phase II skills in settings outside the home, such as when visiting others or at the grocery store.

WHEN TO PROGRESS TO THE NEXT SKILL: BEHAVIORAL CRITERIA

Progression to each new skill in the parent training program is determined by the use of behavioral criteria. The therapist uses the observational data collected during each ses-

---

[1]In the original edition of this manual (Forehand & McMahon, 1981), we referred to clear instructions as "alpha commands." In this edition, we use "commands" and "instructions" to refer to the broad class of directives given by parents to their children. "Clear instructions" refer specifically and only to commands using the criteria specified in the parent training program (see Chapter 7). We continue to use the terms "alpha commands" and "beta commands" in the Behavioral Coding System, which we use in our observations of parent–child interaction (see Chapter 4).

sion to determine if the parent–child pair has attained the behavioral criteria necessary for movement to the next step of the program. The behavioral criteria ensure that the parent has attained an acceptable degree of competence in a particular skill before being taught additional parenting techniques. This is critical, since the parenting skills build on one another. In addition, these criteria allow for the individualization of the program by allocating training time more efficiently. Some parents require more training in some parenting skills than in others. The behavioral criteria allow a flexible approach whereby the therapist can concentrate greater attention on the more serious parenting skill deficiencies. The criteria for each skill are presented in Table 3.3.

STRUCTURE OF SESSIONS

The number of sessions necessary for the completion of each phase of the parent training program depends upon the speed with which the parent demonstrates competence in the skills being taught and the child's response to this intervention. The number of sessions for each family necessary for the completion of the entire parent training program has ranged between 5 and 14 sessions. The average number has been approximately 8–10 intervention sessions. Each 75- to 90-minute session typically consists of the following activities:

TABLE 3.3. Behavioral Criteria for Successful Skill Acquisition

For the relevant parenting skill, the parent is required to complete at least one 5-minute observation (Child's Game or Parent's Game) in which the parent obtains:

Phase I

Attends
- Average of 4 or more attends per minute (i.e., at least 20 attends).
- Average of .4 or fewer commands plus questions per minute (i.e., no more than a total of 2 commands and questions).

Rewards
- Average of 4 or more rewards plus attends per minute (i.e., at least 20 attends plus rewards).
- Of this sum, at least 2 rewards per minute (i.e., at least 10 rewards).

Ignoring
- Successfully ignores 70% of child's inappropriate behavior.[a]

Phase II

Clear Instructions
- Average of 2 or more alpha commands per minute (i.e., at least 10 alpha commands).
- No more than 25% of total commands are beta commands.

Consequences
- 75% child compliance ratio (child compliance/total parental commands plus warnings).
- 60% rewards plus attends ratio (parental rewards plus attends issued within 5 seconds following child compliance to a parental command or warning).

[a]Recommended.

1. A 5-minute data-gathering period in which the therapist observes the parent and child engaged in either the Child's Game (Phase I) or the Parent's Game (Phase II).
2. Discussion with the parent about the use of the relevant parenting skill(s) (attends, rewards, ignoring, clear instructions, TO) during the preceding observation period and at home (which skills are discussed depends on the skill(s) taught to that point).
3. The procedure and rationale for the next skill are explained, and the underlying social learning principles on which the skill is based are briefly presented.
4. The therapist demonstrates the skill via modeling and role playing.
5. The parent practices the skill with the therapist, who role plays the child.
6. The child is taught the skill. First, a developmentally appropriate explanation of the skill is given to the child by the parent and therapist. Then the parent and therapist demonstrate the skill to the child. The child repeats the skill verbally and participates in role plays of situations involving the skill.
7. The parent practices with the child in the intervention setting. The therapist observes and coaches, either through the bug-in-the-ear device or by nonverbal prompts and feedback.
8. The parent practices with the child in the intervention setting but without ongoing feedback from the therapist.
9. Depending upon the parent's progress, the therapist may conduct a 5-minute data-gathering period to determine whether the parent meets the behavioral criteria for that particular skill (see Table 3.3).
10. Parents are given handouts specific to each parenting skill for reference in the home setting.
11. Specific homework is assigned to practice the skills on a daily basis at home, both in structured practice sessions with the child and, later, at various times throughout the day (e.g., in Phase I, the parent develops programs to increase at least three behaviors using the new skills). Parent uses data sheets to record practice sessions and use of the new parenting skills in the home.

TRAINING MATERIALS

In addition to this volume, there are additional materials that therapists may find helpful in learning and implementing this parent training program. A 70-minute videotape (*Parent Training for the Noncompliant Child: A Guide for Training Therapists*; Forehand, Armistead, Neighbors, & Klein, 1994) that demonstrates the intervention procedures and component parenting skills is available for training therapists. It may be obtained from the second author (RLF) at the following address: ChildFocus, 17 Harbor Ridge Road, South Burlington, VT 05403. A supplemental self-guided book for parents that employs similar skills and teaching techniques (*Parenting the Strong-Willed Child*; Forehand & Long, 2002) is available from McGraw-Hill (800-722-4726, ext. 3; *http:// books.mcgraw-hill.com*) (see Chapter 10 for a description). A leader's guide for a 6-week parent class (Long & Forehand, 2000b) based on the Forehand and Long volume is available from Nicholas Long, Department of Pediatrics, UAMS/ACH, 800 Marshall Street, Little Rock, AR 72202.

ETHICAL CONSIDERATIONS

Therapists who plan to use the procedures described in this book should be aware of their ethical obligations when treating child noncompliance. Teaching parents to increase compliance should involve monitoring and training of parents by the therapist with regard to the kinds of commands to be given, the proper use of consequences for compliance and noncompliance, and parental expectations for the level of child compliance (Forehand, 1977). For example, although unlikely, it is conceivable that parents might use the skills taught to them to obtain compliance to deviant or morally undesirable commands. Similarly, regarding the proper use of consequences, parents could effectively reduce noncompliance by leaving a child in TO most of the day. Obviously, this is not an acceptable approach. Regarding parental expectations, parents might expect 100% compliance from their children. The normative developmental data that have been collected (see Chapter 1) make such a goal unrealistic and harmful. Such situations rarely occur; however, the important issue is that therapists should be sensitive to the possibility of their occurrence and incorporate instructional and monitoring procedures into their parent training programs to prevent these situations from happening. Our goal is not to develop quiet, docile children but rather to enhance the pleasure and significance of family interactions for all members of the family (Risley, Clark, & Cataldo, 1976).

ENGAGING FAMILIES IN THE INTERVENTION

For parent training to be successful, families must (1) believe that the intervention is an appropriate and potentially useful one for dealing with their concerns about their child's behavior, (2) become actively involved in the intervention, and (3) complete the program (i.e., not drop out). This process of engagement in parent training has received increased attention in the past several years. Of prime importance has been the development of conceptual frameworks for examining the engagement process in general (e.g., Kazdin, Holland, & Crowley, 1997; Prinz & Miller, 1996; Webster-Stratton & Herbert, 1994) and therapist behavior in particular (e.g., Patterson & Chamberlain, 1994). For example, Prinz and Miller (1996) present four domains that they suggest affect parental engagement in parent training interventions such as ours: (1) parents' personal expectations, attributions, and beliefs (e.g., expectations about the nature of the intervention, attributions about the source of the child's problem and/or about their own self-efficacy); (2) situational demands and constraints (e.g., financial and social stressors, marital and personal adjustment, daily hassles, and competing demands of other activities); (3) intervention characteristics (e.g., group versus individual parent training, home versus clinic delivery, type of intervention, scheduling of sessions, including the child in the session, homework); and (4) relationships with the therapist. These domains have been shown to be associated with engagement in parent training over and above that provided by the child, parent, and family factors described in Chapter 1 (Kazdin et al., 1997; Prinz & Milller, 1994). Furthermore, the greater the number of barriers experienced by the family, the greater the likelihood of subsequent dropout (Kazdin et al., 1997).

Webster-Stratton and her colleagues (e.g., Webster-Stratton & Herbert, 1994) used qualitative research methods to describe the process of intervention from the perspective of the parents. Participants in her parent training program (which, as discussed in Chapter 2, is also derived from the work of Hanf) went through five phases during the course of intervention (Spitzer, Webster-Stratton, & Hollinsworth, 1991). In the first phase (Acknowledging the Family's Problem), parents first had to acknowledge that their child was engaging in behaviors that the parents were unable to control. This was associated with parental anger, fear of losing control, self-blame, and depression. In addition, some parents also expressed concerns about being stigmatized and socially isolated from other parents because of their children's behavior. In the second phase (Alternating Despair and Hope), many parents often experienced immediate relief once they began using the newly acquired parenting skills and experienced some initial success. However, they failed to consider the long-term effort required to sustain these improvements and the "one step forward, two steps back" nature of much child behavior change. In the third phase (Tempering the Dream), apparent setbacks and parental resistance became more common, as progress slowed or regressed. Parents needed to understand that maintenance of improvements in child behavior required a long-term commitment to carrying out the program. In the fourth phase (Making the Shoe Fit), parents were able to adapt the program to fit their own needs. Key components of success in this phase were understanding the parenting techniques and how to implement them in multiple settings and situations above and beyond those directly discussed in the parent training program. In the final phase (Coping Effectively), parents accepted the notion that their children would require intensive efforts over the long term; however, they also were able to develop ways to provide self-reinforcement and support from others in their environment.

THERAPISTS

A single therapist per family is sufficient to conduct the parent training program successfully. However, in settings where therapist training occurs, it can be very helpful to employ two therapists to work with each family. First, it permits trainees to learn from in vivo exposure. As the trainee becomes more experienced and comfortable in the role of cotherapist, he or she can assume a greater proportion of the teaching role. Eventually, this person may function as a primary therapist. A second advantage of employing cotherapists is that it enables the therapists to be more flexible in demonstrating various skills to the parent. In the initial stages of teaching a new skill, one therapist models the skill while the other therapist role plays the child. This allows the parent to devote full attention to the modeling of the parenting skill. However, utilizing two therapists is obviously an expensive procedure in terms of personnel, and whether it is appropriate in a particular setting will depend upon both resources and training goals.

Therapist Relationship Skills

As noted above, the importance of the therapist establishing a collaborative relationship with the parent during parent training has been emphasized (Kazdin et al., 1997; Prinz & Miller, 1996), and therapist activities in such a relationship have been delineated (Sanders & Dadds, 1993; Webster-Stratton & Herbert, 1994). For example, Webster-Stratton and Herbert have described a number of roles for the therapist in the context of her parent training program (Webster-Stratton, 2000) that are clearly relevant to the program described in this volume. These roles include (1) building a supportive relationship through the use of appropriate self-disclosure, humor, optimism, and serving as an advocate for the parent; (2) empowering parents by reinforcing and validating their insights, modifying powerless thoughts, promoting self-empowerment, and building family and group support systems; (3) active teaching, which includes persuading, explaining, suggesting, adapting the concepts and skills to the parent's situation, giving homework assignments, reviewing and summarizing, ensuring generalization, role play and rehearsal, and evaluating parental satisfaction and progress; (4) interpreting through the use of analogies and metaphors, reframing, and making connections between the parents' childhood experiences and those of the child; (5) leading and challenging by setting limits, pacing the session, and dealing with resistance; and (6) anticipating problems and setbacks, predicting parental resistance to change, and predicting positive change/success.

Despite the obvious relevance of these clinical skills to the success of family-based interventions, there has been very little empirical research to evaluate these skills. Patterson and his colleagues have an ongoing program of research that has focused on the role of parental resistance in their parent training intervention. Patterson and Chamberlain (1994) presented a conceptualization of parental resistance that includes both within-session (refusal, stated inability to perform) and out-of-session (homework) resistance. Initial resistance is thought to be a function of the parents' history of parent–child interaction, preexisting parental psychopathology, and social disadvantage, as well as therapist behavior (Patterson & Chamberlain, 1988). Patterson and Chamberlain demonstrated that these contextual variables were associated with parental resistance throughout parent training. According to their "struggle hypothesis," parental resistance is expected to increase initially but then eventually decrease as the parent begins to meet with success.

High levels of resistance in the first two sessions of their parent training program were associated with subsequent dropout (Chamberlain, Patterson, Reid, Kavanagh, & Forgatch, 1984). Directive therapist behaviors of "teach" and "confront" increased the likelihood of parental noncooperative behavior within the session, whereas supportive and facilitative therapist behaviors had the opposite effect (Patterson & Forgatch,

1985). This poses an intriguing paradox for therapists: the directive therapist behaviors that seem to be intrinsic to parent training would also be those that predict parent non-compliance during treatment. Patterson and Forgatch (1985) conclude that two sets of therapist skills are required: "standard" parent training skills and relationship character-istics to deal with parental noncompliance. Growth-curve analyses of parental resis-tance over the course of parent training have shown a pattern of increasing resistance that peaks at about the midpoint, followed by a gradual decrease in resistance (Stoolmiller, Duncan, Bank, & Patterson, 1993). In general, these findings support the struggle hypothesis proposed by Patterson and Chamberlain (1994).

Research with a family-based intervention for adolescents with conduct problems indicated that relationship characteristics such as affect–behavior integration, warmth, and humor accounted for 45% of the variance in predicting treatment outcomes (Alex-ander, Barton, Schiavo, & Parsons, 1976). Structuring skills such as directiveness and self-confidence accounted for an additional 15% of the variance. Additional research from this group suggests that reframing statements are associated with reductions in fam-ily members' defensive statements (Robbins, Alexander, & Turner, 2000) and with more positive within-session attitudes with adolescents (Robbins, Alexander, Newell, & Turner, 1996).

Researchers involved with the Teaching Family Model (Achievement Place) inter-vention for adolescents with conduct problems have also provided data with respect to the relationship of therapist (in this case, teaching-parent) behavior to intervention outcome (see Braukmann, Ramp, Tigner, & Wolf, 1984, for a review). Use of particular teaching behaviors (description, demonstration, use of rationales, providing opportuni-ties for practicing behaviors, providing positive consequences) is positively correlated with higher levels of youth satisfaction and negatively correlated with self-reports of de-linquency. When teaching parents' used relationship-building behaviors, such as joking, showing concern, and enthusiasm, there was an increase in youths' satisfaction with the interactions (Willner et al., 1977).

Although therapist characteristics have not been studied with the HNC parent training program, we believe that those characteristics that have been identified as im-portant in the family intervention programs just reviewed apply to our program as well. That is, successful application of the parent training program with parents of noncom-pliant children will depend, at least in part, on how the therapist relates to, and inter-acts with, the parent and child.

FINAL THOUGHTS

The HNC parent training program is highly standardized, with the parent proceeding through a set sequence of parenting skills taught in a particular manner. Despite this standardization, the program is also quite flexible. For example, the behavioral criteria ensure that the parent will attain a certain level of proficiency in one parenting tech-nique before moving to the next skill. In addition, they make it more likely that training time will be allocated most efficiently. Skills that are acquired more rapidly (i.e., the behavioral criteria are met early on) will consume much less time than those skills with which the parent is having difficulty. It is also important to note that each parent and child "team" presents unique personalities, problems, and strengths. The steps necessary to persuade one parent to try a particular procedure with a child may be quite different from those required to persuade a second parent. Furthermore, some parents present with intense personal problems that may have to receive attention as part of the therapeutic process. Nevertheless, as long as the child's behavior is the primary difficulty, we have found it to be most effective to continue with the parent training program until it is completed, acknowledging and providing assistance where possible with secondary problems. If necessary, the secondary problems can then be addressed (see Chapter 5).

CHAPTER 4

Assessment Methods and Procedures

In this chapter, we describe the assessment methods and procedures in our parent training program. An overview of the assessment procedures is followed by a description of the interview, the direct observation procedures by independent observers in the clinic and home, the questionnaires that are completed by parents, and the parents' recording of child behaviors in the home. The chapter concludes with a discussion of strategies for school-based problems.

Behavioral assessment with children and their families now emphasizes a problem-solving approach that incorporates both developmental and broader ecological considerations ("Behavioral-Systems Assessment"; Mash & Terdal, 1997). Consistent with such an approach, we emphasize the assessment of the noncompliant child and his or her family through the use of multiple procedures. The focus of this chapter is on the methods and procedures that we currently employ in our assessment of noncompliant children and their families. These include interviews, direct observations in the clinic and home by independent observers, parent-completed questionnaires, and parent-recorded data. Although there is some overlap among the various assessment modalities with respect to the type of information they provide, each modality provides unique information on some aspect of child behavior or the parent–child interaction. By assessing the child and parent(s) by multiple procedures, we are more likely to identify the problem behaviors and their controlling events.[1] We also discuss the use of several instruments to assess broader personal, family, and extrafamilial difficulties. In situations in which the presenting problems involve the school setting, siblings, and/or peers, it will be necessary to obtain information concerning those areas as well. Assessment in the school setting is addressed at the conclusion of this chapter.

Initial assessment occurs at the first meeting with the family. The parent is asked to

---

[1] A number of other instruments and procedures for assessing children with conduct problems and their families may also be of interest. Examples are presented in Barkley (1997), Breen and Altepeter (1990), McMahon and Estes (1997), Sanders and Dadds (1993), and Schroeder and Gordon (2002).

note his or her chief concerns about the child on the Parent Behavior Checklist (see Figure 4.1). Most of the initial session consists of the parent interview, which lasts approximately 45 minutes. The remainder of the session is devoted to a brief interview with the child (approximately 5–10 minutes), a brief 10-minute (20 minutes if both parents participate) observation of parent–child interaction, and making arrangements for the remaining assessment procedures (15 minutes). These include the parent's selection of problem behaviors to record in the home, giving questionnaires to the parent to complete at home, and, if possible, arranging a home observation time. Finally, if a child is having behavioral difficulties at preschool or school, written consent to contact the school is obtained. The time required for each segment of the assessment varies, depending upon factors such as the complexity of the presenting problems, age of the child, and intelligence of the parents. We typically allow 1½–2 hours for the initial assessment session. The Assessment Process Checklist (Figure 4.2) presents the key steps in the process.

THE INTERVIEW

Purposes of the Interview

The interview is the first contact the therapist has with the child and his or her parent(s). The primary function of the interview is to identify the behaviors to be targeted for intervention and the conditions (both antecedent and consequent) that are currently maintaining the problem behaviors. The interview focuses on both parent and child behaviors and, more specifically, on the pattern of interaction between the child and parent.

The major purpose of an interview from a behavioral viewpoint is to determine factors currently operating to maintain the problem interactions. However, the initial contact with significant adults in the child's life can have other, quite important functions (Evans & Nelson, 1986; Haynes, 1991). A second purpose of the initial interview is to obtain a developmental history of the problem interactions. A developmental history of the problem parent–child interactions may be helpful in the following ways: (1) it may suggest conditions under which the problem behavior may reappear after successful modification; (2) it may provide information concerning controlling variables; (3) it may promote understanding for the client of how behavior problems begin; and (4) the historical information may be relevant to the development of intervention programs (Haynes, 1991). In addition, a developmental history of the interactional problems provides the therapist with a better understanding of the extent and severity of the problem behaviors. For example, as noted in Chapter 1, factors related to temperament may have produced a problem situation that has existed since the first few months of life.

A third function of the initial interview is to assess both the motivation of the parents for working in therapy and their ability to understand and execute behavioral programs (Evans & Nelson, 1986). This is important, as Patterson and Chamberlain (1994) have documented that parental resistance during parent training is associated with poor skill acquisition and, as a result, less change in child conduct problem behavior. Closely

Check the behaviors below that represent problem areas with your child. Then rank-order the behaviors you checked from primary problem (rank of 1) to least important problem.

_____ 1. Whines

_____ 2. Physically negative (attacks other persons)

_____ 3. Humiliates (makes fun of, shames, or embarrasses others)

_____ 4. Destructive (destroys, damages, or attempts to damage any object)

_____ 5. Teases

_____ 6. Talks smart

_____ 7. Noncompliance (does not do what he or she is told to do)

_____ 8. Ignores (fails to answer)

_____ 9. Yells

_____ 10. Demands attention

_____ 11. Has temper tantrums

FIGURE 4.1. Parent Behavior Checklist.

I. Prior to initial assessment session

_____ Train observers if home observations are to occur.

_____ Request that both parents (if applicable) attend session.

_____ Inform parents that the session will last 1.5–2 hours.

_____ Tell parents to bring the referred child but, ideally, no other children.

_____ Arrange for someone to watch the child during the parent interview.

II. Assessment session: Preliminaries

_____ Greet parents and child.

_____ Introduce person who will watch the child.

_____ Escort parents to the interview room.

_____ Obtain written consent for assessment and treatment, discuss issues regarding confidentiality, present rationale for the session (i.e., assessment occurs in order to guide treatment), provide brief overview of assessment procedures, and obtain demographic information (if not obtained previously).

III. Assessment session: Interviews

A. Parent interview (45 minutes)

_____ Parents complete the Parent Behavior Checklist (Figure 4.1).

_____ Ask the parents, "Tell me what types of problems you have been having with _____."

_____ Examine antecedents, child's behavior, parents' response, and child's reaction to each parent-generated problem situation.

_____ Examine frequency, duration, and historical–developmental aspects of each parent-generated problem situation.

_____ Pose problem situations from Problem Guidesheet (Figure 4.3) and examine nature of each (as above).

_____ Ask the parents, "Tell me what you like about _____. What does he/she do well?"

_____ Obtain brief developmental and medical history.

_____ Ask parents about previous services for child behavior problems and obtain written consent to contact previous service providers.

_____ Ask the parents, "Is there anything else that you feel I should know about _____, you, or your family that might be helpful?"

(continued)

FIGURE 4.2. Assessment Process Checklist.

   B. Child interview (10 minutes)

_____ Ask the child, "Tell me why you are here today."

_____ Explain to child why he or she is at clinic.

_____ Ask child about problem situations identified by parents.

_____ Ask child about family, school, and social activities.

IV. Assessment session: Observation (10–20 minutes)

_____ Child's Game (5 minutes)

_____ Parent's Game (5 minutes)

_____ Repeat observations with second parent (if applicable). Other parent completes questionnaires (see below).

_____ Discuss interactions with parent(s).

V. Assessment session: Concluding the assessment (15 minutes)

_____ Three primary child problems of concern identified by parents on Parent Behavior Checklist (Figure 4.1) are defined and parents asked to record these behaviors during four 24-hour periods on index cards (see Figure 4.9).

_____ Home observations (if these are to occur) are discussed and scheduled; guidelines for home observations (Figure 4.4) are given to parents.

_____ Sets of parent-completed questionnaires (one set for each parent) are given to parents to complete at home and return prior to the feedback session (if not already completed during clinic observations).

_____ Child Behavior Checklist

_____ Beck Depression Inventory

_____ O'Leary–Porter Scale

_____ Knowledge of Behavioral Principles as Applied to Children

_____ Other measures (as indicated)

_____ Obtain written parental consent to contact the school (as needed).

VI. Posttreatment and Follow-Up Assessments

_____ Parents record during four 24-hour periods the three child behaviors originally identified as problems.

_____ Parents complete same questionnaires as at initial assessment plus complete Parent's Consumer Satisfaction Questionnaire (Appendix A).

_____ Home observations occur.

_____ Clinic observations occur.

related to this is the fourth function: clear communication to the parent of the conceptual framework of the therapist and the nature of the intervention process. Some parents may not expect to be involved in intervention. It is important for parents to understand that the therapeutic approach is one in which a therapist teaches them how to interact more effectively with their child and that they will be involved extensively in the intervention.

Fifth, the initial interview is the first, and perhaps most important, opportunity for the therapist to begin to develop a collaborative relationship with both the parent and child. Unless the parent is highly motivated, can understand and execute the program, is receptive to the intervention approach, and has a positive, trusting relationship with the therapist, attempts to implement the parent training program will be futile. Sixth, from the initial interview, the therapist can derive information about the parents themselves (e.g., expectations of the child, and the personal and interpersonal adjustment of the parents) (Evans & Nelson, 1986). Finally, the initial interview can provide the therapist with the opportunity to question the parent about the need for a medical, speech, or auditory evaluation of the child. Neurological difficulties, mild hearing impairments, and language delays occasionally occur in children referred to clinics for the treatment of noncompliance. If the therapist suspects any of these problems, an appropriate referral (i.e., to a physician, speech therapist, or audiologist) should occur prior to the initiation of parent training.

Using the interview as an assessment tool does not end with the first contact but rather continues throughout treatment formulation and implementation (McMahon & Estes, 1997). Interviews can be used to obtain information necessary for the development of intervention procedures (e.g., potential reinforcers and negative consequences), to assess the efficacy of the parent training program as it is being implemented, and to modify the program if necessary.

Preparing for the Initial Assessment Session

There are two considerations concerning the initial assessment session that must be dealt with before the family even walks through the door for the first appointment. The first has to do with who should be present at the session. We always have at least one parent and the referred child (but not siblings) come to the clinic. However, we strongly recommend that both parents (as well as the child) be involved in the initial assessment session—for a number of reasons. First, it allows the therapist to obtain a more complete picture of the patterns of interaction between each parent and the child, the degree of consistency (or, as may more often be the case, inconsistency) between parents in their child-rearing philosophy and behavior, and a behavioral sample of the marital interaction as it relates to child-rearing issues. Each of these areas is important. Consistency between parents is an important determinant of child behavior (Block, Block, & Morrison, 1981), and, as we noted in Chapter 1, marital interactions (particularly conflict between parents in front of children) have a substantial influence on children and their noncompliant behavior. Mothers are more typically involved in parent training than fathers; however, fathers do play a very important, and often unique but neglected, role in the rearing of children (Marsiglio, Amato, Day, & Lamb, 2000; Phares & Compas, 1992). Thus, having both parents attend the initial assessment session is important, as it may provide information critical to the successful implementation of the parent training program.

Beyond the reasons just delineated, another advantage of both parents being present at the assessment session is to provide a "foot in the door" to having the unwilling parent (usually the father) participate in the parenting program. In our experience, many fathers can be persuaded to become involved in the parent training program to at least some degree after they have attended the initial assessment session and after the conceptualization of the presenting problem and the rationale of the program have been presented to them. Many of these fathers are quite pleased to find that the program makes sense to them. In many cases, both parents have reported their relief at finding that the program would not involve "shrink stuff" (e.g., couches) and that it is skill-oriented and "practical." Thus, by having both parents attend the initial assessment session(s), valuable information may be obtained, and, it is hoped, both parents can be persuaded of the importance of having complete parental participation in the program.

The second consideration concerning the initial session that must be dealt with prior to the family's arrival is whether the child will remain in the room during the parent interview. As a general rule, we prefer to interview the parent(s) alone at the initial interview (cf. Schroeder & Gordon, 2002). Although the child's presence provides the therapist with an opportunity to observe the child's behavior and the parents' reaction to it, this information is best gathered in the more standardized setting of the clinic and/or home observations. A "private" session without the child allows the parents to discuss their relationship with their child more freely without fear of the child overhearing. In addition, it precludes the child from disrupting the interview process. When the child's disruptive behavior occurs repeatedly in the early stages of the initial interview, the parent may become quite embarrassed. Such a reaction, as well as the disruptive behavior itself, mitigate against the development of rapport between therapist and parent. This requires that someone watch (and perhaps interview and play with) the child in the waiting room or in an adjacent therapy room. (Children referred for noncompliance and other conduct problems, regardless of age, generally should not be left alone in the waiting room or elsewhere, at least during the first session). The therapist can interview the child (as is described later) following completion of the behavioral interview with the parent.

Occasionally, space and/or personnel limitations require that the child remain in the room during the initial interview. When this happens, toys can be provided, and the child can be instructed by the parent to "play with the toys while I talk to _____." We usually observe how the parent handles the child's positive and negative behaviors during the first few minutes. If the parent has difficulty with the child's behavior (which is why they are at our clinic in the first place!), we generally provide structure and expectations for the child's behavior for the duration of the interview. In this manner, we model for the parent examples of some of the skills he or she will be learning. Obviously, this must be done in a manner that avoids making the parent feel inadequate. A reassuring statement such as "I know it's hard to handle kids when they're in a new place" will usually be sufficient.

THE PARENT INTERVIEW

After the family has arrived but prior to the assessment portions of the session, the therapist obtains written consent from the parent for both the parent and the child to participate in assessment and treatment and then discusses issues related to confidentiality, including limits (e.g., legal mandates for reporting suspected child abuse, threats of harm to self or others). Given the significant amount of time that will be devoted to the collection of assessment data during this session and throughout the program, it is important to present the parent with a rationale for the necessity of obtaining this information (i.e., assessment is necessary to ensure that the most effective treatment possible is utilized). We stress that the assessment data will enable us to direct our intervention to the most appropriate areas and that this information will also be of direct benefit in informing us of the effectiveness of the intervention. We then provide the parents with a brief overview of the assessment procedures. If the receptionist has not already done so, the therapist obtains demographic information concerning the child and family. This includes such data as the child's date of birth, grade in school, and number of siblings, the siblings' sex and grade in school, and the parents' age, education, and occupation. Then the therapist is ready to pursue the major purpose of the initial interview: assessing the nature of the typical parent–child interactions that are problems, the antecedent stimulus conditions under which problem behaviors occur, and the consequences that accompany such behaviors.

The interview itself typically begins with a general question, such as "Tell me what types of problems you have been having with _____" or "What brings you to the clinic?" This provides the therapist with an immediate opportunity to hear the parent's major concerns about the child and to obtain some initial perception as to the type of treatment that the parent is seeking. For example, the "Play-Therapy Parent" (see Chapter 5) may reveal expectations that the child is to be dropped off at the clinic, the therapist will "fix" the problem, and the child can be picked up an hour later.

In our experience, most parents, not surprisingly, respond with generalizations to the question of what types of problems they are experiencing with their children. To structure the interview and the information obtained from the parent concerning current problematic parent–child interactions, the therapist examines:

1. The antecedent conditions of the situation ("What happens just before the problem interaction?")
2. The child's behavior ("What does [child's name] do?")
3. The parent's response ("What do you do?")
4. The child's reaction to the parent's intervention ("What does [child's name] do then?").

The analysis of both the parent's and child's behavior in the problem situation should be continued until the therapist has a clear understanding of the nature and extent of the parent–child interaction. Other relevant information, such as the frequency ("How often . . . ?"), duration ("How long . . . ?"), and historical–developmental questions specific to the problem interaction, also should be gathered.

Following the parents' statements of their primary concerns about the child, the therapist presents a number of situations that may or may not be problem areas in which noncompliance and other inappropriate behaviors exist for the particular family. The parent is asked if the child is noncompliant or disruptive in situations such as the following: bedtime, getting dressed in the morning, mealtimes, bath time, parental telephone conversations, visiting in a friend's home or having visitors, riding in the car, and in public places (e.g., shopping). The therapist also asks for information about whether the child has behavioral or academic difficulties in preschool or school (see below for further information on assessing school problems), and about the child's relationships with other family members (e.g., siblings, other parent or relative) and peers. If the parent reports that a particular behavior or setting is not problematic, the therapist moves to the next situation. If the parent reports that a particular situation is a problem area for him or her, then the therapist, proceeding in a manner similar to that already described, asks about parent and child behaviors that typically occur in the situation. The therapist asks the parent to describe the situation ("What does your child do?"), the frequency ("How often does this occur?" "How many times each day?") and duration ("How long has this been going on?" "How long does it last each time?") of the problem, the parent's response to the child ("What do you do?"), and the child's response to the parent's intervention ("What does your child do then?"). Finally, the therapist questions the parent about the disciplinary procedures he or she is currently using with the child. An openended question ("How do you discipline [child's name]?") is used to initiate questioning in this area. Frequency, duration (if applicable), and parent and child responses to the disciplinary act can be examined.

Figure 4.3 presents a sample Problem Guidesheet for interviewing parents, which is our adaptation of an interview format originally developed by Hanf (1970). In addition to providing a more complete picture of the interaction pattern between parent and child, this interview format also acquaints parents with the social learning orientation of the therapist. (Barkley, 1997, has developed a parent-rating scale version of this interview called the Home Situations Questionnaire.)

The following is a portion of an initial interview to exemplify the analysis of a problem situation.

THERAPIST: Do you have any problems with Mark at bedtime?

PARENT: Oh my gosh, yes. It takes forever for him to go to sleep. He gets out of bed again and again.

THERAPIST: Tell me about your family's routine during the half-hour before Mark's bedtime.

PARENT: At 7:30 I help Mark with his bath. After he brushes his teeth and goes to the

Setting	Description	Frequency	Duration	Parent response	Child response
Bedtime (A.M. and P.M.)					
Mealtime					
Bath time					
On phone					
Visitors at home					
Visiting others					
Car					
Public places (stores, etc.)					
School					
Siblings					
Peers					
Other parent/ relative					
Disciplinary procedures					
Other					

Child: _____   Interviewer(s): _____

Interviewee(s): _____   Date: _____

FIGURE 4.3. Problem Guidesheet.

bathroom, I read him a story. Then Bob and I kiss him goodnight and tell him to stay in bed and to go to sleep.

THERAPIST: OK, then what happens?

PARENT: Well, things are quiet for about 10–15 minutes. Then Mark is up. He gets out of bed and comes into the den where Bob and I are watching TV.

THERAPIST: What does Mark do when he gets up?

PARENT: He usually comes in and climbs in either Bob's or my lap and complains that he can't sleep.

THERAPIST: What do you do then?

PARENT: Sometimes we let him sit with us for a while, but usually I take him back to bed, tell him goodnight again, and tell him to stay in bed.

THERAPIST: What happens then?

PARENT: Mark stays there for a while, but he's soon out again.

THERAPIST: And then what do you do?

PARENT: I may tell him he's being a bad boy. Then I take him back to bed. Usually I read him another story—hoping he'll get sleepy this time.

THERAPIST: Does that work?

PARENT: No, he's up again before I have time to get settled in my chair.

THERAPIST: What happens then?

PARENT: The whole thing repeats itself. I put him in bed, read him another story, and he gets up again.

THERAPIST: How long does this go on?

PARENT: For about 2 or 3 hours—until Bob and I go to bed.

THERAPIST: What happens when you and your husband go to bed?

PARENT: Mark still gets up, but we let him get in bed with us and he goes to sleep then.

THERAPIST: How many nights a week does this happen?

PARENT: Almost every night! I can hardly think of a night's peace in the last few months.

THERAPIST: How long has Mark been doing this?

PARENT: Oh, I would guess for about a year.

THERAPIST: Have you or your husband tried any other ways of handling Mark at bedtime?

PARENT: Sometimes I get angry and yell at him. Sometimes Bob tries spanking him, but then Mark just ends up crying all evening. At least my way we have a little peace and quiet.

In this sample interview, the therapist obtained a description of the events preceding the problem situation fairly quickly. The therapist had to repeat "What happens then?" or some variation thereof several times until a clear description was obtained of the consequent events currently maintaining the problem behavior. Based on this assessment, the problem behavior—noncompliance at bedtime (getting out of bed)—is occurring at a high rate, has been for some time, and appears to be maintained by the parents giving in to the child.

The next sample interview concerns the same problem situation—bedtime—but in this clinical case the antecedent events emerged as important factors maintaining the problem interaction.

THERAPIST: Do you have a problem with Doug at bedtime?

PARENT: Certainly! He's impossible. He starts to scream and cry the minute we put him to bed.

THERAPIST: Tell me about your family's routine the half-hour before Doug's bedtime.

PARENT: Well, Doug takes his bath and puts on his pajamas right after supper. Then we usually watch television together. He knows his bedtime is 8:30, so when the program ends, his father says, "Bedtime." Then the problems begin. Doug tries to stall, begging to see the next show. We ignore this. His father usually just snatches him up and carries him—screaming all the way—to bed. He puts Doug in bed, tells him to stay, turns off the light, and leaves.

THERAPIST: What happens then?

PARENT: He used to get up again and again. Each time we would spank him and put him back to bed. Now, when we put him to bed the first time, we just lock his door. He cries for a while and then drops off to sleep.

THERAPIST: How many nights a week does this happen?

PARENT: Let me see. Nearly all the time.

THERAPIST: Thinking back over the past week, how many nights out of the last seven have you had problems with Doug at bedtime?

PARENT: Hmmm. Four.

THERAPIST: How long has Doug been difficult at bedtime?

PARENT: For the last 6 months.

Based on this interview, the therapist hypothesized that the antecedent events (the abrupt announcement of bedtime and removal of the child to bed) were contributing to the child's problem behaviors at bedtime. This is in contrast to the previous case example in which the parent's giving in to the child appears to be maintaining the bedtime problems.

After the therapist has determined the situations that are currently problems for the parent and child and the antecedent and consequent factors maintaining these problematic parent–child interactions, the therapist then asks the parents to describe their child's positive attributes and strengths. This serves to balance the discussion about the child somewhat and can provide useful information for Phase I of the parent training program, in which the focus is on parental reinforcement of the child's prosocial behavior. It can also provide an indication of the extent of the parents' negative perceptions about the child (i.e., a situation in which the parent is unable to describe any positive attributes or is limited to just one or two descriptors).

A brief developmental and medical history of the child is then obtained. This history should cover difficulties during pregnancy, birth, and early childhood; the ages for developmental milestones, such as sitting, standing, walking, and talking; medical (especially neurological), speech, and hearing problems; and the presence/absence of various toileting problems. (See Barkley, 1997, for one example of a form for collecting such information.) If there are problems in one or more of these areas, an appropriate referral (e.g., physician, audiologist) may need to be made prior to, or concomitant with, intervention.

Given that a "difficult" temperament (Thomas et al., 1968) may be one risk factor for later conduct problem behavior including noncompliance (see Chapter 1), the therapist may choose to inquire as to the existence of such early characteristics. Characteristics of temperament that might be considered include activity level, rhythmicity (regularity of sleeping, eating, etc.), approach to or withdrawal from new stimuli, adaptability to new situations, intensity of reaction, threshold of responsiveness, quality of mood, distractibility, and attention span. The therapist may choose to query the parents about these dimensions in the context of the initial interview or assess them in a more formal manner. (See Slabach, Morrow, & Wachs, 1991, for a discussion of available instruments.)

Finally, the therapist should ask the parents about any previous attempts to deal with these or other child behavior problems. If appropriate, permission to contact previous service providers should be obtained. It is useful to try to ascertain the parents' perceptions of the usefulness and efficacy of these previous treatment encounters, especially if they have been involved in other family-based interventions.

At the end of the parent interview, it is important to ask the parents whether there is any additional information about the child, themselves, or their family that might be helpful in resolving the current situation. This gives the parents permission to discuss matters that they may have been concerned about but were unsure as to their relevance, and it indicates the therapist's willingness and expectation that the parents be open and active participants in the assessment and therapy process.

The therapist's clinical skills are critical in the initial interview. Clearly, the behavioral interview is quite structured, as substantial information is obtained in a brief period of time. However, within this context the therapist must be warm, genuine, sensitive, and responsive to the individual parent's needs. In our experience, the therapist's clinical skills in the initial interview play an essential role in determining whether or not a parent will return for treatment. Furthermore, work by Prinz and Miller (1994) suggests the importance of such skills in maintaining parents' involvement in parent training programs.

Interview with the Child

We have found an individual interview with children under age 6 to be of limited value in providing the therapist with content information. In fact, children below the age of 10 may not be reliable reporters of their own behavioral symptoms (Edelbrock, Costello, Dulcan, Kalas, & Conover, 1985). Even with younger children, however, a few minutes spent privately with the child in a play situation or a walk to the soda machine allows the therapist to obtain a sample of how the child interacts with an unfamiliar adult in a social situation; to assess the child's perception of why the child has been brought to the clinic; to provide a preliminary evaluation of the child's cognitive, affective, and behavioral characteristics; and to begin to develop a relationship with the child (Bierman, 1983; Evans & Nelson, 1986).

With children of all ages, the therapist typically begins with the statement "Tell me why you are here today." We often have been surprised at the range of responses this has elicited, from a realistic appraisal of "So Mommy, Daddy, and I don't fight so much," to the more typical one of "I don't know," to more interesting statements such as "So I'll have someone to play with." After the child has responded, it is helpful (of course, with parental permission) to explain to the child your view of why he or she is at the clinic. The explanation might be: "Your parents are concerned because you and they don't seem to be getting along very well. They came to see us to get some help so things will be more pleasant for you and them at home."

The interview, particularly with older children, can provide the therapist with additional pertinent information. The therapist can ask the child about various situations at home or elsewhere in an attempt to obtain the child's perception about what is happening in these problem situations. Sometimes such questioning is fruitless; at other times, the child's understanding of the situation and the role he or she plays is quite accurate. Such statements as "I know if I say dirty words that Dad goes nuts and then Mom does too" can be quite informative. Other questions to ask the child include those in the following areas:

Family. "What kinds of things do you do with your father/mother/brothers/sisters?"
   "What can you do to make your father/mother happy/mad?"
School. "Tell me about school." "What do you like best at school?" "What do you dislike most at school?"
Social. "Tell me about your friends." "What kinds of things do you do with [friend's name]?"

DIRECT OBSERVATION

Direct behavioral observation by independent, well-trained observers is the most accepted procedure for obtaining a reliable and valid description of current parent–child interactions and for assessing change in those interactions as a function of intervention.

Through the appropriate use of behavioral observation, the therapist can obtain measures of the frequency and duration of child problem behaviors and the relationship between child and parent behaviors and, thus, is able to quantify the problem interactions targeted for intervention. Similar to parent-recorded data, when compared with parental responses in the interview or on the Child Behavior Checklist (CBCL; Achenbach & Rescorla, 2000, 2001), direct observation can provide important information concerning the congruence of parental perceptions of the child's behavior with actual levels of such behavior.

Observations may occur in either the home or the clinic setting (Gardner, 2000). While extremely valuable for assessment and intervention, behavioral observations by independent observers in the home are very expensive and time-consuming. An alternative assessment procedure that reduces the time and cost required for observation in the natural setting is the observation of parent–child interactions in a structured setting in the clinic. Use of a structured clinic observation is advantageous for several reasons: (1) it may efficiently elicit the problematic parent–child interactions; (2) observation can occur unobtrusively through one-way windows; and (3) the standard situation allows the therapist to make within- and between-client comparisons (Haynes, 1991; Hughes & Haynes, 1978; Mash & Terdal, 1997). Unfortunately, parents and children interacting in a clinic situation may change the nature of their interaction (Haynes, 1991). For that reason, the use of both clinic and home observations is optimal. These assessment procedures are described in this section.

Clinic Observations

Following the interview, the parent–child pair is observed in a clinic playroom, preferably equipped with a one-way observation window and wired for sound. The playroom contains various age-appropriate toys, such as building blocks, toy trucks and cars, dolls, puzzles, crayons, and paper. Prior to the clinic observation, the parent is instructed to interact with the child in two different contexts, referred to as the "Child's Game" and the "Parent's Game." In the Child's Game, the parent is instructed to engage in any activity that the child chooses and to allow the child to determine the nature and rules of the interaction. Thus, the Child's Game is essentially a free-play situation. In the Parent's Game, the parent is instructed to engage the child in activities whose rules and nature are determined by the parent. The Parent's Game is essentially a command situation.

Two other clinic analogues can be considered for use: a Clean-Up task (e.g., Eyberg, Bessmer, Newcomb, Edwards, & Robinson, 1994) and the Compliance Test (Roberts & Powers, 1988). In a recent review, Roberts (2001) has suggested that the toy Clean-Up analogue be used in lieu of the Parent's Game, arguing that the former has greater content validity (i.e., instructing the child to clean up toys versus engaging the child in/switching to various play activities). However, given the documented clinical utility of the Parent's Game analogue by ourselves and others (see Roberts, 2001), we do not feel that the Parent's Game should be abandoned. Instead, we suggest that therapists employ either the Parent's Game *or* Clean-Up, or, if time permits, use both (as per Eyberg et al., 1994).

The Compliance Test (Roberts & Powers, 1988) is a chore analogue for 2- to 6-year-olds in which the parent's instruction-giving behavior is completely structured and prompted by the therapist with a radio signaling device. The parent issues 30 two-step commands to the child. The first command instructs the child to pick up a particular toy. The second step command is either "Put it in/on the [container]" if the child complied to the first step, or "Pick up the [toy] and put it in/on the [container]" if the child did not comply to the first-step command. Child compliance and inappropriate behavior are scored similarly to the coding system described later in this chapter. The Compliance Test can be used to identify the extent to which low compliance in the Parent's Game (or Clean-Up) is due to poor parental instruction giving versus deliberate child noncompliance. It may also facilitate diagnostic decision making concerning the presence of ODD (Brumfield & Roberts, 1998).

Sometimes a parent will be hesitant about interacting with the child while being observed. The therapist should assure the parent that these feelings are normal but that it is important to obtain a sample of how the child interacts with the parent. The therapist also tells the parent that he or she recognizes that such an interaction between parent and child will be artificial; nevertheless, it will provide meaningful information. Finally, the therapist discusses the interaction with the parent once the Child's Game and Parent's Game are completed. The therapist needs to query the parent about whether the interaction was typical of those that occur with the child at home and, if not, in what ways it was different. Also, the therapist may need to tell the parent again that it is typical for parents to feel uncomfortable being observed and to reassure the parent that he or she did a satisfactory job. Understanding how the parent may react to the observation and supporting those parental feelings can help the therapist build rapport with the parent.

During the clinic observation, the therapist codes the parent–child interaction from behind a one-way observation window for 5 minutes in both the Child's Game and the Parent's Game. (If a one-way observation window is not available, the therapist can sit in a corner of the playroom and code the interaction.) In a situation in which both parents are present, one parent can participate in the observation with the child while the other parent completes questionnaires in another room. The parents then switch at the end of the first set of observations.

Home Observations

When feasible, observational data also are collected in the home by an independent observer at a time convenient for the parent. This time is typically one in which the parent reports that the child problem behaviors occur frequently. The therapist arranges the time for the first observation at the end of the assessment (interview) session and, if possible, introduces the home observer to the parent. After the first observation, the parent and observer arrange subsequent observation times. In our work, separate sets of four observations occur prior to treatment, after treatment, and at each follow-up assessment. Each observation is 40 minutes in length. Reliability data are obtained for one-fourth of the home observations; on those occasions, two observers score the parent–child interactions.

For each observation, the parent is asked to interact with the child as she or he would normally during that time of day. A number of procedural guidelines have been formulated in an attempt to facilitate the collection of data in the home. The parent is given a written handout describing these guidelines (see Figure 4.4), and the therapist discusses these with the parent near the end of the initial session.

As our coding system only permits the behavior of a single adult to be recorded at a time (see below), observations have typically occurred with just one parent present. However, if it is possible for both parents to participate in observations, the observer can code the behavior of each parent with the child in alternating 5-minute periods. This process can occur for 40 minutes, so that 20 minutes of data are collected for each parent. Alternatively, separate observation periods of 20 to 40 minutes may occur with each parent and the child.

After introducing the concept of home observations to the parent, the therapist may need to deal with the parent's reservations about home observations. The primary issue raised by most parents is the difficulty with following a normal routine when an observer is present. The parent should be assured that it is recognized that the observer's presence and the guidelines set up for the observation are not natural. However, these procedures are at present the most effective method available for obtaining information in the home environment. Parental concerns can be minimized by emphasizing that the information obtained will be used to design an effective intervention program for the child. Finally, the parent can be told that most parents report becoming progressively less aware of and anxious about the observer's presence with each observation.

Home observations are an expensive undertaking, with extensive time and transportation costs. While we value this assessment procedure, we recognize that home observations may not be possible in many settings. Because our assessments in the clinic and in the home have yielded similar results (Peed, Roberts, & Forehand, 1977), data collected during clinic observations by an observer or therapist may serve as an alternative to home observational data.

Coding System

We have developed an observational system for use in both the clinic and home settings. The coding system was designed specifically to tap patterns of parent–child interaction as well as specific parent and child behaviors related to child compliance and noncompliance to parental instructions. The coding manual used to train observers in the Behavioral Coding System (BCS), which was presented in the first edition of this volume (Forehand & McMahon, 1981), is now available at *www.guilford.com*. A simplified version of the BCS (McMahon & Estes, 1994) was developed for use in the Fast Track project (see Chapter 10) and may have particular appeal to clinicians. It is available from the first author (RJM), University of Washington, Department of Psychology, Box 351525, Seattle, WA 98195-1525. The procedure for training observers will be discussed later in this chapter.

As we discussed during our initial meeting, allowing us to see you and your child in a more normal routine will help us to better design treatment and to determine its effectiveness. We appreciate your allowing us into your home.

When the observer arrives, you will see that he or she has a tape recorder and earphone. The observer is *not* recording the observation. The observer is listening to a tape that is cueing him or her when to code information. If you'd like, the observer can let you hear a portion of the tape.

Occasionally, two observers will come to your home. The second observer is there to check the recording accuracy of the first observer, *not* to evaluate your performance.

During each observation, please try to interact normally with your child. Don't feel compelled to do anything you wouldn't ordinarily be doing at this time. Ignore the observer—he or she will try to be as unobtrusive as possible. During the observation, the observer will not be able to interact with you or your child.

It is very important that you follow these guidelines as closely as possible for each home observation. They are designed to help the observer hear and see as much of the observation as he or she can.

- Remain in a two-room area with your child, in view and hearing range of the observer. If your child leaves the observation area, please bring him or her back.
- You may bring any work materials or toys desired into the observation area, with the exception of commercial board games (for example, Candyland, Monopoly) or playing cards. It is a good idea to do this *before* the observation starts. Also, we have found it helpful if you check on your child's bathroom needs prior to the beginning of the observation.
- Do not watch TV or play video games.
- Please don't read to your child.
- It is best if your child does not have friends over during the observation. If brothers or sisters are present at one observation, then they should be at the other observations as much as possible.
- If the telephone rings, talk as briefly as possible, or ask if you may return the call later.
- If you have any questions regarding your appointments at the clinic or concerning the treatment program, please do not ask the observer. Observers are not trained in these matters. If you will call us at the clinic, we will try to answer your questions.

Don't be surprised if you feel a bit awkward at first—everyone does. However, if you just pretend the observer is not there, then you will be more comfortable and will act more naturally. Thank you for your cooperation.

FIGURE 4.4. Parent's guidelines for home observations.

An overview of the BCS will be presented here. There are six parent behaviors and three child behaviors that can be recorded onto the score sheet (see Figure 4.5). The parent behaviors (and coding symbols) are:

1. Rewards (R): praise, approval, or positive physical attention that refers to the child or the child's activity; verbal rewards include both specific (labeled) and nonspecific (unlabeled) reference to "praiseworthy" behavior.
2. Attends (A): descriptive phrases that follow and refer to (1) the child's ongoing behavior, (2) objects directly related to the child's play, (3) his or her spatial position (e.g., "You're standing in the middle of the room"), or (4) the appearance of the child.
3. Questions (Q): interrogatives to which the only appropriate response is verbal.
4. Commands (C):
   a. Alpha commands (clear instructions): orders, rules, suggestions, or questions to which a motoric response (i.e., one eliciting movement) is appropriate and feasible.
   b. Beta commands (unclear instructions): commands to which the child has no opportunity to demonstrate compliance. These commands include parental commands that (1) are so vague that proper action for compliance cannot be determined, (2) are interrupted by further parental verbiage before enough time (5 seconds) has elapsed for the child to comply, or (3) are carried out by the parent before the child has an opportunity to comply. A beta command is also scored if the parent restricts the child's mobility in such a way as to preclude his or her compliance.
5. Warnings (W): statements that describe aversive consequences to be delivered by the parent if the child fails to comply to a parental command.
6. Time out (TO): a procedure used by the parent that clearly is intended to remove the child from positive reinforcement because of the child's inappropriate behaviors (e.g., placing the child in a chair in the corner of the room).

The child behaviors (and coding symbols) are the following:

1. Child compliance (C): an appropriate motoric response initiated within 5 seconds following a parental alpha command.
2. Child noncompliance (N): failure to initiate a motoric response within 5 seconds following a parental alpha command.
3. Appropriateness of child behavior: Child inappropriate (i.e., deviant) behavior (√) may include: (1) whining, crying, yelling, or tantrums; (2) aggression (e.g., biting, kicking, hitting, slapping, grabbing an object from someone, or the threat of aggression); or (3) deviant talk (e.g., repetitive requests for attention, stated refusals to comply, disrespectful statements, profanity, and commands to parents that threaten aversive consequences). The absence of such behaviors is scored as appropriate child behavior by means of a zero (0).

SCORE SHEET   page _____

Child's Name _____   Date _____   Time _____
              Last   First   Coder's Name _____
Parent's Name _____   Session _____ Place _____
              Last   First

1
[grid] ○

2
[grid] ○

3
[grid] ○

4
[grid] ○

5
[grid] ○

6
[grid] ○

7
[grid] ○

8
[grid] ○

9
[grid] ○

10
[grid] ○

ROW 1	ROW 2	ROW 3	CIRCLE	OTHER
C command	C compliance	A attend	√ inappropriate	TO time out
W warning	N noncompliance	R reward	child behavior	
Q question			0 appropriate	
A attend			child behavior	
R reward				

FIGURE 4.5. Score Sheet for the Behavioral Coding System.

The score sheet for recording parent and child behaviors using the BCS is presented in Figure 4.5. Each score sheet contains 10 rectangular blocks, each subdivided into 3 rows and 10 columns, with a circle following each rectangle. Each rectangle represents 30 seconds of observation time; thus, each score sheet contains 5 minutes of data. The three rows represent three categories of behavior: parental antecedents (C, W, Q, A, R) in row 1, child responses (C, N) in row 2, and parental consequences (A, R) in row 3. The behaviors recorded within a single column indicate a sequence of related behaviors, or an interaction. The columns also denote the order of occurrence of these interactions.

Notice two points about the rectangles. First, within any given rectangular block typically not all of the columns are scored. Up to 10 interactions may be scored each 30 seconds (1 per column); only rarely will 10 or more scorable behavioral interactions occur during a 30-second interval. Second, all three categories (rows) in the rectangle need not be scored in any given interaction (column). The following rules determine which categories of behavior are scored for any given interaction.

1. The occurrence of any of the five parental antecedents (C, W, Q, A, R) is recorded in row 1, unless all 10 columns in the rectangle have been used before the 30-second interval is completed. Parental antecedents are recorded in order beginning in the far-left column. A parental antecedent is the cue that initiates the start of an interaction.
2. A child response of compliance (C) or noncompliance (N) may be scored in row 2 if and only if the recorded parental antecedent in row 1 was a command (C) or a warning (W). If a child response does not occur, the next recording will be a parental antecedent placed in row 1 of the next column to the right.
3. A parental consequence (A, R) may be scored in row 3 if and only if the recorded child response in row 2 was compliance (C). If the child response was noncompliance (N), the next scoring will again be a parental antecedent in row 1 of the next column (unless TO is initiated).
4. TO is scored in row 3 or below the rectangle, depending upon how the parent implements the procedure. (See the BCS for details.)

In summary, each rectangle marks a 30-second interval, each row indicates a different category of parent or child behavior, and each column contains an interaction consisting of a sequence of one to three behaviors. The rules for scoring an interaction or sequence of behaviors specify that any recordable parental antecedent, up to 10 per rectangle, is always scored. A score for row 2 (child responses of compliance or noncompliance) depends on the occurrence of a specific type of parental antecedent (command or warning) in row 1. A score for row 3 (parental consequences of rewards or attends) depends on the occurrence of a specific child response (compliance) in row 2. TO may be scored in either row 3 or in the margin below the rectangle.

The circle on the score sheet is used to record an additional category of child behavior (appropriateness of child behavior) on an interval sampling basis. Each circle is scored for the same 30-second interval as the rectangle that precedes it. The rule for scoring inappropriate child behavior is simply that at least one of the three forms of inappropriate behavior occurred at some point during the interval. Inappropriate child behavior is recorded at the time that behavior occurs during the 30-second interval. However, inappropriate child behavior may be recorded only once per circle regardless of subsequent occurrences during the remainder of the interval. If child behavior is appropriate for the *entire* 30-second interval, appropriate child behavior is recorded in the circle at the conclusion of the interval. Therefore, the marking of a checkmark or zero in the circle denotes the presence or absence of at least one inappropriate behavior.

During observations, an audiotape cues observers at the end of each 30-second interval to shift to the next rectangle and circle.

With respect to reliability, we have typically obtained average interobserver agreement above .75 for each of the parent and child behaviors that are coded (e.g., Forehand, Lautenschlager, Faust, & Graziano, 1986; Forehand, Wells, & Griest, 1980; McMahon, Forehand, & Griest, 1981). The coding system possesses adequate test–retest reliability as well. Data from repeated observations of nonintervention parent–child interactions are stable and consistent (Peed et al., 1977).

With respect to validity, significant differences in compliance between clinic-referred and nonreferred (i.e., "normal") children have been found using this coding system (Forehand, King, Peed, & Yoder, 1975; Forehand, Sturgis, et al., 1979; Griest, Forehand, Wells, & McMahon, 1980). The observation procedure is also sensitive enough to measure significant treatment effects and maintenance of treatment effects in the clinic and at home with clinic-referred populations (e.g., Baum & Forehand, 1981; Forehand, Griest, & Wells, 1979; Forehand, Sturgis, et al., 1979; Humphreys, Forehand, McMahon, & Roberts, 1978; Peed et al., 1977). In other studies, parent–child interactions in the clinic have been shown to be similar to those observed in the home (Peed et al., 1977) and to predict child behavior in the home (Forehand, Wells, & Sturgis, 1978). Treatment effects observed in the clinic coincide with treatment effects observed in the home (Peed et al., 1977).

Following the clinic observation, the therapist summarizes the data from the Child's Game and the Parent's Game on the Observation Data Summary Sheet— Clinic Observations (see Figure 4.6). (The observer summarizes the data from each set of home observations in a manner similar to that for the clinic observation data. Figure 4.7 presents an Observation Data Summary Sheet—Home Observations for this purpose.)

For the Child's Game, the rates per minute of the parent behaviors of total commands, questions, attends, and rewards are of particular interest, as is the percentage of intervals of child inappropriate behavior. For the Parent's Game, several parent and child behaviors are of particular interest. These include parent behaviors expressed as rates per minute of total commands, alpha commands, beta commands, warnings, questions, attends, and rewards. In addition, the percentage of parental attention contingent upon child compliance (i.e., rewards plus attends emitted within 5 seconds following child compliance) and the total number of TOs are computed. Child behaviors include percentage of child compliance to alpha commands, percentage of child compliance to total commands, and percentage of child inappropriate behavior.

Observation Data Summary Sheet—Clinic Observations

Child's Name _____   Date of Observation _____

Parent's Name _____

Therapist's Name _____

Session: Pre, Post, or Follow-up (circle one)

CHILD'S GAME or PARENT'S GAME (circle one)   Data Tallied by _____

Behaviors   Total

Row 1
  Attends   = (a) _____
  Rewards   = (b) _____
  Questions   = (c) _____
  Warnings   = (d) _____
  Total commands   = (e) _____
    Beta commands   = (f) _____
    Alpha commands   = (g) _____
Row 2
  Compliances to commands   = (h) _____
  Compliances to warnings   = (i) _____
  Noncompliances to commands   = (j) _____
  Noncompliances to warnings   = (k) _____
Row 3
  Attends   = (l) _____
  Rewards   = (m) _____

Other
  Time outs (TO)   = (n) _____
  Inappropriate behavior   = (p) _____

Data Summary
 (a + l) ____ ÷ 5   ____ Attends per minute (p.m.)
 (b + m) ____ ÷ 5   ____ Rewards p.m.
 (a + l + ____ ÷ 5   ____ Attends + rewards p.m.
 b + m)
   (c)   ____ ÷ 5   ____ Questions p.m.
   (d)   ____ ÷ 5   ____ Warnings p.m.
   (e)   ____ ÷ 5   ____ Total commands p.m.
   (f)   ____ ÷ 5   ____ Beta commands p.m.
   (g)   ____ ÷ 5   ____ Alpha commands p.m.
   (h)   ____ ÷ (g)   ____ × 100 = ____ % Compliance to alpha commands
   (h)   ____ ÷ (e)   ____ × 100 = ____ % Compliance to total commands
   (j)   ____ ÷ (e)   ____ × 100 = ____ % Noncompliance to total commands
   (i)   ____ ÷ (d)   ____ × 100 = ____ % Compliance to warnings
   (k)   ____ ÷ (d)   ____ × 100 = ____ % Noncompliance to warnings
 (l + m) ____ ÷ (h + i) ____ × 100 = ____ % Contingent attention
   (p)   ____ ÷ 10   ____ × 100 = ____ % Intervals inappropriate behavior
                              (n)   ____ # Time outs

FIGURE 4.6. Observation Data Summary Sheet—Clinic Observations.

Observation Data Summary Sheet—Home Observations

Child's Name _____   Dates of Observations _____

Parent's Name _____

Therapist's Name _____

Session: Pre, Post, or Follow-up (circle one)   Data Tallied by _____

Behaviors	Observations					Total
	1	2	3	4		
Row 1						
Attends	____	____	____	____	= (a)	____
Rewards	____	____	____	____	= (b)	____
Questions	____	____	____	____	= (c)	____
Warnings	____	____	____	____	= (d)	____
Total commands	____	____	____	____	= (e)	____
Beta commands	____	____	____	____	= (f)	____
Alpha commands	____	____	____	____	= (g)	____
Row 2						
Compliances to commands	____	____	____	____	= (h)	____
Compliances to warnings	____	____	____	____	= (i)	____
Noncompliances to commands	____	____	____	____	= (j)	____
Noncompliances to warnings	____	____	____	____	= (k)	____
Row 3						
Attends	____	____	____	____	= (l)	____
Rewards	____	____	____	____	= (m)	____
Other						
Time outs (TO)	____	____	____	____	= (n)	____
Inappropriate behavior	____	____	____	____	= (p)	____

Data Summary

(a + l) ____ ÷ 160   ____ Attends per minute (p.m.)
(b + m) ____ ÷ 160   ____ Rewards p.m.
(a + l + ____ ÷ 160   ____ Attends + rewards p.m.
b + m)

(c) ____ ÷ 160   ____ Questions p.m.
(d) ____ ÷ 160   ____ Warnings p.m.
(e) ____ ÷ 160   ____ Total commands p.m.
(f) ____ ÷ 160   ____ Beta commands p.m.
(g) ____ ÷ 160   ____ Alpha commands p.m.
(h) ____ ÷ (g)   ____ × 100 =   ____ % Compliance to alpha commands
(h) ____ ÷ (e)   ____ × 100 =   ____ % Compliance to total commands
(j) ____ ÷ (e)   ____ × 100 =   ____ % Noncompliance to total commands
(i) ____ ÷ (d)   ____ × 100 =   ____ % Compliance to warnings
(k) ____ ÷ (d)   ____ × 100 =   ____ % Noncompliance to warnings
(l + m) ____ ÷ (h + i)   ____ × 100 =   ____ % Contingent attention
(p) ____ ÷ 320   ____ × 100 =   ____ % Intervals inappropriate behavior
                            (n)   ____ # Time outs

FIGURE 4.7. Observation Data Summary Sheet—Home Observations.

Figure 4.8 shows a sample data sheet from the observation of the parent–child interactions during a Parent's Game session in the clinic. The data from the sample observation are summarized at the bottom of the table (this information would be obtained from the Observation Data Summary Sheet—Clinic Observations, Figure 4.6). As can be seen, the child engaged in inappropriate behavior (e.g., whining, crying, hitting) in 40% of the ten 30-second observation intervals. Compliance to the total number of commands given by the parent was 19%. However, compliance to clear, direct commands (alpha commands) was much higher (75%). The parent provided positive consequences to only 17% of the child's compliant responses. Differentiating child compliance to alpha and total commands provides the therapist with information concerning the antecedent events maintaining child noncompliance. In this example, the large difference between the percentage of compliance to alpha commands and to total commands indicates that modification of the parent's command behavior is essential to treatment success. Based on this observation, the treatment goals would be: (1) to teach the parent to give clear instructions (i.e., alpha commands); (2) to decrease the number of unclear instructions (i.e., beta commands); (3) to increase the parent's positive consequences (i.e., rewards and attends) for child compliance; and (4) to decrease the child's inappropriate behavior by teaching the parent a TO procedure.

Observer Training

Training observers in the reliable use of a complex coding system can be a difficult and time-consuming task (Margolin et al., 1998). In this section, we describe briefly some of the procedures we use. Although the focus here is on training independent observers to conduct home observations, the procedures are also applicable to therapists learning the BCS for coding the clinic analogues (i.e., the Child's Game, the Parent's Game).

Our observers typically are undergraduate psychology majors who are selected as observers because of their interest in child psychology. We attempt to select individuals who are highly motivated and are seeking a relevant field experience. The observers typically receive course credit for participation in an independent study course for their participation.

We train observers in groups of four or five. Initially, they are instructed to read the BCS manual (Forehand & McMahon, 1981; *www.guilford.com*). We then discuss the general framework within which the coding is done, the setting in which behavior is coded, and the individual behavior categories. Subsequently, we present each behavior category and its general coding procedure. Actual training is then initiated. We teach one behavior at a time. A behavior is selected; the definition is presented; the trainer models several examples of the behavior; and observers, enacting the parts of parent and child, take turns role playing the behaviors with available toys while remaining observers code the occurrence of the behavior being taught. Following each role play, the trainer and observers compare their recorded frequency of occurrence of the behavior. Agreements and disagreements are discussed.

SCORE SHEET page _____

Child's Name _Begood,_ _____ _Jack_ _____ Date _9/17/01_ Time _5:30_ _____
          Last   First   Coder's Name _JKL_ _____

Parent's Name _Begood,_ _____ _Lois_ _____ Session _1_ _____ Place _Clinic_ _____
          Last   First

1

C	C	A	C	C					
			N	C					

(O)

2

A	A	C	C	Q	C				
					C				

(O)

3

C	C	Q	Q	C	C				
					C				

(√)

4

R	C	C	C	Q					
			N						

(√)

5

C	C	Q	A	C	C				
	C								

(O)

6

C	C	Q	C	C	C				

(√)

7

A	A	R	C	C					
				C					

(O)

8

C	C	C	Q	W					

(O)

9

Q	A	Q	C	C					
			C						
			R						

(O)

10

C	C	Q	Q						

(√)

ROW 1	ROW 2	ROW 3	CIRCLE	OTHER
C command	C compliance	A attend	√ inappropriate	TO time out
W warning	N noncompliance	R reward	child behavior	
Q question			0 appropriate	
A attend			child behavior	
R reward				

32/5 = 6.4 Total commands/min.   11/5 = 2.2 Quest./min.   6/8 = 75% Compliance to
 8/5 = 1.6 Alpha commands/min.   7/5 = 1.4 Attends/min.   alpha commands
24/5 = 4.8 Beta commands/min.   3/5 = .6 Rewards/min.   6/32 = 19% Compliance to
 1/5 = .2 Warnings/min.   total commands
                                                 1/6 = 17% Contingent
                                                     attention
                                                  4/10 = 40% Inappropriate
                                                        child behavior

FIGURE 4.8. Sample Score Sheet for the Parent's Game.

After we have taught one behavior, a second behavior is then taught similarly. Subsequently, role playing occurs in which both behaviors are modeled and recorded by observers. In addition, we use written exercises to provide the observers with exposure to making various subtle discriminations (e.g., between a question and a question command). We teach each new behavior in this manner. New behaviors are continually taught until observers can code all behaviors simultaneously in the role-played vignettes.

From this point on, training occurs primarily through the use of videotaped interactions. These may be tapes of simulated parent–child interactions employing the trainers or of actual parent–child interactions. The advantage of the former is that specific discriminations or types of interactions may be presented. They are usually presented in the earlier stages of training. The tapes of actual parent–child interactions provide a more realistic approximation to what the observer will experience in the home setting and are employed more frequently in the later stages of training.

Training continues until the observers have attained an acceptable level of skill in using the coding system. We have operationally defined this level as that of obtaining a total reliability coefficient of 80% on a prescored 10-minute videotape of an actual parent–child interaction. The reliability coefficient for any one behavior is calculated by first computing the number of agreements between a prescored protocol and the trainee and the number of agreements plus disagreements for each 30-second interval. Each of these figures is summed across 30-second intervals, and the total number of agreements between the trainee and the protocol is divided by the total number of agreements plus disagreements to obtain a reliability coefficient. It typically takes 20 to 25 hours of training for observers to reach this level of skill.

Training sessions occur two or three times weekly, and each lasts 1–1½ hours. In the initial stages of training, sessions occur more frequently than they do in later stages. This is done in order to provide a more intensive exposure to the coding system early in the training sequence. After observers are trained and are doing observations, we hold weekly group practice sessions in order to ensure that reliable scoring continues and to prevent observer drift.

An important aspect of training observers is teaching them about appropriate professional behavior. This is done prior to their first home observation. The importance of being prompt for observations is noted. Although we instruct the observers to be courteous and polite at all times, we request that they not socialize with parents. We stress the confidentiality of the information gathered during the observations. Parents' questions regarding treatment or their children's problems are to be referred to the therapist. Under no circumstances are observers to give advice or suggestions on how to manage children.

An experienced observer accompanies new observers on their first home observation. We have found that this minimizes much of the anticipatory anxiety the new observer may have and provides a model of appropriate professional behavior. In these situations, reliability data are collected as well. (Reliability checks are usually conducted during one of the later observation sessions to allow the parent to get used to the primary observer's presence.)

PARENT-COMPLETED QUESTIONNAIRES

Questionnaires that parents complete as part of the assessment process can give the therapist additional information beyond that obtained in the interview. For example, the therapist may not be able to explore all relevant areas in an interview because of time constraints. Questionnaires completed by parents allow the therapist to examine some of these areas without any time commitment from the therapist (Evans & Nelson, 1986). The therapist gives questionnaires to the parent at the end of the initial interview and asks the parent to complete and return them prior to the feedback session. If both parents attend the initial interview, then each parent can work on the questionnaires while the other parent is participating in the Child's Game and the Parent's Game observations with the child. The therapist can explore any areas of concern from the parent's responses on the questionnaires at the beginning of the feedback session. This is particularly true for parental personal and marital adjustment. As the initial interview focuses on parent–child problem interactions, the personal and marital adjustment of the parent may not be examined. Questionnaires concerning such adjustment can provide the therapist with important information for discussion in subsequent sessions and may help the therapist decide if parent training is the most appropriate intervention (see Chapter 5).

Behavioral rating scales completed by the parents concerning the child's behavior are very useful as screening devices, both for covering a broad range of conduct problem behaviors in addition to noncompliance and for screening for the presence of other child behavior disorders (McMahon & Estes, 1997). Behavioral rating scales are currently regarded as excellent measures of parental perceptions of the child, and when examined in the context of information from other assessment data (i.e., behavioral observations, parent and child interviews), they can be important indicators as to whether the parent appears to have a bias in his or her perceptions of the child. For example, behavioral observations may indicate that a child is not noncompliant and deviant; however, the parent may report on a behavioral rating scale that the child is perceived as noncompliant and deviant at home. This suggests to the therapist that it may not be the child's behavior but rather the parent's expectations that need to be changed. Alternatively, in some cases (e.g., when the child is referred by the school), it may be that parental perceptions are biased in the opposite direction (i.e., the parent does not view the child as noncompliant and deviant). In addition, having each parent complete the behavioral rating scale independently can assist in the identification of incongruities between parents as to their perceptions of their child's behavioral adjustment.

Behavioral rating scales that tap parental perceptions of the child also provide valuable information concerning the social validity of the parent training program (McMahon & Estes, 1997) in terms of whether the child's behavior is considered to be improved after treatment by significant individuals in the child's environment (see Chapter 2). Chapter 10 describes our empirical examination of the social validity of HNC.

We use parent-completed questionnaires to assess four areas: (1) parental perceptions of child adjustment; (2) parental perceptions of their own personal and marital adjustment; (3) parental knowledge of social learning principles; and (4) parental satisfaction with treatment. Questionnaires in the first three areas usually are given to the parent to complete at the end of the initial assessment session. They should be returned to the clinic (by the parent or home observer, or by mail) *prior to* the next session so that the therapist can determine whether additional assessment in these areas is warranted. These questionnaires, as well as the one assessing parental satisfaction with treatment, also can be given to the parent to complete after treatment is terminated and at follow-up assessments. Because of the young age of the children who participate in the parent training program, we do not have them complete questionnaires.

If possible, both parents should complete the questionnaires. Areas of discrepancy and mutual agreement between parents are an important source of data, whether they concern perceptions of the child's behavior or the marital relationship. In addition, responses to questionnaires by both parents may suggest different therapeutic goals for the two parents. For example, treatment for depression concomitantly with parent training might be necessary for the father, while extensive training in social learning principles might be beneficial for the mother.

It is important to have each parent complete the questionnaires separately. This is both to maintain independence of responding and to provide confidentiality, a particular concern with the measures of personal adjustment and marital satisfaction. For these two types of measures, the therapist should tell the parents that some of the questions touch on personal matters and, consequently, the therapist will not share the responses with the other parent (i.e., confidentiality will be provided).

Parent Perceptions of Child Adjustment

We currently utilize the CBCL (Achenbach & Rescorla, 2000, 2001) to assess parent perceptions of their child's adjustment.[2] The CBCL is a widely used checklist that has national norms and excellent reliability and validity data. The CBCL family of instruments (Achenbach & Rescorla, 2000, 2001) currently consists of parallel forms for parents, teachers and caregivers (e.g., day care providers), youth (aged 11 years and older), interviewers, and direct observers. We focus on the parent form here (the teacher/caregiver versions of the CBCL are described below).

The parent form of the CBCL currently consists of two newly revised scales: one completed by parents of children aged 6 to 18 (CBCL/6–18; Achenbach & Rescorla, 2001) and one completed by parents of children aged 1½–5 (CBCL/1½–5; Achenbach & Rescorla, 2000). The CBCL/6–18 includes both Competence (e.g., sports in which

---

[2]In addition to the CBCL family of instruments (Achenbach & Rescorla, 2000, 2001), the Eyberg Child Behavior Inventory (ECBI) and the Sutter-Eyberg Student Behavior Inventory—Revised (SESBI-R) (Eyberg & Pincus, 1999), which focus only on conduct problem behaviors, have also been recommended for use with parents and teachers of young children referred for noncompliance (McMahon & Estes, 1997).

In the first edition (Forehand & McMahon, 1981), we described our extensive use of the Parent Attitudes Test (PAT; Cowen, Huser, Beach, & Rappaport, 1970) as a measure of parental perceptions of the child's behavior. The limited psychometric data on this measure and the presence of more psychometrically sound and broadly focused alternatives such as the CBCL (Achenbach & Rescorla, 2000, 2001) led us to discontinue its use.

the child participates, success in school) and Problem items, while the CBCL/1½–5 includes Problem items and a Language Development Survey. The forms can be completed in 10–20 minutes. The Problem scales of the CBCL/6–18 consist of 120 items. There are separate norms for boys and girls at two age levels (6–11 and 12–18). The instrument yields Total, Internalizing (e.g., withdrawn/depressed, somatic complaints, anxious/depressed), and Externalizing (e.g., aggressive and rule-breaking behavior) broad-band scores. Furthermore, eight narrow-band subscales can be tabulated: Anxious/Depressed, Withdrawn/Depressed, and Somatic Complaints (which comprise the Internalizing broad-band scale); Social Problems, Thought Problems, and Attention Problems; and Rule-Breaking Behavior and Aggressive Behavior (which comprise the Externalizing broad-band scale). The Aggressive Behavior subscale is of particular interest because it includes items that assess aspects of noncompliance (e.g., disobedient at home, stubborn, argues) and items which frequently accompany noncompliance (e.g., fights, screams, temper). The CBCL/6–18 also yields six DSM-oriented scales, including scales labeled Oppositional Defiant Problems and Conduct Problems.

The CBCL/1½–5 consists of 99 Problem items and yields Total, Internalizing, and Externalizing broad-band scales. There are seven narrow-band subscales: Emotionally Reactive, Anxious/Depressed, Somatic Complaints, and Withdrawn (which comprise the Internalizing broad-band scale); Sleep Problems; and Attention Problems and Aggressive Behavior (which comprise the Externalizing broad-band scale). Similar to the CBCL/6–18, the Aggressive Behavior scale is particularly relevant for children referred for noncompliance. The CBCL/1½–5 also yields five DSM-oriented scales, including the scale labeled Oppositional Defiant Problems.

Substantial research now suggests that various child psychological disorders frequently overlap (e.g., Angold, Costello, & Erkanli, 1999). Children referred for noncompliance and other conduct problems are particularly likely to meet criteria for coexisting (i.e., comorbid) ADHD (see Chapters 1 and 9). The Attention Problems scale on the CBCL/1½–5 and the CBCL/6–18 (Chen, Faraone, Biederman, & Tsuang, 1994) can be used as a screen for ADHD. Comorbid internalizing problems such as anxiety and depression can also be screened using the CBCL.

The availability of equivalent forms of the CBCL for parents and teachers can maximize the amount of information about the child and permits comparisons across informants (parents and teachers) and settings (home and school). If parent and teacher perceptions about the child's behavior are congruent, this provides some support for the veracity of the parent's report and may suggest that the child has progressed further along the early starter pathway of conduct problems described in Chapter 1. Elevations on the teacher versions of the CBCL (Achenbach & Rescorla, 2000, 2001), with or without comparable elevations on the parent version of the CBCL, indicate that the child's behavior in school should be more thoroughly assessed (see below). It is important to note, however, that disagreement between parents or between parents and teachers is not necessarily a problem, as it may be due to the situational specificity of the child's behavior (i.e., the child's behavior is a problem with only one adult or in one setting). This, of course, has important implications for treatment planning.

Manuals describing the various forms of the CBCL, blank rating scales, and the scoring keys can be obtained from ASEBA, Research Center for Children, Youth, and Families, Room 6436, 1 South Prospect Street, Burlington, VT 05401-3456; *www.aseba.org.*

As noted above, one advantage of using well-standardized behavioral rating scales such as the CBCL is the opportunity to compare parental perceptions of the child's behavior to that of a normative sample on a variety of factor-analytically derived sub-scales. Therapists would do well to heed the advice of Breen and Altepeter (1990), who recommend that interpretation of behavioral rating scales also include an inspection of the individual items endorsed by parents on these scales. Their point is that some items that statistically load on a particular factor may have only minimal clinical relevance to the labeled factor.

Parents' Perceptions of Personal Adjustment and Interparental Conflict

Parental personal adjustment, particularly depressive symptomatology, and conflict be-tween parents have been two areas of family functioning found repeatedly to be related to child behaviors such as noncompliance. Thus, we always assess these two areas through parent-completed questionnaires.

The Beck Depression Inventory (BDI; Beck, Rush, Shaw, & Emery, 1979) has been our primary measure of parental perceptions of personal adjustment, while the O'Leary–Porter Scale (OPS; Porter & O'Leary, 1980) is the instrument we now use to measure interparental conflict. Both measures are readily administered and scored.

Substantial research has demonstrated that the BDI is reliable and valid (e.g., for reviews, see Beck, Steer, & Garbin, 1988; Kendall, Hollon, Beck, Hammen, & Ingram, 1987). Furthermore, parents of clinic-referred children score higher on this measure than parents of nonclinic children (Griest et al., 1980), and, relative to other types of measures (e.g., behavioral observations of child behavior), the BDI has been found to be the best predictor of maternal perceptions of clinic-referred noncompliant children (Forehand, Wells, McMahon, Griest, & Rogers, 1982; Griest, Wells, & Forehand, 1979). The BDI has changed in a positive direction following completion of our parent training program (Forehand et al., 1980) and has predicted dropouts from treatment as well (McMahon, Forehand, Griest, & Wells, 1981).

The BDI consists of 21 items, each of which is scored on a 4-point scale. Higher scores indicate greater depressive symptomatology. Scores of 10–20 are indicative of mild depression, scores of 20–30 are indicative of moderate depression, and scores of greater than 30 are indicative of severe depression (Kendall et al., 1987). The question-naire is presented in Beck and colleagues (1979), and is available from The Psychologi-cal Corporation, P.O. Box 839954, San Antonio, TX 78283-3954; *www.PsychCorp.com.*

One aspect of the marital relationship that is particularly detrimental for children is conflict between parents in front of a child (Davies & Cummings, 1994; Emery & Forehand, 1994). The O'Leary–Porter Scale (OPS; Porter & O'Leary, 1980) examines such conflict. Higher scores on this 10-item instrument have been shown repeatedly to relate negatively to child behavior problems (e.g., Forehand, McCombs, Long, Brody, &

Fauber, 1988). The OPS can be obtained from the second author (RLF) of this volume at the Department of Psychology, University of Vermont, Burlington, VT 05405.

Optional Instruments for Assessing Other Family (and Related) Problems

Beyond utilizing the BDI to assess depressive mood and the OPS to assess conflict between parents, we often employ other instruments to assess the factors that fall under the rubric of behavioral family therapy. Our approach in the assessment of these areas of family functioning has been to employ the instruments on an "as needed" basis. That is, when we believe there may be a problem in a particular area, we assess that area. We briefly describe instruments in several potentially relevant areas: parental antisocial behavior, alcohol use, stress, general marital satisfaction, and insularity.

Parental antisocial behavior can be assessed with structured diagnostic interviews or the Minnesota Multiphasic Personality Inventory (MMPI; Butcher, Dahlstrom, Graham, Tellegen, & Kaemmer, 1989). However, given the time and expense involved, their use in this limited fashion does not seem warranted. An alternative is the Antisocial Behavior Checklist (Zucker & Fitzgerald, 1992), which is a 46-item self-report rating scale that has been shown to be consistent with DSM criteria for APD.

Research has not been undertaken to examine the extent to which parent alcohol consumption influences the referral of children for treatment. However, in some families this may be an important area and, thus, one to potentially assess for in the initial interview. This can be done during the interview by asking parents about drinking patterns and their estimation of the extent to which drinking is related to their child's inappropriate behavior or interferes with their parenting. Ideally, each spouse's view of his or her own drinking behavior and the other spouse's drinking behavior should be assessed. Some of the more frequently employed screening instruments that may prove useful in assessing parents' drinking patterns are the short version of the Michigan Alcoholism Screening Test (SMAST; Selzer, Vinokur, & van Rooijen, 1975) and the Alcohol Use Disorders Identification Test (AUDIT; Saunders, Aasland, Babor, de la Fuente, & Grant, 1993).

General measures of stress (e.g., life event scales) and specific measures of parenting-related stress have been employed with parents of children with conduct problems. An example of the former is the Life Experiences Survey (Sarason, Johnson, & Siegel, 1978). Measures specific to parenting-related stress include Parenting Daily Hassles (Crnic & Greenberg, 1990) and the Parenting Stress Index (Abidin, 1995). The Parenting Stress Index has been extensively employed with parents of children with conduct problems (e.g., Abidin, Jenkins, & McGaughey, 1992; Kazdin, 1990; Ross, Blanc, McNeil, Eyberg, & Hembree-Kigin, 1998; Webster-Stratton, 1994), and is available from Psychological Assessment Resources, 16204 N. Florida Avenue, Lutz, FL 33549; *www.parinc.com.*

Earlier in the chapter, we indicated that we use the OPS (Porter & O'Leary, 1980) to assess conflict between parents. A measure of general marital satisfaction that also can be used in the Dyadic Adjustment Scale (DAS; Spanier, 1976).[3] The DAS, which is a 32-item scale, has been used extensively in marital research and treatment during the past 25 years (e.g., Beach, Sandeen, & O'Leary, 1990; Fincham, 1998; Margolin, 1990). The DAS yields a global marital adjustment score and four subscale scores. Because the four subscales have not always been replicated (see Fincham, 1998), the global score is best used as an overall index of marital adjustment. Spanier (1976) reported a Cronbach's alpha value of .96 for the global score and presented validity (content, criterion-related, and construct) data.

On the basis of normative data presented by Spanier (1976), Jacobson and Anderson (1980) suggested that a cutoff score of 97, which corresponds to one standard deviation below the mean of Spanier's normative sample, be used to classify individuals as maritally distressed. The mean of Spanier's normative sample (115) would seem to be a conservative cutoff score for maritally nondistressed couples. However, Bond and McMahon (1984) adopted a score of 107 as a cutoff for classifying mothers as maritally nondistressed, based on the mean score of 107.34 obtained by Houseknecht (1979) for a sample of 50 mothers. The DAS is available from Multi-Health Systems, Inc., 908 Niagara Falls Blvd., North Tonawanda, NY 14120-2060; *www.mhs.com*.

While we have not systematically assessed for insularity, the notion of looking beyond the family for stressors that may disrupt parenting may be important for therapists to consider with some families. Support from extended family and friends, social support from the community (e.g., church groups, civic organizations), and employment-related support and stress can be ascertained in the interview process. The Community Interaction Checklist (CIC; Wahler, Leske, & Rogers, 1979) can be utilized to assess insularity, which is operationalized as the number of persons with whom a parent interacts on a given day and the valence (i.e., whether the interaction is positive or negative) of each interaction. The CIC has adequate reliability and validity data (Cerezo, 1988). The CIC is usually administered by an observer after each home observation; thus, multiple administrations of the CIC are the norm. Mothers are categorized as insular if they report at least twice as many daily contacts with relatives and/or helping agency representatives as with friends and if at least one-third of the daily contacts are reported as neutral or aversive (Dumas & Wahler, 1983, 1985). The CIC is available from Robert G. Wahler, Department of Psychology, University of Tennessee, Knoxville, TN 37996.

Parent Knowledge of Social Learning Principles

We administer a slightly abridged version of the Knowledge of Behavioral Principles as Applied to Children test (KBPAC; O'Dell, Tarler-Benlolo, & Flynn, 1979) to determine the parents' knowledge of social learning principles. Parents who receive formal instruction in the social learning principles underlying our parent training program tend to be more satisfied with the intervention, generalize their skills more effectively, and perceive their children more positively than parents who are not explicitly taught the principles (McMahon, Forehand, & Griest, 1981) (see Chapters 8 and 10). The KBPAC provides a basic measure of the level of sophistication about social learning

---

[3]The modified form of the Marital Adjustment Test (Kimmel & Vander Veen, 1974), which we have employed in some of our clinical research studies, is another alternative.

principles the parent brings to the parent training program and can help the therapist determine to what extent social learning principles need to be presented to the parent.

The abridged KBPAC consists of 45 multiple-choice questions, most of which present practical problem situations.[4] Each question has four possible answers. The parent is asked to select the response that is the most likely to produce the desired effect. A total score is obtained by summing the number of items answered correctly. O'Dell and colleagues (1979) presented some reliability and validity data. The KBPAC has been shown to be sensitive to change as a function of social learning-based intervention (e.g., McMahon, Forehand, & Griest, 1981).

The KBPAC and scoring key are presented in O'Dell and colleagues (1979). Administration time is approximately 30 minutes. Other investigators have developed short forms of the instrument, although none of them has been evaluated with parents (Furtkamp, Giffort, & Schiers, 1982; McKee, 1984). McKee developed a 16-item version of the KBPAC that is psychometrically stronger than the 10-item versions described by Furtkamp and colleagues (1982). Administration time is less than 10 minutes.

Parent Satisfaction with Treatment

We developed and employ the Parent's Consumer Satisfaction Questionnaire (PCSQ) to measure parental satisfaction with our parent training program at termination and follow-up. Several investigators (see Jensen & Haynes, 1986; McMahon & Forehand, 1983) have suggested that consumer satisfaction with a particular treatment strategy or an entire treatment approach, which is one form of social validity, is likely to be a factor in the ultimate effectiveness of the intervention. We (McMahon, Forehand, & Griest, 1981) have found that parents perceive the program positively and that this satisfaction is maintained at 2-month (McMahon, Tiedemann, Forehand, & Griest, 1984) and 1–4½ year (Baum & Forehand, 1981) follow-ups (see Chapter 10). The PCSQ consists of 42 items that sample parent satisfaction with the overall program (partially derived from Eyberg's [1993] Therapy Attitude Inventory), the teaching format, the specific parenting techniques that are taught, and the therapists. Items examining both the usefulness and difficulty of the teaching format and specific parenting techniques are included. In all of the areas, parents respond to items on a 7-point Likert-type scale. Parents also can reply to several open-ended questions concerning their reactions to the parent training program. The PCSQ and a key for scoring are presented in Appendix A.

PARENT-RECORDED BEHAVIOR

One approach to obtaining information about child noncompliant and inappropriate behaviors is to have the parent observe and record the frequency of the behaviors in the home. Parental recording of the child's behavior offers several advantages over other assessment procedures. First, it gives more precise information about the child's behavior

---

[4]Five items are omitted from the original KBPAC in our abridged version: 14, 24, 26, 35, 38.

than an interview or parent-completed questionnaire. Second, it is more efficient than behavioral observations completed by independent observers. Third, it may be the only way to obtain information on the occurrence of low-rate behaviors such as stealing and fire setting (McMahon & Estes, 1997). Fourth, comparison of these data with parental reports of child behavior in the interview or on the CBCL may provide some clues as to whether the parents' perceptions of the child's behavior are congruent with the child's actual behavior.

At the beginning of the initial interview, the parent completes the Parent Behavior Checklist, which is presented in Figure 4.1. The 11 problem behaviors listed on the Checklist were initially identified as aversive child behaviors, as determined by parental ratings and the parental consequences applied to the behaviors, in research by Adkins and Johnson (1972). We have found that parents of young noncompliant children still report similar problems.

As indicated in the instructions to the Checklist, the parent checks the behaviors that present problem areas with the child and then ranks the problem behaviors that are of the most concern to him or her in order of severity. The information can be used in the interview as an additional problem guide. At the conclusion of the interview, the behaviors ranked in the top three are carefully defined jointly by the therapist and parent. As indicated in the instruction sheet presented in Figure 4.9, the therapist then asks the parent to record the frequency of each of the three selected problem behaviors during four consecutive 24-hour periods. (If home observations are to be conducted, then the parent records the behaviors during the 24-hour period prior to each of the four home observations.) For recording purposes, the parent is given index cards that list the three behaviors. The completed cards are put in an envelope, and the parent returns the envelope to the therapist prior to the feedback session.

The therapist can use this information to identify the frequency of the reported problem behaviors. The information can also be used in subsequent sessions with the parent to discuss particular incidents of child problem behaviors, as well as the relevant antecedent conditions and consequences. The same parent-recorded data can be collected after treatment and at follow-ups to assess changes resulting from treatment.

Forehand and colleagues (1979) reported that the parent-recorded data during a 24-hour period did not correlate significantly with observer measures of child compliance and child inappropriate behavior during a 40-minute observation occurring in the 24-hour period. This suggests that the two methods of data collection provide different snapshots of the child's problem behavior.

ASSESSMENT OF SCHOOL PROBLEMS

In our experience, approximately one-half of the children referred for problems with noncompliance in the home also demonstrate problems in the preschool or school setting. These difficulties typically include noncompliance and other acting-out problems. Academic difficulties also may be evident. As noted above, initial assessment of preschool or school problems occurs during the interview with the parents. If the parents

One of the things we have asked you to do is to keep track of several of your child's behaviors for 4 days. As we explained, this will help us to design a better treatment program for you and help determine its effectiveness. Therefore, it is very important that you try to be as accurate as possible. The attached index cards are numbered 1 to 4. Also, note that each index card lists three behaviors. These are the behaviors that you listed earlier as being of primary concern to you. We would like you to do the following:

1. For 4 consecutive days, keep a running tab of the number of times your child does each of these three behaviors. (If we will be conducting home observations, record these behaviors for the 24-hour period before each of the home observations.) Most parents find that carrying the index card in a pocket or putting it in a conspicuous place (for example, on the refrigerator door) is a good way to remind themselves to record this information. Simply put a slash or a number down on the card each time the behavior occurs. An example of Day 3's results might look like this:

		3
1. Temper Tantrums	I I I	
2. Noncompliance	I I I I I I	
3. Physically Negative	I I I I	

   Try to make sure the time period for which you record is 24 hours—no more, no less.
2. Place the four cards in the envelope and seal it.
3. Return the envelope to your therapist *prior* to the next session at the clinic. (If you are having an observer come to your home, please give him or her the envelope at the end of the final observation.)

Thanks!

FIGURE 4.9. Counting Your Child's Behavior.

indicate that the child has problems in the preschool or school setting, the therapist follows up this question by asking about the nature of the difficulties. If difficulties are behavioral, the therapist can ask about specific behavior problems (e.g., noncompliance to teacher requests or classroom rules, peer difficulties, aggression toward teachers or peers). If difficulties lie in the academic area, the therapist inquires about difficulties in areas such as reading, spelling, arithmetic, and writing. If the parents report behavioral or academic difficulties in school, the therapist emphasizes the importance of a thorough assessment of the child. If the parents agree, the therapist obtains consent to contact the preschool or school.

An assessment of school problems should utilize methods similar to those outlined above for assessment in the home: an interview with the teacher, behavior rating scales, and observation. (For more extensive discussions of assessment of child conduct problems in the school setting, see Breen & Altepeter, 1990; McMahon & Estes, 1997; Walker, 1995.)

The interview with the teacher follows the same format as the parent interview. The situations to be covered can be based on Barkley's (1987, 1997) School Situations Questionnaire (see Figure 4.10) and on Wahler and Cormier's (1970) Pre-Interview Checklist. Scoring guidelines and normative data for the School Situations Question-

Child's name _____ **Date** _____

Name of person completing this form _____

Instructions: Does this child present any problems with compliance to instructions, commands, or rules for you in any of these situations? If so, please circle the word Yes and then circle a number beside that situation that describes how severe the problem is for you. If this child is not a problem in a situation, circle No and go on to the next situation on the form.

		If yes, how severe?
Situations	*Yes/No*	Mild Severe
When arriving at school	Yes No	1 2 3 4 5 6 7 8 9
During individual desk work	Yes No	1 2 3 4 5 6 7 8 9
During small group activities	Yes No	1 2 3 4 5 6 7 8 9
During free playtime in class	Yes No	1 2 3 4 5 6 7 8 9
During lectures to the class	Yes No	1 2 3 4 5 6 7 8 9
At recess	Yes No	1 2 3 4 5 6 7 8 9
At lunch	Yes No	1 2 3 4 5 6 7 8 9
In the hallways	Yes No	1 2 3 4 5 6 7 8 9
In the bathroom	Yes No	1 2 3 4 5 6 7 8 9
On field trips	Yes No	1 2 3 4 5 6 7 8 9
During special assemblies	Yes No	1 2 3 4 5 6 7 8 9
On the bus	Yes No	1 2 3 4 5 6 7 8 9

FIGURE 4.10. School Situations Questionnaire. From Barkley (1997). Copyright 1997 by The Guilford Press. Reprinted by permission.

naire can be found in Altepeter and Breen (1992), Barkley (1997), and Barkley and Edelbrock (1987). Areas to cover in the interview with the teacher include school arrival, individual desk work, small-group activities, recess, lunch, field trips, assemblies, free time in class, and, if the child is beyond preschool, particular academic topics (e.g., math, social studies). If the teacher indicates that a particular situation is a problem, then the therapist should obtain a description of the situation ("What is the class doing?"), the child's behavior ("What does the child do?"), the teacher's response to the child ("What do you do?"), and the child's response to the teacher's intervention ("What does the child do then?"). The frequency and duration of the problem, as well as the role of other children in escalating or inhibiting the problem, also should be addressed. Contextual factors, such as classroom rules of conduct, teacher expectations, and the behavior of other children in the classroom, are important to assess as well.

In addition, a focus on behaviors that create challenges to classroom management can provide useful information. Typical questions include: "Does the child leave his or her desk inappropriately?"; "Does the child bother classmates while they are working?"; "Does the child talk out of turn?"; "Does the child demand excessive teacher attention?"—and so forth. Once a particular rule violation has been identified, then questions concerning antecedent events (e.g., "In what situation is the child more likely to hit another student?"), the exact behavior of the child, the teacher's response, and the child's response to the teacher's interventions can be asked. In talking with the teacher, the therapist is also interested in understanding exactly what the teacher considers appropriate student behavior in each of the problem situations; potential reinforcers that can be used in the classroom; and the teacher's willingness, motivation, and ability to work with the therapist in carrying out an intervention program.

The teacher also can be asked to complete the Teacher's Report Form (TRF; Achenbach & Rescorla, 2001), which is a parallel form of the parent-completed CBCL/6–18. (The TRF also yields a ninth narrow-band subscale—Hyperactivity–Impulsivity.) By the parent and teacher completing similar forms, comparisons of their perceptions of the child's behavior problems can occur. However, it is important to note that the TRF is utilized only for children aged 6 years and above. For younger children, either the new Caregiver–Teacher Report Form for Ages 1½–5 (C-TRF; Achenbach & Rescorla, 2000), which is a parallel form for the parent-completed CBCL/1½–5 (Achenbach & Rescorla, 2000), or the SESBI-R (Eyberg & Pincus, 1999), which is a parallel instrument to the parent-report ECBI (Eyberg & Pincus, 1999), can be utilized. The SESBI is designed to assess disruptive classroom behavior of children as young as 2 years of age (see McMahon & Estes, 1997, for a review of the SESBI). Having access to the teacher-completed behavior rating scale prior to the interview with the teacher allows the therapist to provide focus to the interview and to make the most of the usually limited time available to meet with the teacher (Breen & Altepeter, 1990).

If the presenting problems at school concern behavior, observation will likely be beneficial. However, it is important to note that direct observations in the school have the same practical problems as those noted for home observations. The BCS can be modified for use in the classroom to assess teacher–child interactions. One such modification that obtained adequate interobserver agreement was described by Breiner and

Forehand (1981). McMahon and Estes (1997) describe several other possible coding systems for observation in the school.

Walker (1995) presents guidelines and examples of simple observation procedures appropriate for use by teachers (and observers) in the classroom. For example, academic engaged time (AET) is the amount of time that a child is appropriately engaged in on-task behavior during class time (Walker, Colvin, & Ramsey, 1995). Walker and colleagues (1995) have developed a simple stopwatch recording method for assessing AET in which children are observed for two 15-minute periods. AET has been shown to correlate positively with academic performance and to discriminate boys at risk for conduct problems from boys not at risk (e.g., Walker, Shinn, O'Neill, & Ramsey, 1987).

The Revised Edition of the School Observation Coding System (REDSOC; Jacobs et al., 2000) is an interval coding system that is based partly on the coding system described in Forehand, Sturgis, and colleagues (1979) and that also includes Walker and colleagues' (1995) AET. It focuses on noncompliant, inappropriate, and off-task behaviors. Three classroom observations occur over a 2-week period, and 30 minutes of data are gathered on the target child. To control for the highly variable nature of different classroom environments, observations are also conducted with three "control" children of the same sex in the classroom. Psychometric properties based on observations of 3- to 6-year-old clinic-referred children with ODD and nonreferred children in preschools and kindergarten classrooms suggest that the REDSOC may be particularly appropriate for classroom observations of young noncompliant children.

Although interviews, observations, and behavioral rating scales are important sources of information concerning the child's behavioral and academic problems, additional evaluation in the form of intelligence and achievement tests may be indicated to determine whether the child has learning problems as well. Lyon (1994) provides a complete review of assessment strategies with which to evaluate learning problems, and Walker (1995) discusses the use of a standardized method for retrieving and using school records (School Archival Records System; Walker, Block-Pedego, Todis, & Severson, 1991) with children with conduct problems.

POSTTREATMENT AND FOLLOW-UP ASSESSMENTS

Assessment procedures similar to those described above (i.e., parent-completed questionnaires, parent-recorded data, clinic [and home] observations) should be employed at the completion of the parent training program (and at relevant follow-up assessments as applicable). In addition, the parents should complete the PCSQ (Appendix A) at these assessments.

CHAPTER 5

The Feedback Session and Sample Program Outline

In this chapter, we first describe how the therapist provides feedback on assessment information, case conceptualization, and treatment recommendations to the parents. We then describe how the therapist presents the rationale, overview, and mechanics of the parent training program. The next section of the chapter presents a session-by-session example of the HNC parent training program in outline form. Reference is made in parentheses to sections of the text where the material is discussed in detail. (It is important to note that the actual content of individual sessions and the length of the program itself will vary according to the progress of the particular parent.) The chapter concludes with descriptions of some commonly encountered problems and solutions for them.

THE FEEDBACK SESSION

Overview

Once the assessment is completed, the therapist reviews the data and meets with the parent(s) to provide (1) summary feedback about the assessment, (2) a conceptualization of the child's noncompliance and other inappropriate behaviors in the context of the parent–child interaction, and (3) recommendations for intervention. The therapist usually presents this material in a subsequent session so that the therapist has had time to review the information from the questionnaires, parent-recorded data, and the home observations (if conducted). The child is not present for the meeting. Assuming that the HNC parent training program has been recommended as an appropriate intervention, the therapist then presents a rationale for the HNC program and an overview of the content and teaching methods. This process is summarized in Figure 5.1.

Preparing for the Feedback Session

Prior to meeting with the parents for the feedback session, the therapist reviews the various assessment data to assist in the conceptualization of the child's noncompliance and to guide selection of the most appropriate intervention(s). Our therapeutic approach

I. General considerations

_____ Usually a separate session.

_____ Child not present.

II. Feedback from assessment

_____ Summarize assessment information from all sources (Chapter 4).

_____ Summarize situations in which noncompliance and problem behaviors occur (Chapter 5).

_____ Ask parents whether summary is accurate, and provide opportunities for parents to provide additional information and ask questions.

III. Conceptualization of child noncompliance and other behavior problems

_____ Describe coercive nature of parent–child interaction (Chapter 1).

_____ Ask parents whether this process seems applicable to current situation with their child.

IV. Recommendations for intervention

_____ Present recommendations for intervention.

_____ If HNC is recommended, provide rationale and overview of content and teaching methods (Chapter 5).

_____ Rationale of program (Chapter 5).

_____ Behavior is learned and can be changed.

_____ Focus is on changing child noncompliance.

_____ Distinction between "OK" and "not OK" behaviors.

_____ Draw and explain child behavior graphs (Figure 5.2).

_____ Present two approaches to decreasing noncompliance.

_____ Decreasing noncompliance directly through punishment.

_____ Increasing compliance through reinforcement.

_____ Overview of HNC program (Chapter 5).

_____ Program is divided into two phases.

_____ Phase I increases compliance ("OK" behavior).

_____ Phase II decreases noncompliance ("not OK" behavior).

_____ Stress importance of consistency.

(continued)

FIGURE 5.1. Assessment Feedback Session Checklist.

_____ Mechanics of HNC program (Chapter 5).

    _____ Give overview.

        _____ HNC program is active.

        _____ Parent is primary agent in changing child behavior.

        _____ Parent learns number of skills for interacting with child.

    _____ Describe teaching procedures.

        _____ Explain.

        _____ Demonstrate.

        _____ Role play with parent.

        _____ Teach child the skill.

        _____ Practice with child in clinic (therapist feedback).

        _____ Practice with child in clinic (no therapist feedback).

        _____ Give handout.

        _____ Assign homework.

    _____ Behavioral criteria determine rate of progress.

V. Concluding the Feedback Session

    _____ Ask parent(s) to consider recommendations. (If two-parent family, request that parents be sure to discuss with each other.)

    _____ Ask parent(s) to notify therapist within 1 week about decision as to whether to participate in parent training program.

begins with the assumption that parent training is the treatment of choice for noncompliance and other child behavior problems. Primary indicators of the appropriateness of a parent training intervention include evidence of significant familial influences on the development or maintenance of the child's conduct problem behavior and parental recognition of the child's problem and willingness to participate in the intervention (Sanders & Dadds, 1993).

It is also important for the therapist to be aware of cultural and ethnic differences. Families with backgrounds (e.g., with respect to ethnicity, minority status, SES) that differ from that of the therapist may have different child-rearing attitudes and practices. Unless a therapist is aware of these potential differences, the feedback provided to the family may not be sensitive, resulting in their feeling alienated (for a thorough discussion of these issues, see Forehand & Kotchick, 1996; Kotchick & Forehand, 2002; Kotchick et al., in press).

Once it has been determined that a parent training approach is indicated, then the therapist must be concerned with several additional treatment selection issues, such as: (1) whether parent training alone is likely to be sufficient; (2) whether to intervene in additional areas such as other child disorders; in other settings, such as the school; and in familial and extrafamilial difficulties, such as parental personal or marital adjustment, child or parent perceptual biases, and/or extrafamilial functioning (e.g., insularity); and (3) if intervention is to take place in one or more of these areas, whether it should occur before, after, instead of, or concurrently with a parent training type of intervention (McMahon, 1987). We discuss two treatment selection issues in detail below.

Intervention for Behavior Problems in the School

In addition to determining whether to recommend parent training as an intervention, the therapist also needs to consider whether intervention concerning the child's behavior in the school is indicated. The teacher interview, teacher-completed behavior rating scale, and school observation are used to make this decision (see Chapter 4). The data can guide the therapist in choosing among three options. First, if there is no evidence of school behavior problems, based on the parent's report or the more extensive assessment outlined in Chapter 4, a school intervention obviously is not necessary. However, even in this case, the therapist should monitor or have the parent or teacher monitor the child's behavior in the school setting during and after intervention. This will allow the detection of any behavioral difficulties that may arise and also provides the opportunity to see if the child's behavior improves with parent training. Second, if behavioral difficulties exist in the school setting but they are not severe, the therapist may choose to implement parent training and monitor the child's behavior in the school setting. There have been reports of some positive effects of parent training in the school setting (e.g., McNeil, Eyberg, Eisenstadt, Newcomb, & Funderburk, 1991; Serketich & Dumas, 1996; Webster-Stratton, 1998), although we have not found systematic changes in school behavior with HNC (Breiner & Forehand, 1981; Forehand, Sturgis, et al., 1979) (see Chapter 10). Monitoring the child's behavior in the school setting will enable the therapist to determine whether generalization is occurring for that particular child. When generalization does occur, intervention in school may not be necessary. However, if generalization to the school setting does not occur, then intervention can be implemented at school. Third, if severe behavior difficulties exist in the school setting, the therapist will likely need to recommend intervention simultaneously in the home and school settings. When intervention in the school is necessary, the therapist may choose to implement an in-class intervention (e.g., Walker & Walker, 1991), a home-based reinforcement program (e.g., Kelley, 1990; Walker & Walker, 1991), or both.

Parent Training versus Intervention for Familial and Extrafamilial Stressors

Another issue for therapists involved in parent training is when to initiate or continue parent training versus when to focus on significant familial or extrafamilial stressors that may be occurring. As we have noted in earlier writings (McMahon & Forehand, 1988), a few investigators have described preliminary formulations for matching clinic-referred families with specific interventions (e.g., Blechman, 1981; Embry, 1984). However, we are still of the opinion that it may be premature to utilize such algorithms. It has only been in recent years that the influence of various stressors has been delineated, and, as we have noted, the interrelationships of these stressors are only now beginning to be understood. For example, if a child is referred for noncompliance problems and a parent has both depressive symptoms and low marital satisfaction, does the therapist focus on child noncompliance, parental depressive symptoms, or the marital differences? While some research (e.g., Beach & Jones, 2002) is beginning to address such issues, the picture is far from clear. Nevertheless, it is possible to present some guidelines.

It is important to recognize that some children may be referred for treatment of noncompliance when, in reality, their behavior is not deviant; instead, the parent has distorted perceptions or unrealistic perceptions of the child because of the parent's depressive symptoms (e.g., Dumas & Serketich, 1994). If the parent's BDI score is elevated, the therapist should look for discrepancies between the parent-reported data (e.g., CBCL, interview) and behavioral observations. If the parent's report suggests that the child is deviant but the observations do not, sharing information about child development norms with the parent is indicated. In addition, the therapist should discuss with the parent the therapist's concern about the self-reported depressive symptoms and how they can influence perceptions of the child, parenting behavior, and child behavior. The depressive symptoms also may need to become a target for intervention.

In most cases, we assume that parent training is the treatment of choice for noncompliance and other child behavior problems. However, if one or more of these other areas is compromised, then based on the initial assessment of the child and family, a decision has to be made about whether to initiate parent training or, instead, to focus on one or more of the other areas. The interview with the parent(s) and examination of self-report measures of personal adjustment and marital conflict can be especially helpful in this regard. Such decisions always should be made in collaboration with the parent(s). Again, exact guidelines are not available for indicating when other areas, such as parental depression or marital conflict, are sufficiently severe to rule out parent training initially. In essence, this is a decision that the therapist has to make after taking into account the particular situation for that particular family.

It is also important to note that the decision does not have to be an "either–or" one. That is, in collaboration with the parent, a decision may be made to intervene first with parent training to address the child's noncompliance. If the parent does not respond to this intervention with improvements in parenting skills and perhaps in other personal or familial risk factors, then adjunctive interventions that directly address these other risk factors can be considered (Sanders et al., 2000). Examples of available interventions to address these issues are presented in Table 5.1 (also see Chapter 8). This approach is based on empirical evidence that indicates that some parents report improvements in their personal (e.g., depressive symptoms) and/or marital adjustment after participating in parent training (see Chapter 10; Sanders et al., 2000). Alternatively, the decision may be to simultaneously begin parent training and intervention focusing on the other family issue(s) that need to be addressed. If the other family issues are not severe, intervention might include one or more of the modules in the Parent Enhancement Therapy adjunct to the parent training program (Griest et al., 1982; see Chapter 8). However, if the family issues are severe, it is our experience that it is best to keep the two interventions separate. Parent training sessions and sessions for the treat-

TABLE 5.1. Examples of Interventions to Address Parental Personal Adjustment and Marital and Extrafamilial Difficulties

Area of difficulty	Intervention	Source
Parental perceptions/expectations	Parent enhancement therapy[a]	Griest et al. (1982)
Depression	Cognitive therapy	Beck, Rush, Shaw, & Emery (1979)
	Marital therapy	Beach & Jones (2002)
Alcohol problems	Coping skills training	Monti, Abrams, Kadden, & Cooney (2002)
	Self-change programs	Sobell & Sobell (1983)
	Marital therapy	O'Farrell (1993)
Parental stress	Stress management	Sanders, Markie-Dadds, Tully, & Bor (2000)
Marital conflict/discord	Integrative couple therapy	Jacobson & Christensen (1996)
	Creating connections	Johnson (1996)
	Cognitive behavior therapy	Epstein & Baucom (2002)
Divorce	Making divorce easier	Long & Forehand (2002a)
	Children of divorce	Stolberg, Zacharias, & Camplair (1991)
	Parenting through change	Forgatch (1994)
Stepfamilies	Parenting for stepfamilies	Nicholson & Sanders (1999)
Insularity	Synthesis teaching	Wahler, Cartor, Fleischman, & Lambert (1993)

[a]See Chapter 8.

ment of other family problems should be at separate times and perhaps conducted by separate therapists. This prevents other family problems from interfering with the tasks to be accomplished during the parent training sessions.

If parent training is initiated and progress is not occurring, a decision has to be made about whether to continue this treatment. The therapist may decide to continue parent training alone, continue parent training and have a second separate treatment for the other family issue(s) implemented, or terminate parent training and focus treatment on the other family issues. The severity of the other issues and the nature of the lack of progress in parent training (e.g., parents not utilizing skills, parents not completing homework) should be considered in making the decision, which should occur in collaboration with the parents.

Conducting the Feedback Session

Giving Feedback

The therapist begins the feedback session by briefly summarizing the situations in which noncompliance and related problem behaviors occur, using the data gathered from the various interviews, questionnaires, clinic and home observations, and parent-recorded data. The therapist notes the extent to which the child's behavior is generally problematic (and in which settings), as well as the accuracy of parents' perceptions of the child's behavior. Special attention is given to the coercive nature of parent–child interactions, and its significance is explained. As the assessment summary and conceptualization are being presented, it is critical that the therapist frequently ask the parent(s) whether the information makes sense to them and is consistent with what they know about the child and his or her behavior. Parents should be given the opportunity to provide additional information and to ask questions. Parental agreement with the therapist on the nature and causes of the child's behavior problems should facilitate parental engagement in intervention (Sanders & Lawton, 1993). Once agreement is reached, the therapist can provide recommendations for intervention.

Assuming that the parent training program is the recommended intervention, the therapist then provides a rationale for the HNC program and an overview of the content and teaching methods.

Providing the Rationale

The therapist covers the following key points in the rationale. First, much of a child's behavior is learned. As such, the best approach for changing the child's inappropriate behavior is to teach the child more acceptable behaviors. Since young children are most influenced by their parents, then the purpose of these sessions is to teach the parent effective ways to interact with the child.

The therapist then tells the parent that the HNC program is designed to deal specifically with noncompliance. It is pointed out that noncompliance was indicated as a primary problem during the assessment. Most child behavior problems can be viewed as a failure to comply to some instruction or rule that is in effect; therefore, they can also be successfully treated within this framework.

We have found it useful to refer to "OK" behaviors and "not OK" behaviors in our discussions with parents about compliance and noncompliance. We operationally define an "OK" behavior as any child behavior that the parent would like to see continue or to occur more frequently. A "not OK" behavior is one that the parent would like to see decrease in frequency or be eliminated. Compliance and noncompliance are the major "OK" and "not OK" behaviors that we focus on in the HNC parent training program. This distinction is a useful way to facilitate individualization of the parent training program to individual parental preferences and cultural norms.

At this point, the therapist draws the two bar graphs in Figure 5.2 for the parent and, pointing to the first bar graph, says:

> "This graph shows a large amount of 'not OK' behavior (that is, noncompliance) and a much smaller amount of 'OK' behavior (that is, compliance). This is the situation that we have with Greg right now."

Pointing to the second bar graph, the therapist says:

> "This graph shows a more preferable situation. Here, there is more 'OK' behavior than 'not OK' behavior. This graph shows a situation in which Greg is behaving positively most of the time, with occasional noncompliance and limit testing. This is what we want from him."

The therapist then notes that there are two major approaches for reducing noncompliant, or "not OK," behavior. The first approach focuses on lowering noncompliance directly. We tend to do this by punishment of one sort or another (e.g., spanking, loss of privileges). Unfortunately, while that particular "not OK" behavior may decrease in frequency temporarily, punishment does not necessarily increase the amount of compliance, or "OK" behavior. This is because most types of punishment fail to provide an alternative appropriate behavior to take the place of the "not OK" behavior. In other words, punishment tells the child what *not* to do but does not teach the child an appropriate behavioral alternative. In this situation, the child may substitute a different "not OK" behavior for the punished behavior. The therapist also points out that if the initial focus is on reducing "not OK" behavior by punishment, then the parent will have to punish the child frequently (because of the relatively high proportion of inappropriate child behavior). Although punishment is necessary on certain occasions, excessive punishment is distressing for both the parent and the child and may cause guilt in the parent and anxiety in the child.

The therapist states that, for these reasons, greater progress can be made by initially focusing on increasing compliance (i.e., "OK" behavior) directly. This approach lets the child know exactly what "OK" behavior is expected. Also, when compliance increases, then noncompliance automatically decreases! This is explained to the parent by noting

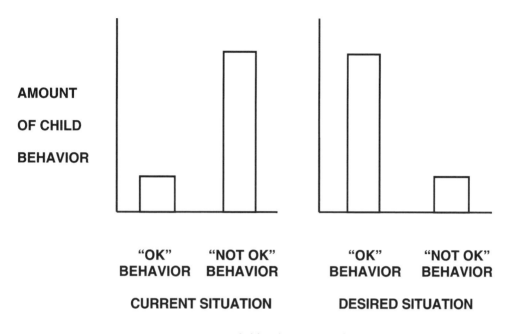

FIGURE 5.2. Child Behavior Graphs.

that the more time the child spends doing "OK" behaviors, then naturally less time is available to engage in "not OK" behaviors. We usually provide the following example:

> "Let's say that Greg is awake 16 hours each day. And let's suppose, for example, that right now he spends 12 hours doing 'not OK' behaviors and the remaining 4 hours are spent doing 'OK' behaviors. If we were somehow able to get him to increase the time he spends each day in 'OK' behaviors to 12 hours, then there are only 4 hours left during the day in which he can do 'not OK' behaviors. So, the 'not OK' behaviors automatically go down. Note, too, that the opposite situation doesn't work the same way: decreasing a 'not OK' behavior doesn't automatically mean that the 'OK' behavior will increase. Another 'not OK' behavior might take its place."

The major advantage of a focus on increasing compliance directly is that it lets the child know exactly what behavior he or she is to substitute for noncompliance. The therapist tells the parent that this focus remedies many child behavior problems and is a necessary first step in the treatment of all of them. A side benefit is that, by decreasing noncompliance, punishment can be used much less frequently but in a more effective manner. Finally, a focus on increasing child compliance makes for a much more pleasant family life, since the parent's positive influence on the child is increased and a positive parent–child relationship is facilitated.

However, it is also important to stress to the parents that some "not OK" behaviors will need to be dealt with directly. Thus, the HNC program also includes ways for parents to directly decrease noncompliance, including a mild form of punishment.

Overview of the Program and Discussion of Teaching Methods

Next, the therapist provides a general overview of the HNC program. The overview begins with the therapist stating that the parent training program will help the parent learn two sets of skills: those for increasing compliance and those for decreasing noncompliance. The therapist notes that the program is divided into two phases. In Phase I, the parent will learn specific ways to increase the child's positive ("OK") behavior. The therapist emphasizes to the parent that Phase I is considered to be the most important part of the program, since it is critical for a positive parent–child relationship. In addition, the therapist explains that this phase serves as the foundation upon which the effectiveness of the other parenting skills is based. The therapist states that many of the high-rate coercive behaviors associated with noncompliance are significantly reduced during Phase I. The therapist then tells the parent that in Phase II he or she will learn how to deal with noncompliance directly. The parent is told that he or she will learn how to give clear instructions to the child and how to provide appropriate consequences for the child's compliance or noncompliance to these instructions and to rules. Finally, the therapist emphasizes the need for consistency in dealing with the child. The therapist explains that consistency provides a more secure environment for the child and one in which he or she will have to test limits less frequently.

Once the overview of the HNC program has been presented and the parents' questions answered, the therapist then describes the mechanics of the parent training program. The therapist first stresses that this is an active program, with the parent serving as the primary agent in changing the child's behavior. The importance of the parent–child interaction in changing the child's behavior is reiterated. The therapist then tells the parent that he or she will be learning a number of parenting skills that have been shown to be highly effective in interacting with children and improving their behavior. The therapist describes the training format for each skill in the following way.

The parent is told that he or she will proceed through each skill or set of skills in a number of small steps during the sessions. The therapist explains that this procedure is used to maximize the parent's learning and to make the parent feel more comfortable. The therapist then tells the parent that the following procedures will be used in teaching each skill:

- The therapist will explain the procedure and rationale for each skill.
- The therapist will demonstrate the skill through modeling and role playing.
- The parent will practice the skill with the therapist role playing the child.
- The therapist and parent will teach the skill to the child. They will provide an explanation and demonstration of the skill to the child. The child will repeat the skill verbally and will participate in role plays of situations involving the skill.
- The parent will practice with the child during the session. The therapist will observe and coach (either from within the room or from behind the one-way window with the bug-in-the-ear. If using the bug-in-the-ear, the device should be demonstrated to the parent.)
- The parent will practice with the child during the session but without ongoing feedback from the therapist.
- The parent will receive a handout describing the skill.
- Specific homework will be assigned to practice the skills at home. The parent records practice sessions and use of skills at home on data sheets.

The therapist notes that the program is geared to the parent's own rate of progress. The parent is assured that training in a particular skill will continue until he or she is comfortable with that skill and has met set behavioral criteria found to be necessary if the parenting skills are to be used for maximum benefit. The therapist tells the parent that brief 5-minute observations at the beginning of each session and at other times will be conducted. The purpose of these observations is not only to assess the behavioral criteria for each skill but also to provide important data for discussion.

In this section, we have described the parent training sessions as involving only one parent. We will continue to describe the program in this way in the sample outline presented in this chapter and in the next two chapters. However, when two parents do attend, the teaching procedures are identical except in the steps that involve practice. During these steps, the two parents take turns practicing the skill with the therapist or child. Each parent separately practices the skills with the child at home.

Concluding the Feedback Session

The therapist does *not* ask the parent for a decision concerning whether he or she wants to participate in the intervention during the feedback session. Instead, the therapist asks the parent to think over the various options and to discuss the decision with his or her partner, as appropriate. The therapist then asks the parent to call and notify the therapist of the parent's decision within a week. There are several reasons for this approach: (1) it relieves the parent of feeling pressure to make a decision within the feedback session; (2) it allows the parent time to process the information concerning the assessment, case conceptualization, and parent training recommendation (and to do so in consultation with her or his partner); and (3) it increases the likelihood that if the parent does elect to participate in the parent training program, he or she will enter with a stronger and more genuine commitment.

SAMPLE OUTLINE OF THE PARENT TRAINING PROGRAM

Session 1

    I. Therapist gives setting instruction (i.e., to play quietly and not interrupt) to child (Chapter 6).

        A. Therapist and parent reinforce appropriate child behavior.

        B. Therapist prompts parent to reinforce child throughout session.

        C. Therapist and parent ignore child, as necessary.[1]

    II. Phase I (Chapter 6).

        A. Therapist presents rationale and overview.

            1. Purposes.

                a. Change coercive cycle of parent–child interaction.

                b. Enhance positive quality of parent–child relationship.

                c. Make parent skilled in use of differential attention to manage child's behavior.

            2. Explain two assumptions on which Phase I is based.

                a. Positive Reinforcement Rule.

                b. Attention Rule.

            3. Discuss the Attention Table (Chapter 6, Figure 6.1).

                a. "Catch your child being good."

                b. Ignore minor "not OK" behavior.

                c. Avoid the "criticism trap."

                d. Avoid ignoring "OK" behavior.

---

[1] As noted in Chapter 6, it may be necessary to teach the ignoring skill earlier in the program if the child is engaging in moderate levels of inappropriate behavior in the playroom (e.g., ignores the setting instruction to play quietly and not interrupt). Since the ignoring procedure can be taught independently of the positive attention skills, it may be taught out of sequence. Parent Handout 6: Ignoring (Appendix B) should be given when ignoring is taught.

       4. Phase I parenting skills.
         a. Positive reinforcement skills (attends and rewards).
         b. Extinction procedure (ignoring).
       5. Teach Phase I skills in context of Child's Game.
   B. Introduce attends.
       1. Define.
       2. Cite advantages.
       3. Discuss Child's Game.
       4. Therapist demonstrates skill for 10 minutes.
         a. Parent plays part of child.
         b. Therapist gives feedback.
       5. Parent role plays attending (briefly) with therapist.
       6. Explain/demonstrate attending to child.
       7. Parent practices attending with child and receives prompts and feedback from therapist.
       8. Parent practices attending with child (no feedback from therapist).
       9. Parent and therapist discuss interaction.
 III. Therapist gives Parent Handout 1: Introduction to Phase I and Parent Handout 2: Attends and the Child's Game (Appendix B).
 IV. Assign homework (Chapter 6).
   A. Therapist assigns daily 10- to 15-minute homework in which parent is to practice attending during Child's Game.
   B. Therapist gives Parent Handout 3: Parent Record Sheet: Child's Game (Appendix B) for recording homework.

Session 2 (Chapter 6)

    I. Therapist observes parent and child interacting in Child's Game and counts attends, rewards, commands, and questions.
   II. Parent gives setting instruction to child.
     A. Therapist reminds parent to reinforce child throughout session.
     B. Therapist reminds parent to ignore "not OK" behavior.
  III. Therapist and parent discuss interaction.
  IV. Therapist and parent discuss homework.
     A. Did parent practice daily?
     B. How did child respond to attending?
    V. Therapist reviews attending.
   VI. Therapist models attending.
  VII. Parent role plays attending with therapist.
 VIII. Parent practices attending with child and receives prompts and feedback from therapist.
   IX. Parent practices attending with child (no feedback from therapist).
    X. Parent and therapist discuss interaction.

   XI. Therapist observes parent and child interacting in Child's Game and counts attends, rewards, commands, and questions.
        A. Discuss interaction.
  XII. Assign homework.
        A. Parent continues to practice and record attending during Child's Game at home.

Session 3 (Chapter 6)

     I. Repeat Session 2 with modifications unless the parent meets behavioral criteria for attends in either final observation of Session 2 or initial observation of Session 3 (Chapter 6).
    II. Discuss homework.
        A. Did parent practice daily?
        B. Did child respond to attending?
   III. Reduce time spent on reviewing attending and demonstrating the skill.
   IV. Increase time spent on parent practicing attending with child.
    V. Observe parent and child interaction in Child's Game at end of session to determine whether parent meets behavioral criteria for attends.
        A. Discuss interaction.
   VI. Instruct parent to continue to practice attending during Child's Game at home.

Session 4 (Chapter 6)

     I. Repeat Session 3 unless the parent meets behavioral criteria for attends in either final observation of Session 3 or initial observation of Session 4.
    II. Discuss rewards if parent meets criteria for attends.
        A. Using types of rewards.
           1. Physical
           2. Unlabeled verbal
           3. Labeled verbal
        B. Learning to reward.
           1. Specific
           2. Immediate
           3. Focus on improvement
           4. Consistent
        C. Employing attends in conjunction with rewards.
   III. Therapist demonstrates three types of rewards and intermixing of rewards and attends.
   IV. Parent role plays rewards and intermixing of rewards and attends.
    V. Explain/demonstrate to child.
   VI. Parent practices attends and rewards with child with feedback from therapist.
  VII. Parent practices attends and rewards with child (no feedback from therapist).

VIII. Parent and therapist discuss interaction.
  IX. Therapist observes parent and child in Child's Game and counts attends, rewards, commands, and questions to determine whether parent meets behavioral criteria for rewards (Chapter 6).
    A. Discuss interaction.
   X. Therapist gives Parent Handout 4: Rewards (Appendix B).
  XI. Assign homework (Chapter 6).
    A. Therapist assigns daily 10- to 15-minute homework in which parent is to practice attending and rewarding during Child's Game.
    B. Therapist asks parent to bring in list of three "OK" child behaviors that parent would like to increase (Parent Handout 5: Parent Record Sheet: Identifying "OK" Behaviors to Increase; Appendix B).

Session 5 (Chapter 6)

   I. Therapist observes parent and child interacting in Child's Game and counts attends, rewards, commands, and questions to determine whether parent meets behavioral criteria for rewards.
  II. Parent gives setting instruction to child.
 III. If parent meets behavioral criteria for rewards or met them in Session 4, session proceeds as follows. (If not, continue to practice rewards.)
    A. Discuss interaction.
    B. Discuss Child's Game homework.
  IV. Therapist introduces ignoring and discusses it as an *active* procedure.
    A. Decreasing significantly the child's "not OK" behavior is a goal.
    B. Learning to ignore requires the following:
      1. No eye contact or nonverbal cues.
      2. No verbal contact.
      3. No physical contact.
      4. Start ignoring with onset of "not OK" behavior.
      5. Stop ignoring shortly after child resumes an "OK" behavior.
    C. Ignoring always combined with positive attention (differential attention).
    D. Not used if potential danger to people or property.
   V. Therapist models ignoring "not OK" behavior.
  VI. Parent role plays ignoring.
 VII. Explain/demonstrate ignoring to child.
VIII. Parent practices attends, rewards, and ignoring with the child and receives prompts and feedback from therapist.
  IX. Discuss parent's list of three "OK" child behaviors to increase.
    A. Discuss ways to use attends and rewards at home to increase desirable behavior.
    B. Assist parent in setting up programs using differential attention for one or two of the "OK" behaviors parent wishes to increase (Chapter 6).

1. Four-step plan.
   a. Identify "not OK" behaviors to ignore.
   b. Identify incompatible "OK" behaviors.
   c. Explain/demonstrate the differential attention plan to the child.
   d. Implement the plan at home.
2. Therapist takes major responsibility for setting up first program.
3. If time allows and first program is not too complex, parent takes major responsibility for setting up a second program.

X. Parent practices Phase I skills with child in clinic.

XI. Therapist observes parent and child interacting in Child's Game and counts attends, rewards, ignoring, commands, and questions to determine whether parent meets recommended behavioral criteria for ignoring (and continues to meet criteria for attends and rewards).
A. Discuss interaction.

XII. Therapist gives Parent Handout 6: Ignoring and Parent Handout 7: Combining Positive Attention and Ignoring (Differential Attention) (Appendix B) to parent.

XIII. Assign homework (Chapter 6).
A. Parent continues with daily Child's Game sessions at home.
B. Parent to implement programs to increase "OK" behavior listed on Parent Handout 5: Parent Record Sheet: Identifying "OK" Behaviors to Increase (Appendix B).

Session 6

I. Therapist observes parent and child interacting in Child's Game and counts attends, rewards, ignoring, commands, and questions. Therapist also notes whether recommended criteria for ignoring are met.

II. Parent gives setting instruction to child.

III. If recommended criteria for ignoring have been met in Session 5 or at the beginning of Session 6, session proceeds as follows. (If not, continue to practice ignoring skills, unless opportunities for the parent to ignore are not occurring.)
A. Discuss interaction.
B. Discuss homework.
   1. Daily Child's Game practice sessions.
   2. Differential attention program(s) for increasing "OK" child behaviors.
   3. Program(s) modified, if necessary.
   4. Parent program(s) continued.

IV. Therapist introduces Phase II of program (Chapter 7).
A. Review the two approaches to dealing with "not OK" child behavior (Chapter 5, Figure 5.2).
B. Parent is to use Phase II skills in conjunction with skills learned in Phase I.
C. Primary focus of Phase II skills is on parent behaviors to increase child compliance through use of the clear instructions sequence.

       1. Antecedent behaviors: how to give clear instructions.
       2. Consequent behaviors.
          a. Reinforcing compliance.
          b. Applying a TO procedure for noncompliance.
    D. Teach skills in context of Parent's Game.
 V. Introduce training in clear instructions.
    A. Emphasize that how parents give commands to their child is important in determining whether or not the child will comply.
    B. Discuss types of unclear instructions.
       1. Chain commands ("Pick up toys, straighten table, brush teeth, and go to bed")
       2. Vague commands ("Be careful")
       3. Question commands ("Would you like to pick up your toys?")
       4. "Let's . . . " commands ("Let's clean up the yard")
       5. Commands followed by rationale or other verbalizations ("Please put your clothes away. We're having guests tonight, and your room is a mess")
          a. Actual command is obscured.
          b. Rationale is fine, so long as it precedes the command.
    C. Present qualities of clear instructions.
       1. Get child's attention.
          a. Move close.
          b. Say child's name.
          c. Establish eye contact.
       2. State the instruction clearly.
          a. Give one instruction at a time.
          b. Use a firm voice.
          c. Use "do" commands rather than "stop" commands whenever possible.
          d. Use simple language.
          e. Use gestures to further explain the command.
          f. Rationale (if given) *precedes* the clear instruction.
       3. Clear instruction is followed by 5 seconds of quiet by parent in order to allow child time to initiate compliance.
          a. Parent counts silently from 1 to 5.
    D. Give a clear instruction only if you are willing to follow through with it.
 VI. Therapist models a mix of individual clear and unclear instructions.
    A. After each instruction, therapist asks parent whether it was a clear or unclear instruction, and why. Parent rephrases each unclear instruction into a clear instruction.
VII. Introduce consequences for compliance.
    A. Reinforce child with positive attention (attends and rewards) if child initiates compliance within 5 seconds of clear instruction.
    B. Reinforce child upon completion of compliance.
    C. Use attends and rewards as child continues to comply to an extended task.
    D. Emphasize that labeled rewards are especially important.

VIII. Draw diagram of Path A of clear instructions sequence (parent clear instruction, child complies, parent positive attention) (Chapter 7, Figure 7.2).

IX. Demonstrate Path A of clear instructions sequence.

X. Parent role plays Path A.

XI. Explain/demonstrate Path A to child.

XII. Parent practices Path A with child.
   A. Tell parent to issue clear instructions to child and reinforce compliance but to ignore noncompliance at present time.
   B. Deliver prompts and feedback to parent.

XIII. Therapist observes parent and child interacting in Parent's Game and counts alpha and beta commands to determine whether parent meets behavioral criteria for clear instructions and to provide ongoing feedback about use of positive attention for child compliance.
   A. Discuss interaction.

XIV. Therapist gives Parent Handout 8: Introduction to Phase II and Parent Handout 9: The Clear Instructions Sequence: Path A (Appendix B).

XV. Assign homework (Chapter 7).
   A. Instruct parent to monitor and record frequency of clear and unclear instructions.
   B. Present child with clear instructions with which he or she is likely to comply.
      1. Compliance receives positive attention.
      2. Noncompliance is ignored.
   C. Give Parent Handout 10: Parent Record Sheet: Clear Instructions and Child Compliance (Appendix B).
      1. Parent records use of two clear instructions per day and positive attention (rewards, attends) for compliance.
      2. Parent records unclear instructions and notes alternative clear instructions.
   D. Continue with the differential attention programs to increase "OK" behaviors.

Session 7 (Chapter 7)

I. Repeat Session 6 unless the parent meets behavioral criteria for clear instructions in either final observation of Session 6 or initial observation of Session 7.

II. Parent gives setting instruction to child.

III. If criteria for clear instructions are not met, session proceeds as follows.
   A. Discuss interaction.
   B. Discuss homework (including differential attention programs for "OK" child behaviors).
   C. Repeat training in clear instructions, as covered in Session 6, focusing on role playing and practice with child.

IV. If criteria for clear instructions are met, session proceeds as follows.
   A. Discuss interaction.

B. Discuss homework (including differential attention programs for "OK" child behaviors).

C. Introduce Path B (Chapter 7).

   1. Child noncomplies to clear instruction.

   2. Warning ("If . . . then" statement)

      a. TO is specified as a consequence for noncompliance to warning.

      b. Wait 5 seconds.

   3. Positive attention (rewards, attends) for compliance to warning.

D. Draw diagram of Path B of clear instructions sequence (Chapter 7, Figure 7.2).

E. Model Path B sequence.

F. Parent role plays Path B sequence.

G. Explain/demonstrate Path B sequence to child.

H. Parent practices Paths A and B with child.

   1. Tell parent to issue clear instructions to child, reinforce compliance, and issue warnings as needed.

   2. Parent ignores noncompliance to the warning for the time being.

   3. Deliver prompts and feedback to parent.

V. Therapist observes parent and child interacting in Parent's Game and counts alpha and beta commands to determine whether parent continues to meet behavioral criteria for clear instructions.

VI. Therapist gives Parent Handout 11: The Clear Instructions Sequence: Path B (Appendix B).

VII. Assign homework.

A. Parent to continue practicing Path A of the clear instructions sequence.

   1. Give clear instructions to which child is likely to comply.

   2. Reinforce compliance.

   3. Ignore noncompliance (for now).

   4. Parent should *not* employ Path B (i.e., warning for noncompliance) at home at this point.

   5. Continue recording on Parent Handout 10: Parent Record Sheet: Clear Instructions and Child Compliance (Appendix B).

B. Parent to continue differential attention programs for "OK" child behaviors.

Session 8 (Chapter 7)

I. Therapist observes parent and child interacting in Parent's Game and counts alpha and beta commands to determine whether parent continues to meet behavioral criteria for clear instructions.

II. Parent gives setting instruction to child.

III. Discuss interaction.

IV. Discuss homework (including differential attention programs for "OK" child behaviors).

V. Review Paths A and B with parent and child.

   VI. Introduce Path C (Chapter 7).

      A. Child noncomplies to clear instructions *and* to warning.

      B. TO for noncompliance to warning.

         1. Child stays in TO chair.

      C. Return to original clear instruction situation.

  VII. Draw diagram of Path C of clear instructions sequence (Chapter 7, Figure 7.2).

 VIII. Help parent choose appropriate TO area in the home.

   IX. Parent role plays all three paths of the clear instructions sequence with therapist, and therapist discusses and models when necessary.

    X. Review Paths A and B of the clear instructions sequence with child (by using verbal instruction, modeling, and role playing).

      A. Explain/demonstrate Path C sequence to child.

   XI. Parent practices all three paths of the clear instructions sequence with child and receives prompts and feedback from therapist.

  XII. Discuss practice period with parent.

 XIII. Assign homework.

      A. Parent to continue practicing Path A of the clear instructions sequence.

         1. Give clear instructions to which child is likely to comply.

         2. Reinforce compliance.

         3. Ignore noncompliance (for now).

         4. Parent should *not* employ Paths B or C for noncompliance at home at this point.

         5. Continue recording on Parent Handout 10: Parent Record Sheet: Clear Instructions and Child Compliance (Appendix B).

      B. Parent to continue differential attention programs for "OK" child behaviors.

Session 9 (Chapter 7)

    I. Therapist observes parent and child interacting in Parent's Game and counts alpha and beta commands to determine whether parent continues to meet behavioral criteria for clear instructions.

   II. Parent gives setting instruction to child.

  III. Discuss interaction.

  IV. Discuss homework (including differential attention programs for "OK" child behaviors).

   V. Review all paths of the clear instructions sequence.

  VI. Parent practices all three paths of the clear instructions sequence with child and receives prompts and feedback from therapist.

 VII. Discuss practice period with parent.

 VIII. Therapist presents and demonstrates challenges in the use of the clear instructions sequence.

  IX. Therapist and parent role play various challenges.

   X. Explain and demonstrate challenges to child.

  XI. Parent and child practice challenges with feedback from therapist.

XII. Therapist observes parent and child interacting in Parent's Game and counts parental alpha and beta commands, child compliances and noncompliances, parental attends, rewards, warnings, contingent attention, and TO to determine whether parent meets behavioral criteria for consequences segment of Phase II (Chapter 7).

   A. Discuss interaction.

XIII. Give Parent Handout 12: The Clear Instructions Sequence: Path C and Parent Handout 13: Challenges in the Use of the Clear Instructions Sequence (Appendix B).

XIV. Assign homework.

   A. If parent can use procedures correctly in clinic and child remains in chair during TO, assign homework of selecting one noncompliant situation, using clear instructions, reinforcing compliance, and using TO (if necessary).

      1. Ask parent to record clear instructions and warnings, consequences for compliance, and use of TO on Parent Handout 14: Parent Record Sheet: Clear Instructions Sequence (Appendix B).

   B. If parent cannot use procedures correctly or child will not remain in chair during TO, repeat homework assignment from Sessions 7 and 8.

   C. Parent to continue use of differential attention programs for "OK" child behaviors.

Session 10 (Chapter 7)

   I. Therapist observes parent and child in Parent's Game and counts parental alpha and beta commands, child compliances and noncompliances, parental attends, rewards, warnings, contingent attention, and TO to determine whether parent meets behavioral criteria for consequences segment of Phase II.

   II. Parent gives setting instruction to child.

   III. If behavioral criteria for consequences segment of Phase II are not met or child will not remain in chair during TO, the session proceeds as follows.

   A. Discuss interaction.

   B. Discuss homework (including differential attention programs for "OK" behaviors).

   C. Repeat Session 9.

   IV. If criteria for consequences segment of Phase II are met (or were met at the end of Session 9) and child will remain in chair during TO, session proceeds as follows.

   A. Discuss interaction.

   B. Discuss homework.

   C. Parent practices Child's Game with child for brief period as prelude to Parent's Game.

   D. Parent switches to Parent's Game.

      1. Parent practices all three paths of the clear instructions sequence with child.

      2. Role play and practice challenging situations in use of the clear instructions sequence (Chapter 7, Figure 7.6).

   V. Therapist observes parent and child in Parent's Game and counts parental alpha and beta commands, child compliances and noncompliances, parental attends, rewards, warnings, contingent attention, and TO to determine whether parent meets behavioral criteria for consequences segment of Phase II.

  VI. Assign homework.

     A. Depending on parent's progress, either assign homework from Session 9 or have parent employ TO for all instances of noncompliance at home.

     B. Parent records on Parent Handout 14: Parent Record Sheet: Clear Instructions Sequence (Appendix B).

     C. Parent to continue with differential attention programs for "OK" child behaviors.

Session 11 (Chapter 7)

    I. If criteria for consequences phase of Phase II have not been met or child will not remain in chair during TO, the session proceeds as follows:

     A. Therapist observes parent and child in Parent's Game and counts parental alpha and beta commands, child compliances and noncompliances, parental attends, rewards, warnings, contingent attention, and TOs to determine whether parent meets behavioral criteria for consequences segment of Phase II.

     B. Parent gives setting instruction to child.

     C. Discuss interaction.

     D. Discuss homework (including differential attention programs for "OK" behaviors).

     E. Repeat Session 10.

   II. If criteria for consequences segment of Phase II have been met and child remains in chair during TO, the session proceeds as follows.

     A. Therapist observes parent and child in Child's Game and counts attends, rewards, ignoring, commands, and questions.

     B. Therapist observes parent and child in Parent's Game and counts parental alpha and beta commands, child compliances and noncompliances, parental attends, rewards, warnings, contingent attention, and TO.

  III. Parent gives setting instruction to child.

  IV. Therapist discusses preceding interactions and homework.

   V. Therapist introduces standing rules as a supplement to clear instructions sequence.

     A. "If . . . then" statement.

     B. Once stated, continuously in effect.

     C. TO is consequence for breaking the rule.

     D. After TO, parent rehearses rule with child.

  VI. Parent generates one or two standing rules.

 VII. Therapist and parent role play and practice standing rule(s).

VIII. Explain and demonstrate standing rule to child.

IX. Parent and child practice standing rule in session with therapist feedback.
X. Therapist gives Parent Handout 15: Standing Rules (Appendix B).
XI. Assign homework.
   A. Parent implements one or two standing rules.
   B. Parent to complete Parent Handout 16: Parent Record Sheet: Standing Rules (Appendix B).
   C. Parent to continue employing all three paths of the clear instructions sequence with child.
      1. Parent records on Parent Handout 14: Parent Record Sheet: Clear Instructions Sequence (Appendix B).
   D. Parent to continue with differential attention programs for "OK" child behaviors as needed.

Session 12 (Chapter 7)

   I. Therapist observes parent and child in Child's Game and Parent's Game.
   II. Parent gives setting instruction to child.
   III. Therapist discusses preceding interaction and homework.
   IV. If necessary, continue with additional practice with parent and child concerning standing rules.
   V. Therapist discusses appropriateness of Phase I and Phase II skills to situations outside of the home.
   VI. Parent identifies at least one situation outside the home that is of concern.
      A. Therapist and parent identify strategy for dealing with the situation.
      B. Therapist and parent role play planned solution.
      C. Explain and demonstrate plan to the child.
      D. Parent and child practice, with feedback from therapist.
   VII. Give Parent Handout 17: Dealing With Situations Outside the Home (Appendix B).
   VIII. Assign homework.
      A. Parent to hold at least one practice session with child in the identified situation.
      B. Parent to gradually implement plan.
      C. Parent to continue with differential attention programs, use of the clear instructions sequence, and standing rules as needed.

Session 13 (Chapter 7)

   I. Therapist observes parent and child in Child's Game and Parent's Game.
   II. Parent gives setting instruction to child.
   III. Therapist discusses preceding interaction and homework.
   IV. If necessary, proceed with additional practice with parent and child concerning situations outside the home.
   V. Therapist and parent discuss any problem behaviors that are continuing.

VI. Emphasize consistency as key to program.
   A. Child will not need to test limits as much if parent is consistent.
   B. If parent is consistent, number and intensity of problems will be reduced.
VII. Note that, although program is not a cure-all, it will make family interactions more positive and enjoyable.
VIII. Emphasize continued use of Phase I skills.
IX. Encourage parent to contact therapist if difficulties arise.

COMMONLY ENCOUNTERED PROBLEMS

The parent training program is relatively straightforward. However, there are a number of situations that may arise that can impede the engagement process, interrupt progression through the program, or which deserve special mention. The purpose of this section (and similar sections in Chapters 6 and 7) is to present some of these situations and the solutions we employ for resolving them.

The Play-Therapy Parent

Occasionally, a parent will not want to be part of the intervention but instead wants the therapist to treat only the child. This is the parent who would like to drop the child off at 4:00 P.M., have the child "fixed," and pick up the child at 5:00 P.M. Our approach to this type of parent is to explain that we believe the problem is not the child's or the parent's per se but rather the parent–child interaction. Therefore, it is necessary for both parent and child to be a part of the intervention process. Furthermore, we point out to the parent that since the child is with the parent the majority of the time, the most efficient and effective procedure is to teach the parent how to deal with the problems that are occurring. Even if we could effect some change in the child in a 1-hour individual therapy session, it is doubtful that the improvement would generalize to the home situation, where all other aspects of the environment, such as the parent's behavior, remain the same. By working through the parent, it is possible to achieve a more durable and effective change in the child's behavior.

This approach typically is effective in convincing the parent of the need for involvement. If the parent still does not wish to participate in intervention, we recommend a therapist who works individually with children.

The Guilty Parent

At the other end of the continuum of perceived responsibility is the "Guilty Parent." Throughout the HNC program, emphasis is placed on the fact that much of a child's behavior is learned and that the parent can change the child's undesirable behavior. Some parents immediately assume that the child's problems are solely their responsibility. These parents frequently wish to focus on a series of unpleasant past interactions between the child and parent.

It is important to acknowledge and respond empathetically to the parent's feelings of guilt concerning past interactions with the child. However, we do not make these feelings a focus of the parent training program. Instead, we respond in several ways. We first reassure the parent that he or she is not to blame for the child's problems. We then note that it is not possible to look back into the past and accurately identify the causes of the child's problems. Even if possible, this knowledge would be of minimal assistance in resolving current problems. Instead, we remind the parent of the reciprocal nature of the coercive processes that gradually evolved over time. We encourage the parent to not worry about the past but, starting now, to work with the therapist to make some changes that will improve the interaction between parent and child. (While we have generally been successful with this approach, it is important to note that, for some parents, this self-blaming may be a sign of concurrent depression, which may have to be dealt with separately.)

The Shy Parent

Some parents have difficulty practicing the skills taught in the program in front of the therapist. This may occur in role playing with the therapist or in practice sessions with the child. These parents frequently state that they can use the skills effectively at home but that they are too shy to try them in front of the therapist. Our approach is to stress to the parent in the initial intervention session that practicing the skills in the session is an important part of the intervention process. With this initial statement, most parents are able to engage in the skills when the time arrives. We also tell the parent that there are usually three steps to beginning a new routine: "awkward" to "aware" to "automatic" (McMahon, Slough, & the Conduct Problems Prevention Research Group, 1994). When we try something new or unfamiliar, we initially feel awkward. As we get more familiar with the routine, we become aware of what is required, but it still takes a lot of work. With enough practice, the routine finally becomes almost second nature. The parent also tends to feel less inhibited in the role play and practice activities after observing the therapist become involved in them as well. Once the parent starts to engage in the role playing, we elicit personal feelings about the activity, note progress, and again offer support. Appropriate reinforcement from the therapist for progress is usually effective in relieving the parent's performance anxiety.

CHAPTER 6

Phase I: The Skills of Differential Attention

In this chapter, we first provide a description of the procedures we employ to facilitate child cooperation and participation during the intervention sessions through the use of setting instructions. We then present a rationale and overview of Phase I. This is followed by descriptions of each of the three parenting skills that are taught during this phase. The use of these skills in the form of differential attention is then presented. We next describe the various homework assignments that are made during Phase I and then present a sample Phase I session. Finally, we delineate commonly encountered challenging problems and recommended solutions.

FACILITATING CHILD COOPERATION AND PARTICIPATION DURING THE FIRST INTERVENTION SESSION: THE USE OF SETTING INSTRUCTIONS

The first intervention session, which begins Phase I, usually presents a powerful opportunity for demonstrating the effectiveness of social learning procedures in general, and Phase I skills in particular, to the parent. We typically have the child present in the playroom with the parent throughout the program while the therapist and parent are discussing and practicing the parenting skills. It is an excellent opportunity to demonstrate the relevant skills to the parent and demonstrate how quickly they can be effective. It seems that a stranger (in this case, the therapist) is often able to elicit appropriate behavior from children more readily than their parents can. In fact, data from several studies (e.g., Dumas & LaFreniere, 1993; Landauer, Carlsmith, & Lepper, 1970) indicate that children are more compliant to strangers than to parents. The therapist can make use of this phenomenon by demonstrating the appropriate parenting skills within the session with the child. This is most beneficial in the first intervention sessions, when the parent may be a bit skeptical that social learning techniques can be effective with his or her child. By seeing them successfully employed in a "real life" situation, probably quite similar to one experienced at home, the parent can be persuaded of the efficacy of the procedures early on.

An additional structuring strategy can be essential to increasing the probability that the session will proceed without interruption. Prior to beginning the first treatment session, the therapist should ask the parent to make sure that the child has taken care of any bathroom needs. In subsequent sessions, the therapist checks to make sure that the parent has taken the child to the bathroom prior to the beginning of the session.

When the family enters the room at the beginning of the first treatment session, the therapist models an appropriate setting instruction to the child for the parent. The therapist takes the child to the area of the playroom where the toys are located. The therapist tells the child, " [Name], your Mom and I are going to be talking over here. Here are some toys for you to play with. We have lots of work to do, so please don't interrupt us. If you do, we will ignore you." For younger children, the therapist adds an explanation, such as "That means that we will turn away and not look at you or talk to you."

The therapist then returns to the parent and tells the parent that this setting instruction should be repeated at the beginning of all further sessions by the parent. The therapist then presents the rationale for Phase I of the parent training program (see below). After a few minutes have elapsed, the therapist interrupts the presentation of the rationale and says to the parent, "Since [name] has been playing quietly, I am going to let him [or her] know we appreciate that." The therapist walks over to the child and praises him or her by saying, "Thanks for playing by yourself over here. We like it when you do that." The therapist then returns to the parent and resumes the presentation. This procedure should be repeated at variable intervals throughout the session, but with the parent providing the positive attention to the child. Since the relevant parenting skills have not been covered, at first the therapist tells the parent exactly what to say and when to say it. As the parent becomes more proficient, the therapist encourages the parent to interrupt the therapist at appropriate intervals to reinforce the child for appropriate behavior. When the parent does this correctly within the session, the therapist reinforces this behavior. Throughout the program, and especially during Phase I, the parent is encouraged to apply this "interrupting" procedure in the home when alone with the child or when interacting with a spouse, a friend, and so forth.

At some point during the first session, the therapist and/or parent is likely to have occasion to ignore the child's inappropriate behavior as well. This behavior is most likely to take some form of attention seeking, such as attempting to interrupt the therapist or parent. Quite often this occurs soon after the child has been reinforced for appropriate behavior. This is because the child has not yet determined the reinforcement contingencies for particular behaviors. The child only knows that he or she likes the attention from the adults and, therefore, seeks more. When this inappropriate attention-seeking behavior occurs, the therapist again instructs the parent in the appropriate response—in this case, ignoring. As the parent and therapist are ignoring the child (with a great deal of verbal direction and support from the therapist), the therapist can provide the rationale for this active ignoring procedure (see below).

The key here is that the child begins to learn that the therapist and parent will follow through on the setting instruction established at the beginning of the session. By using positive attention and, when necessary, in combination with ignoring (i.e., differential attention), the therapist is also demonstrating to the parent that these skills have practical value and, more importantly, that they are effective. By having the parent state the setting instruction in subsequent sessions and take increasingly greater responsibility for deciding when to provide positive attention to the child for appropriate in-session behavior, the therapist is able to gradually shift control to the parent.

RATIONALE AND OVERVIEW OF PHASE I

The purposes of Phase I are to (1) change the coercive cycle of interaction between parent and child, (2) reestablish more prosocial patterns of parent–child interaction and enhance the overall quality of the parent–child relationship, and (3) help the parent to become skilled in the use of differential attention to the child's behavior. Through parental use of differential attention, the child's appropriate ("OK") behavior will increase, and his or her own inappropriate ("not OK") behavior will decrease. Differential attention is the "application of adult attention following the occurrence of a desired behavior and the removal of an adult's attention after an undesired behavior" (Sajwaj & Dillon, 1977, p. 303).

Three parenting skills are taught in Phase I. These include two types of positive reinforcement skills (attends and rewards) and an extinction procedure (ignoring). They will be described more fully later in this chapter. It is important to note that the positive reinforcement skills include only social types of positive reinforcement (i.e., positive attention from the parent). Although we do occasionally find it necessary to establish behavior management programs that employ material reinforcers (stars, tokens, money), we have found social reinforcement to be at least as effective, more developmentally appropriate for children in this age range, and more versatile. Parents will not run out of social reinforcers, as may happen with material reinforcers. In addition, use of social reinforcers obviates the need for later transfer of training from material to social reinforcement. Finally, social reinforcers tend to be more effective in maintaining appropriate behavior.

By the time most parents and children seek assistance from a mental health professional, they can see few if any positive aspects to the other's behavior. The parenting skills taught in Phase I help the parent to observe the child's behavior more closely. Many parents are surprised to discover that their child already engages in a fair share of positive behaviors. The task of Phase I then becomes increasing the frequency of those positive behaviors.

As a side benefit of Phase I, the parent slows down, enjoys the child, and relates to the child on the child's level. As the parent shows interest in the child and his or her activities, the child begins to enjoy interactions with the parent, and the parent's value as a source of reinforcement increases. In essence, time spent with each other becomes "quality" time.

Teaching the Parent about Reinforcement: The Positive Reinforcement Rule and the Attention Rule

Phase I is formulated on two assumptions.[1] The first is the "Positive Reinforcement Rule," which states that when a behavior receives positive consequences immediately after it occurs, that behavior is more likely to occur in the future. This rule is very important in starting and maintaining "OK" child behavior. The therapist provides parents with a scenario such as the following:

> "Suppose I was to tell you that every time you raised your hand to ask a question in these sessions, I would give you a $5 bill. You would probably be quite skeptical, but you also might give it a try. And, sure enough, I give you the $5. Do you think that you would be more or less likely to raise your hand in the future?"

Assuming the parent answers affirmatively, the therapist then moves on to the second rule. The second rule, which is a corollary of the positive reinforcement rule, is the "Attention Rule." It states that attention from others, especially parents, is a very powerful reinforcer to children in this age range (i.e., 3–8 years). The attention can be either positive (e.g., praise) or negative (e.g., yelling, criticism, scolding) in nature. If the child is not receiving positive attention, then that child will work to receive negative attention, which he or she considers to be better than no attention at all. Therefore, because the parent's attention serves as a very powerful reinforcer to the child, it can be used to change behavior.

The therapist then draws or shows the parent the 2 × 2 table presented in Figure 6.1. The therapist states that a major focus of Phase I is to use positive parental attention to increase positive "OK" child behaviors (upper left quadrant of Figure 6.1). Too often as parents we tend to take good behavior for granted because we expect children to behave or because "OK" behavior does not grab our attention in the dramatic way that "not OK" behavior does. The therapist tells the parent that, instead, the object should be to "catch your child being good" (Becker, 1971). The flip side of this approach is that the parent also can decrease many "not OK" behaviors by withholding attention from the child (i.e., ignoring) (lower right quadrant of Figure 6.1). That will also be a focus of Phase I.

Pointing to the two remaining quadrants in Figure 6.1, the therapist states that there are two additional situations that must be considered when using parental attention to influence child behavior. The first is referred to as the "criticism trap," and describes the situation in which the parent provides negative attention (in the form of nagging, scolding, or yelling) to the child after the child engages in some form of "not OK" behavior. It is a trap because, although the negative attention may stop the "not OK" behavior temporarily, in the long run, it actually *increases* the "not OK" behavior!

The second situation is when the child is engaged in an "OK" behavior but the parent ignores it. Parents often justify this approach by stating that they do not want to dis-

---

[1] We are indebted to Thomas R. DuHamel, PhD, for this formulation.

	"OK" CHILD BEHAVIOR	"NOT OK" CHILD BEHAVIOR
PARENT ATTENTION (Increases Behavior)	+ **POSITIVE ATTENTION** "CATCH YOUR CHILD BEING GOOD" (Positive Behavior Increases)	− "CRITICISM TRAP" (Negative Behavior Increases)
NO PARENT ATTENTION (Decreases Behavior)	− "LET SLEEPING DOGS LIE" (Positive Behavior Decreases)	+ **IGNORE** (Negative Behavior Decreases)

FIGURE 6.1. The Attention Table.

turb the child when he or she is behaving, since they believe that the child will then demand attention continually. This parental attitude toward positive child behavior can be described as "let sleeping dogs lie" or "leave well enough alone." Unfortunately, the effect of such an approach is that the child's "OK" behavior will occur less often—and may even disappear—because of this lack of positive attention.

The therapist then illustrates this last point by saying to the parent, "You know, Nick has been playing quietly with the toys for the past few minutes, and we've essentially ignored him. Based on this chart, what should we be doing?" Hopefully, the parent will realize that playing quietly is an "OK" behavior, and that the child should be receiving positive attention. The therapist says, "Go over to Nick and say 'Nick, thanks very much for playing so quietly with the toys. I really appreciate it!' Then come back over here without saying anything else to him." The therapist observes the parent and provides assistance as needed to make sure that the interaction with the child is limited to this brief statement of positive attention. When the parent returns, the therapist praises the parent and states that, from this point on, the parent should look for opportunities in the sessions to provide positive attention to the child. As noted above, the therapist encourages the parent to interrupt the therapist at any time to provide positive attention to the child for "OK" behavior. The therapist prompts the parent to repeat this activity a few minutes later (and throughout the sessions) if the parent does not initiate this action. Parents eventually become very proficient at this activity. The therapist points out that this situation is analogous to those that commonly occur at home when the parent is having a conversation with another adult and wants to decrease the likelihood of being interrupted by the child.

The therapist gives Parent Handout 1: Introduction to Phase I (Appendix B) to the parent at the end of the session in which the rationale and overview of Phase I are presented.

PARENTING SKILLS

Attends

Defining Attends

This procedure is a high-rate form of positive attention in which the parent provides an ongoing verbal description of the child's activity (e.g., "You're putting all the toys into the cabinet"). The essential features of attends are presented in Figure 6.2. Attends are essentially a running commentary (a "play-by-play" account, if you will) on the child's activity and, as such, provide a more constant source of attention than rewards (i.e., praise statements), which tend to be more discrete. There are two basic types of attends: those that simply describe overt behavior ("You're stacking the blocks" or "Here comes the truck") and ones that may be used to emphasize a desired prosocial behavior ("You're playing all by yourself" or "You're talking in a regular voice").

A major effect of using attends is that it helps the parent to relate to the child on his or her level (because the child is directing the play, not the parent). Children in the

- Follows, rather than leads, the child's activity (by a running verbal commentary).
- Used only to reinforce "OK" behaviors.
- Two basic types:
  - Describe overt behavior ("You just put the red block on top of the green block").
  - Emphasize desired prosocial behavior ("You're talking in a regular voice").
- "Volume control" feature allows parent to raise or lower the intensity and frequency of the positive attention.

- Do *not*:
  - Ask questions.
  - Give commands.
  - Try to teach.

FIGURE 6.2. The skill of attends.

3- to 8-year age range enjoy this type of interaction tremendously, because it clearly demonstrates that the parent is interested in what the child is doing. Opportunities for children in this age range to "be in charge" of an interaction with a parent are relatively rare. When children are given this opportunity in the context of the Child's Game, they tend to respond quite positively. As a result, an overall effect is that there is an increased likelihood of inducing a more positive mood in the child (Lay, Waters, & Park, 1989) and reciprocal cooperation between parent and child (Parpal & Maccoby, 1985).

Teaching Attends to Parents

The Phase I parenting skills, starting with attends, are taught within the context of the Child's Game. As noted in Chapter 4, the Child's Game is essentially a free-play situation in which the parent is instructed to engage in any activity that the child chooses and to allow the child to determine the nature and rules of the interaction. The Child's Game is used not only in the playroom setting but is also employed as a homework assignment throughout Phase I. Its use in the latter context is described later in this chapter.

In order to attend properly, the parent must first be able to *follow* the child's behavior; that is, the parent must be interested enough in the child's activity to observe what the child is doing in a relatively sustained manner. An occasional glance from behind the evening paper is not really following! We describe this to the parent as "tailgating" the child. The parent then provides a running commentary on the child's activity, using attending statements. We tell the parent to imagine being a radio announcer, and the parent's job is to provide a play-by-play account of the child's activity.

There are also certain types of verbal behavior that should *not* be intermixed with attends. First of all, the parent should eliminate questions (see Chapter 9 for an exception with respect to children with language disabilities) or commands directed to the child. Questions and commands interrupt and/or structure the child's activity. Furthermore, the parent should refrain from turning the Child's Game into a teaching session ("Tell me what color this block is"). When the purpose of a parent–child interaction is to increase the child's appropriate behavior, it is best not to teach the child or test the child's knowledge. In a similar manner, the parent should not attempt to direct the child's play. Participation in the activity is certainly appropriate and may include cooperative or parallel play (e.g., by handing materials to the child, taking a turn, or imitating the child's play). However, during such play, the parent should be reminded to continue to attend to the child's activity as opposed to his or her own.

It is also important to stress that attending is to be used only to describe appropriate ("OK") child behavior. Although this point seems obvious, many parents who are novices at attending inadvertently reinforce their children's inappropriate ("not OK") behavior by attending to it. We have heard more than one parent say to a child, "Now you're throwing the blocks against the wall," or some other comment on the child's inappropriate behavior. After the parent has become relatively proficient at attending to the therapist role playing the child, the therapist should "sneak in" a minor inappropriate behavior (e.g., rough play with the toys, whining) during the role play in order to see whether the parent attends to it or correctly determines that it is a "not OK" behavior that should be ignored.

As noted above, attends can be employed as a more or less constant form of attention. In essence, the parent is equipped with a "volume control" to raise or lower the intensity and frequency of the positive attention. Therefore, attending is especially helpful when the parent is attempting to establish a new behavior in the child's repertoire or to maintain continued compliance to an extended activity. For example, a problematic situation that is commonly reported by parents is the child's failure to pick up toys after use. Even if the child has made some initial effort toward this goal, parents often report that the task is rarely completed. Attending may be used to maintain such activity by providing it on a constant basis as the child picks up the toys (see the example in Chapter 7, "Positive Attention for Child Compliance [Path A]"). Once the extended compliance is well established, the parent fades the frequency of attending to a more intermittent schedule.

When the Child's Game is being explained to the parent, the therapist should acknowledge the artificial nature of a play setting in the clinic. However, the therapist also should note that the playroom presents an excellent setting for the parent to acquire and practice the parenting skills. The parent should be reassured that the actual problem behaviors that are of particular concern will also be addressed.

It is not unusual for a parent to feel uncomfortable at first in using attends with the child. This is understandable since the parent is not used to this style of interacting and because the therapist is prompting and encouraging the parent to use attends at a very high rate. This is done because we realize that the rate of attends is likely to be substantially lower in the natural environment; therefore, we have the parent overlearn the skill in the intervention session to ingrain the skills as much as possible. One strategy that we have found to be effective in helping parents who are first learning to attend get started is to have the parent silently ask himself or herself the question "What is [child's name] doing now?" as the parent follows the child's behavior. The parent then answers the question out loud (e.g., "You're pushing the race car underneath the chair"). By repeating this "silent question—verbal answer" procedure many times in succession, the parent's rate of attending rapidly increases. We also find that the parent's initial awkwardness diminishes significantly as the parent practices attending in a variety of situations. The therapist may choose to use the "awkward—aware—automatic" description of steps to beginning a new routine (McMahon et al., 1994) that was presented in Chapter 5, page 105, as a way to both acknowledge the parent's initial discomfort and to show anticipation of improvement and mastery in the use of attends.

When the parent first begins to practice attending, he or she may give a relatively high proportion of rewards (e.g., praise statements). This is because such praise statements are more familiar to the parent than attends, and the parent feels more comfortable using them. The therapist should encourage the parent to focus on attends to the exclusion of rewards initially so that he or she will become more proficient at, and comfortable with, this style of interacting with the child. Later in Phase I, the parent learns how to combine attends and rewards in the most effective manner.

The novelty of being attended to, particularly with a high schedule of attends in the intervention session, sometimes leads the child to state "You're talking funny" or "Why are you talking like that?" The therapist should instruct the parent to respond by saying, "I'm just interested in what you're doing," and to ignore repeated questions by the child. This response is usually sufficient. Younger children (3 to 6 years of age) rapidly acclimate to this new way of interacting with their parents and appear to enjoy the high rate of parental attention. These children will often engage in a discrete behavior (e.g., putting a block on top of another) and then look expectantly at the parent to see what he or she will say. However, in the event that the child is continually questioning the parent about attending, the parent would do well to examine the style and quality of attending and modify it as necessary. With older children (7 or 8 years of age), it is often necessary to have the parent use more varied attends and/or reduce the rate of attends during the practice session. This has handled the problem in nearly all cases. Interestingly, parents report that older children appear to enjoy the attends at home—perhaps because of their lower rate of occurrence.

The therapist gives Parent Handout 2: Attends and the Child's Game (Appendix B) to the parent at the end of the session in which attends are introduced.

Goals for Attends: Behavioral Criteria

The behavioral criteria for the parent's successful completion of the attending segment of Phase I involve at least one 5-minute observation of the Child's Game in which the parent employs (1) an average of 4 or more attends per minute and (2) an average of .4 or fewer commands plus questions per minute. After parents meet these criteria, they begin learning the skill of rewards. Training in the attending segment of Phase I is typically limited to no more than four sessions.

Rewards

Defining Rewards

The second positive reinforcement skill concerns the use of praise and positive physical contact and is taught in the latter part of Phase I (see Figure 6.3). The therapist notes that there are three types of rewards. "Physical rewards" include various kinds of physi-

- Three types:
  - Physical rewards (e.g., hug, kiss, pat on the back)
  - Unlabeled verbal rewards (e.g., "Great!" "Nice job!")
  - Labeled verbal rewards (e.g., "Thank you for picking up the toys like I asked")

- Guidelines for using rewards:
  - Be specific.
  - Give immediately.
  - Focus on improvement.
  - Use consistently.

FIGURE 6.3. The skill of rewards.

cal affection, such as a hug, kiss, pat on the back, and the like. The second type of re-ward is an "unlabeled verbal reward." These rewards include praise statements that, while positive in evaluation, do not tell the child exactly which behavior is being rein-forced. Examples of unlabeled verbal rewards are the following: "Terrific!," "I liked that," and "Very nice." While nearly all parents are accustomed to providing these first two types of rewards, at least on an occasional basis, they rarely employ the third cate-gory of rewards. "Labeled verbal rewards" are praise statements that specifically describe the particular child behavior that the parent is reinforcing. Examples include "Thank you for picking up the toys" and "I really like it when you do what Mom says." The ad-vantage of this type of reward is that it teaches the child exactly which of several ongo-ing behaviors is being specifically reinforced. For example, if a parent walked through a room in which the child was playing quietly and gave an unlabeled verbal reward such as "That's nice," the child might attribute that praise to the tower of blocks he or she has just built, the quiet play, or the interesting mural the child has just drawn on the new wallpaper (out of sight, of course). Thus, we strongly emphasize the use of labeled verbal rewards as a means of positive parent attention. As a teaching aid, it is helpful to instruct the parent to pair an unlabeled verbal reward with an appropriate attend (e.g., "Good job! You're playing carefully with Patrick's toys"). This ensures the labeling of the child's behavior.

Teaching the Parent to Reward

It is also necessary to teach the parent how to reward the child. The therapist empha-sizes four general guidelines. First, as noted above, rewards should be *specific* (i.e., use a labeled verbal reward such as "You did a good job of playing nicely with your sister"). Second, the parent should give a reward *immediately* after the "OK" behavior or while it is ongoing. This helps the child make the connection between the "OK" behavior and the positive attention from the parent. Third, use rewards to focus on *improvement* by giving them for steps along the way to completing a task. For example, if the child is cleaning up his or her room, use labeled verbal rewards for putting the books on the shelf, putting the blanket on the bed, etc. Fourth, it is important to use rewards *consis-tently*. When the child is first learning an "OK" behavior, such as compliance to parental commands, the parent should reward this behavior every time that it occurs. Once the behavior is well established, the parent can adjust the frequency of rewards to a more intermittent basis.

The therapist also emphasizes that the parent must be sincere in the expression of rewards and must also be sure that the reward she or he provides is one that is socially reinforcing to the child. A reward offered in either a diffident or overly enthusiastic manner will likely have the opposite intended effect on the child's behavior. Likewise, a big hug and kiss for a 7-year-old boy in front of his peers may be the "kiss of death" in that context.

Finally, the therapist stresses that rewards are not intended to replace attends. Rather, the two skills are most effectively employed in conjunction with each other. The therapist advises the parent that attending is a more versatile technique that can be applied in most situations and for longer periods of time, whereas rewards can be utilized best to selectively evaluate particular child behaviors in a positive manner. As a rough rule of thumb, the therapist should suggest to parents that they provide at least three to four attends for every reward. After presentation and discussion of the didactic material concerning rewards, the focus of demonstration, role playing, and practice is on the integration of rewards and attends (as opposed to rewards alone).

The therapist gives Parent Handout 4: Rewards (Appendix B) to the parent at the end of the session in which rewards are introduced.

Goals for Rewards: Behavioral Criteria

The behavioral criteria for the successful completion of the rewards segments of Phase I are at least one 5-minute observation of the Child's Game in which (1) the parent employs an average of four rewards plus attends per minute; (2) of this sum, at least two rewards per minute are required; and (3) the parent must also use an average of .4 or fewer commands plus questions per minute. Training in the use of rewards is typically limited to no more than two sessions.

Ignoring

Defining Ignoring

The third skill that is taught in Phase I—ignoring—can be used to reduce or eliminate many types of inappropriate, "not OK" child behaviors, especially those that are attention seeking in nature (e.g., whining, nagging, temper tantrums, interruptions). The essential features of ignoring are presented in Figure 6.4.

Teaching the Parent to Ignore

The therapist tells the parent that ignoring is a major way to decrease the child's "not OK" behavior and that it is much easier to use than punishment. Behavior tends to decrease when it does not receive attention. The therapist stresses that ignoring should

- Attention-seeking behaviors (e.g., whining, nagging, temper tantrums, interrupting) can be ignored. Behaviors that are potentially harmful to people or property (e.g., fighting) should *not* be ignored.
- Ignoring is an active process.
  - Decide ahead of time which "not OK" behaviors to ignore.
  - When ignoring, actively avoid giving attention to the child.
- Three components of ignoring:
  - No eye contact or nonverbal cues ("Don't look!")
  - No verbal contact ("Don't talk!")
  - No physical contact ("Don't touch!")
- Ignoring *starts* as soon as the "not OK" behavior begins. Ignoring *stops* soon after (10–15 seconds) the "not OK" behavior ceases.
- The "not OK" behavior must be ignored *every* time that it occurs; otherwise, the behavior will get worse instead of better.
- Ignoring is never used alone. It should always be combined with positive attention (attends and rewards) for the alternative "OK" behavior.

FIGURE 6.4. The skill of ignoring.

never be used alone; instead, it should always be combined with positive attention (attends and rewards) to increase "OK" behaviors that are incompatible with the "not OK" behaviors. The therapist tells the parent that this differential attention procedure will be covered a bit later in the program.

The therapist notes that there are some situations in which ignoring should *not* be employed. The guideline is that ignoring should not be used whenever children's behavior is harmful to, or has the potential to harm, themselves, others, or property. In that situation, a more active intervention (e.g., TO) should be utilized.

Most parents readily accept the rationale for utilizing an ignoring procedure with the child. However, parents also frequently report that they have tried ignoring and that it did not work. Children's "not OK" behavior typically *escalates* when it is first ignored, making consistent application of ignoring difficult for many parents. For this reason, we have devised a series of component skills that make up an effective, *active* ignoring procedure. Ignoring is active in that (1) the parent has decided ahead of time which behaviors are ignorable, and (2) when the parent is engaged in ignoring, the parent is actively avoiding giving any attention to the child. The components of the ignoring procedure are as follows.

1. *No eye contact or nonverbal cues ("Don't look!").* Unfortunately, often when a child is engaging in "not OK" behaviors that the parent would like to eliminate, it is very difficult to ignore the activity. The child may anger the parent, or may even be rather cute. Whatever the reason, parents often reinforce this "not OK" behavior inadvertently by a brief smile, a frown, or even a glance at the child. For this reason, we instruct the parent to turn at least 90° (and preferably 180°) away from the child. The child will then be less likely to notice any inadvertent facial responses that might rein-

force inappropriate behavior. This turning away also sends a very clear message to the child that the parent is *actively* ignoring the child's "not OK" behavior.

2. *No verbal contact ("Don't talk!")*. The therapist instructs the parent to refrain from any verbal contact with the child while the child is engaging in the "not OK" behavior. This usually presents a problem to the parent in at least two ways. The first has to do with whether the parent should provide a rationale or explanation to the child for ignoring him or her. A second, but related, way in which verbal contact with the child may occur is by the child asking the parent why he or she is being ignored. If the parent responds to the child's query, then by definition the parent is no longer ignoring! It is imperative that the parent not have any verbal contact with the child once the ignoring procedure has started. The appropriate time to provide a rationale for ignoring is when the child is behaving appropriately. Verbal contact at any other time is simply reinforcing the child's "not OK" behavior.

3. *No physical contact ("Don't touch!")*. The child will often attempt to initiate physical contact with the parent once the parent has started to ignore. The child may tug on the parent, attempt to sit on the parent's lap, or, in rare instances, become aggressive. It is a good idea to have the parent stand when ignoring the child. This prevents the occurrence of lap-sitting, and it also provides another discriminative cue to the child that the parent is actively ignoring as opposed to simply being engrossed in some other activity.

The therapist can also tell parents that in more severe cases they may find it necessary to leave the room in order to avoid reinforcing the child's "not OK" behavior. This "TO procedure in reverse" is useful, but it does have two serious shortcomings. As noted below, it is important that ignoring be terminated soon after the cessation of the child's inappropriate behavior, but the parent may not be aware that the "not OK" behavior has ceased if she or he is in another room. In addition, the parent's ability to monitor the child's activity (especially important for younger children) is impaired. Thus, this solution is not the most desirable one.

The ignoring procedure should begin as close to the onset of the child's inappropriate behavior as possible. When the "not OK" behavior has stopped, the parent waits for a brief period (e.g., 10–15 seconds) and then uses attends and rewards to describe the child's appropriate behavior. It is critical that the "not OK" behavior be ignored every time that it occurs and for the duration of the episode. Otherwise, the behavior will get worse instead of better. For example, a parent begins to ignore the child's whining. The child does not like being ignored, so he or she increases the frequency and intensity of the whining. If the parent stops ignoring at this point and provides attention of any sort (e.g., criticism, scolding), then the child has learned that the key to getting the parent's attention is to engage in more intensive levels of whining. Thus, in future attention-seeking attempts, the child will start at the higher level of whining intensity. Furthermore, the behavior will be that much more firmly entrenched and will require more intensive parental intervention to decrease or eliminate it. The good news is that if the parent can use the ignoring procedure consistently, the child's attention-seeking behavior will decrease dramatically.

Teaching the Child about the Ignoring Procedure

After the therapist has modeled the ignoring procedure for the parent and the parent has role played it with the therapist, the therapist has the parent explain the ignoring procedure to the child in the session. The sophistication of the explanation varies depending upon the age of the child, but the explanation generally consists of a verbal statement, such as:

> "Colleen, I am going to ignore you when you [*specify 'not OK' behavior*]. That means I am going to turn away and not *look* at you, *talk* to you, or *touch* you. When I am ignoring you, it means that I don't like what you are doing. As soon as you stop [*specify 'not OK' behavior*], then I will stop ignoring you."

The parent then demonstrates the ignoring technique to the child, with the therapist role playing a child. It is important to enlist the child's cooperation in the practice. The therapist says: "Colleen, would you be willing to help me practice this with your Mom? We're going to pretend that I'm a kid about your age and I'm doing some 'not OK' behaviors with your Mom like whining." [Parent and therapist play with toys on the floor of the playroom.] The therapist starts to whine: "Mommmm! I'm tired of this. Can we go home now? Can we? Can we?" The parent says to the child: "Dr. McMahon is whining. Is that something I want to see more of?" The child says, "No." The parent replies, "That's right. So we're going to ignore him." The parent and child both ignore the therapist. While ignoring, the parent says as an aside to the child, "I'm going to keep ignoring him until he talks in a regular voice." The therapist continues to whine for another 10 seconds or so, then stops. While being ignored, the therapist should verbalize statements such as "I don't like this. Why won't you pay attention to me? I know—I'll just whine louder. No, that didn't work. . . . Maybe I'll stop whining and see what happens." Finally, the therapist should stop the "not OK" behavior (in this case, whining) and talk in a regular tone of voice. The parent says to the child, "Now he's playing nicely again and talking in a regular voice. We can stop ignoring." The parent turns to the therapist and begins playing with the toys. The parent says, "Thank you for talking in a regular voice. I appreciate that."

During the demonstration, the therapist (in his or her role play as the child) should make sure to engage in behaviors that are ignorable (e.g., attention seeking), as opposed to behaviors that present a danger to people or property (and which are not ignorable).

After the demonstration, the therapist asks the child a series of questions to make sure that the child understands the ignoring procedure. These include "Why did your Mom ignore me?" "What did your Mom do when she ignored me?" "Do you think that I liked being ignored?" "How did I get your Mom to stop ignoring me?" Alternatively, if there is a cotherapist, the role play can be repeated, and the cotherapist asks the child these questions at the appropriate points in the role play.

The therapist gives Parent Handout 6: Ignoring (Appendix B) to the parent at the end of the session in which ignoring is introduced.

Goals for Ignoring: Behavioral Criteria

We have not typically utilized a specific behavioral criterion for successful demonstration of ignoring, since the base rate for inappropriate child behavior during the Child's Game is usually quite low. However, a suggested guideline would be that the parent successfully ignores 70% of the child's inappropriate behavior in at least one 5-minute observation of the Child's Game. Training in the use of ignoring is usually limited to no more than the equivalent of a single session. As noted earlier, ignoring occasionally has to be taught simultaneously with, rather than after, attending or rewarding when a child is excessively disruptive in a session.

COMBINING PHASE I SKILLS: DIFFERENTIAL ATTENTION

The positive attention skills of attends and rewards can be employed alone and in combination to increase child "OK" behaviors. We tell parents to use attends and rewards whenever they see a child behavior that they want to encourage. As noted earlier, ignoring, which is used to decrease inappropriate "not OK" child behaviors, should never be used alone. While it provides the child with feedback about what not to do, ignoring does not provide the child with information about the alternative "OK" behavior. Ignoring should *always* be used in combination with the positive attention skills of attends and rewards. This differential attention procedure can be a very powerful procedure for changing children's behavior when it is employed correctly.

The therapist presents the parent with a four-step plan for using differential attention (see Figure 6.5). First, the parent identifies a "not OK" child behavior that he or she wishes to decrease, using ignoring. The therapist may need to remind the parent that differential attention, because it employs ignoring, is not to be used for child behaviors that are risky to the child, other people, or property. Second, the parent identifies at least one alternative "OK" behavior that the parent would like to see instead of the "not OK" behavior identified in the first step. (There may be a number of "OK" behaviors that can be identified.)

The third step is for the parent to inform the child of the differential attention plan. This can be done during the session or at home. In either case, it should be done at a time when the child is not engaging in the "not OK" behavior. For example, one very common situation that parents identify as problematic and that is very appropriate for the use of differential attention procedures is the child attempting to interrupt the parent when the parent is on the telephone. In this case, the parent might say to the child:

- Identify a "not OK" behavior to ignore.
- Identify at least one "OK" behavior that is incompatible with the "not OK" behavior.
- Explain and demonstrate the differential attention plan to the child.
- Implement the plan at home.

FIGURE 6.5. Differential attention.

"Laura, I get really frustrated when I'm on the phone and you interrupt me. From now on, I will ignore you when you interrupt me while I'm on the phone. Instead of interrupting me, I want you to play quietly or watch TV until I'm off the phone. I'll watch for you to do that, and I'll be sure to let you know that I appreciate that."

In the telephone example presented above, the therapist might set up a role play in which the parent is talking on the phone and the therapist plays the part of the child. The therapist attempts to interrupt the parent while he or she is talking on the phone. The parent ignores the therapist's attempts to interrupt, and, after 30 seconds or so, the therapist begins to play quietly with the toys. The parent ends the call about 30 seconds later and provides positive attention to the therapist for engaging in the "OK" behavior of playing quietly with the toys (e.g., "Thanks for playing quietly for most of the time that I was on the phone"). The child would then be given the opportunity to participate in a practice with the parent, with the therapist providing support and feedback to both the parent and child throughout the procedure.

The fourth step is for the parent to implement the plan at home. The parent should ignore the "not OK" behavior whenever it occurs and provide positive attention (attends, rewards) whenever the child engages in the "OK" behavior. The therapist should emphasize that it is the juxtaposition of the ignoring and positive attention procedures that makes differential attention effective. In the example described above, the therapist might suggest that the parent arrange one or two "fake" phone calls in order to practice the procedure with the child at home. When beginning this procedure, the parent may want to "interrupt" the phone call a few times in order to go to the child and provide positive attention for "OK" behavior. (This is similar to what is done in the parent training sessions with the setting instruction described earlier.) This can be phased out over the course of several calls until finally the parent will be able to complete the call before going to the child and providing positive attention.

We would like to describe an additional strategy that combines Phase I skills and is very helpful in decreasing persistent child disruptive behavior during ignoring. This strategy can be employed both during the session and at home. It involves the therapist or parent making statements about the child's behavior or the contingencies that are in effect for the child's behavior, either to someone else in the room (e.g., therapist, parent, sibling) or to him- or herself. These statements are ostensibly directed to that person, but, in fact, are a way of reminding the child who is being ignored about the "OK" behavior that is required for the procedure to end. The statements are *not* directed to the child, because doing so would be providing attention for the child's "not OK" behavior. For example, if the therapist and parent have been ignoring the child's persistent whining for several minutes, the therapist might say to the parent (without looking at the child), "When Patrick is quiet for a few seconds, then we can play with the toys again." The therapist is talking to the parent, but the child who is whining is really the intended target of the statement. Alternatively, the therapist and parent might move over to the toys and begin playing with them, with the parent attending to the therapist (or vice versa, depending on the parent's skill level). The therapist would say, "When

Patrick is quiet again, then he can play with the toys too." When the parent is faced with such a situation alone, then the parent can go to the toys and start attending to him- or herself (e.g., "Now I'm driving the cars down the road. . . . Now I'm pulling into my house. . . . Hey, everybody! I'm home . . . "). Finally, this approach can also be implemented very effectively when interacting with multiple children (e.g., two siblings) (see Chapter 7, "The Role of Siblings, " pp. 154–155).

The goals of these strategies are (1) to increase the probability that the child will stop engaging in the "not OK' " behavior long enough so that the parent can begin using positive attention for incompatible positive behaviors and (2) to model preferred "OK" behaviors. As always, this positive attention can be provided to the child in the form of labeled rewards (e.g., "I really like playing with you when you talk in a regular tone of voice") and attends ("Now you're moving the dump truck down the driveway . . . ," etc.).

The therapist gives Parent Handout 7: Combining Positive Attention and Ignoring (Differential Attention) (Appendix B) to the parent at the end of the session in which differential attention is introduced.

HOMEWORK ASSIGNMENTS

Child's Game

The major homework assignment during Phase I is the daily practice of the Child's Game. The parent is asked to conduct the Child's Game with the child once a day for 10–15 minutes. If possible, these sessions should be scheduled at the same time each day. Toys and games similar to those employed in the clinic playroom should be used (see Chapter 3). There are two primary goals of these daily Child's Game sessions. The first purpose is to allow the parent to have repeated intensive practice in the use of the various Phase I skills, primarily attends and rewards. The idea is that, once the parent has attained a degree of skill and confidence in employing the Phase I skills with the child in a positive setting at home, the parent will be better equipped to apply the same skills to more problematic situations as part of later homework assignments. The parent is asked to begin the Child's Game assignment as soon as attending has been practiced in the clinic setting (during the first or the second session). Thus, the earlier assignments involve only attends. Later, the parent is asked to incorporate rewards and ignoring into the practice sessions after they have been taught in the clinic. The parent is given the Parent Record Sheet: Child's Game, on which he or she is asked to record the time of day, activity, and child's response for each practice session (see Appendix B, Parent Handout 3). This record sheet is brought to each session and discussed with the therapist.

A sample record sheet that has been completed for 1 week is presented in Figure 6.6. In reviewing this record sheet, the therapist noted that the parent had held six sessions of the Child's Game on 5 days. However, the parent had held only one Child's Game session over the past 3 days. The sessions were 10–15 minutes in duration, as requested, and were generally held during the same time each day (except for the weekend

Parent Handout 3: Parent Record Sheet: Child's Game

Date	Time spent	Activity	Child's response
Wed 8/23	5:25–5:40	Legos, racing cars	Patrick liked it
Th 8/24	5:05–5:20	Racing cars	"Oh, it was OK"
Fri 8/25	5:30–5:45	Legos, blocks	He really enjoyed it
Sat 8/26	9:30–9:45	Coloring books	Got bored toward the end
Sat 8/26	3:00–3:15	Legos	"Play longer, Mom"
Tues 8/29	5:30–5:40	People and dollhouse	"Good"

Date	Time spent	Activity	Child's response

FIGURE 6.6. Sample Parent Handout 3: Parent Record Sheet: Child's Game.

sessions). The parent and child played with a variety of toys. The child seems to have responded very positively to the Child's Game sessions, although the parent reported that the child was bored at the end of one of the sessions. The therapist would use the information on the record sheet to reinforce the parent for carrying out the homework assignment so successfully. In addition, the therapist would inquire as to why the Child's Game sessions had been held less frequently over the past few days.

The second purpose of the Child's Game exercise is to enrich the overall quality of parent–child interaction. Not only is this an important goal in its own right, but establishing this positive, responsive context facilitates the likelihood of cooperative behavior from the child in subsequent parent–child interactions (e.g., Lay et al., 1989; Parpal & Maccoby, 1985). Parents have come to realize that this format is an excellent way to share "quality" time with their children. The high intensity of parental attention and interest that this exercise requires ensures that children genuinely enjoy their "special time." This fact has served as a prompt for the parents to do their homework assignment, since the children are sure to remind the parents that the Child's Game is past due. Nearly all parents, and especially those who are single and/or working and who are not able to spend great quantities of time with their children, have found the Child's Game to be quite helpful. Not only can the parent be guaranteed a positive interaction with the child but the termination of the exercise also serves as a discriminative cue for the parent's own "private time" in which time can be spent with a partner, reading the paper, relaxing, and so forth. For these reasons, we recommend that the parent continue the daily practice of the Child's Game into Phase II and even after the program has officially terminated. Finally, when there is more than one child in the family within the 3- to 8-year range, it is advisable for the parent to conduct separate Child's Game sessions with each child. In this manner, each child is assured of individual time with the parent, and jealousy between the siblings can be minimized. (See Chapter 7, "The Role of Siblings.")

Occasionally, the child will engage in inappropriate ("not OK") behavior during a Child's Game session at home. In these situations, the parent should ignore the "not OK" behavior. If the child's inappropriate behavior continues or is not ignorable, then the parent should end the Child's Game session for that day. The therapist tells parents to matter-of-factly state, "Since you are ["not OK" behavior], we will have to stop our playtime. We can try again tomorrow." Not infrequently, children want to continue with the Child's Game past the allotted time. If the parent is agreeable, that is fine. In other cases, the therapist tells the parent to state that the Child's Game is over for that day and that they will have another session tomorrow. The parent then leaves the situation. (The child may continue playing alone if he or she wishes.)

Specific "OK" Behaviors to Increase

Typically, in the final session of teaching rewards, the parent is asked to generate a list of three "OK" behaviors that he or she would like to see the child engage in more frequently and bring it to the following session, in which the ignoring skill is taught (see Parent Handout 5, Parent Record Sheet: Identifying "OK" Behaviors to Increase, in Appendix B, and Figure 6.7). At that time, the therapist first reviews the behaviors with the parent. In our experience, parents frequently bring in a list of negative ("not OK") child behaviors that they want to see less of. In order to decrease the likelihood of this happening, Parent Handout 5: Parent Record Sheet: Identifying "OK" Behaviors to Increase allows parents to first identify "not OK" behaviors they want to see less of and to then identify alternative "OK" behaviors. Nevertheless, some parents may need additional assistance from the therapist. The therapist uses this worksheet to help the parent to convert the list from "not OK" child behaviors that the parent wants to decrease (e.g., "Stop interrupting me when I'm on the phone, quit arguing with his sister, and stop whining") to "OK" child behaviors that the parent wants to increase (e.g., "Play quietly with toys while I'm on the phone, play nicely with his sister, and talk in a regular voice"). By making the assignment one of increasing "OK" behaviors, the therapist gives the parent practice in conceptualizing behavioral goals as positive events. Examples of goals that are frequently cited by parents during this part of the program are having the child pick up toys, get dressed promptly in the morning, play quietly alone, interact appropriately with siblings or peers, or go to bed when requested.

The therapist then assists the parent in setting up programs for one or two of the

Parent Handout 5: Parent Record Sheet: Identifying "OK" Behaviors to Increase

On the right-hand side of the page, please list three "OK" behaviors that you would like your child to do more often. Sometimes it may be easier to first identify a "not OK" behavior that your child is doing and then identify the "OK" positive behavior that you would like to see instead of the "not OK" behavior. If that is the case, list three "not OK" behaviors on the left-hand side of the page first. (Be sure that the "not OK" behaviors that you list are *not* ones that involve risk to people or property. We will deal with those types of problems later in the program.)

"Not OK" Behaviors I Want to See Less Of	**"OK" Behaviors I Want to See More Of Instead** (There can be more than one "OK" behavior for each "not OK" behavior that is listed.)
1. Stop interrupting me when I'm on the phone	1. Play quietly with toys while I'm on the phone
2. Quit arguing with Colleen	2. Play nicely with Colleen
3. Stop whining	3. Talk in a regular voice

FIGURE 6.7. Sample Parent Handout 5: Parent Record Sheet: Identifying "OK" Behaviors to Increase. Remember: The focus is on "OK" behaviors that you want to see happen more often!

"OK" child behaviors that the parent wishes to increase. The programs involve the use of the differential attention techniques. We recommend that the therapist select the least difficult behavior first in order to increase the likelihood of potential success in a reasonably brief time frame. The first program generally requires a moderate degree of direction from the therapist. The parent is encouraged to assume more responsibility in designing subsequent programs for the other child behaviors using these skills. The therapist asks the parent to keep a daily record of these programs and to bring it to each session. As the parent becomes more proficient at employing the Phase I skills in the natural environment, the therapist encourages the parent to apply these skills to other problematic child behaviors. The work on these programs continues throughout Phase II.

The therapist also encourages the parents to apply the Phase I skills outside of the Child's Game sessions. First, the therapist tells the parent to check on the child's behavior at frequent intervals throughout the day as a way to "catch the child being good." When observing the child engaging in a particular behavior, the parent asks himself or herself, "Do I want this behavior to occur more often, or at least stay the same?" If the answer is "yes," then this is an "OK" behavior; if the answer is "no," then it is a "not OK" behavior. If the child is behaving appropriately, then the parent should provide positive attention to the child, using attends and rewards. If it is a "not OK" behavior, the parent can either ignore it (if there is no risk to people or property) or intervene in some other fashion.

Thus, the parent moves from employing discrete parenting skills in the Child's

Game in the clinic to using differential attention in the home as a means of dealing with specific problem behaviors, and developing a more positive pattern of interaction with the child. Successful use of Phase I skills will reduce the frequency and intensity of child problem behaviors; increase the frequency of prosocial, positive child behaviors; *and* improve the parent–child relationship.

SAMPLE SESSION

The following is an example of a session occurring during Phase I. In prior sessions, the mother, Mrs. M, had been taught attending, rewarding, and ignoring skills. This session initially consisted of a 5-minute assessment observation of Mrs. M and her 4-year-old son, John, engaging in whatever activity the child wished (the Child's Game). During the observation, Mrs. M emitted 21 praise statements, 10 attending statements, 1 command, and no questions. Subsequent to the observation, Mrs. M instructed John to play with the toys by himself while she talked with the therapist. The therapist discussed Mrs. M's use of attending and praise statements during the immediately preceding observation. Mrs. M reported that she believed she had attended to or praised most of John's desirable behaviors. The therapist agreed and commended Mrs. M for her performance. At this point, Mrs. M went over to John, who was playing quietly with the toys at the end of the room. She attended to his play for about 5 seconds and then praised him for playing quietly and not interrupting her while she and the therapist were talking. She then returned to her seat. The therapist praised Mrs. M for remembering to reinforce John's appropriate behavior. Mrs. M repeated this "interrupting" procedure several additional times throughout the session.

The therapist then asked Mrs. M about her use of reinforcement with John at home. She gave the therapist her Parent Handout 3: Parent Record Sheet: Child's Game, which indicated that she and John had engaged in the Child's Game on a daily basis since the end of the last session. Mrs. M reported using attending and reward statements frequently in other situations as well, and indicated that John appeared to be responsive to such statements, as his behavior was becoming less aversive to her. She also reported that she had been able to ignore most of John's whining and demanding attention.

At the previous session, the therapist asked Mrs. M to identify three "OK" behaviors that she would like to see John do more frequently. She was given Parent Handout 5: Parent Record Sheet: Identifying "OK" Behaviors to Increase. The therapist reviewed this record sheet with Mrs. M and decided to focus on a single "OK" behavior in the session. Mrs. M had indicated that she wanted to increase the length of time that John remained in his room and did not demand attention by asking for various items during a 1-hour rest and quiet-play period after lunch. The therapist asked Mrs. M how she might accomplish such a goal by her use of attends, rewards, and ignoring. She replied that she could use positive attention to reinforce John for periods of time that he did not demand attention and remained quietly in his room. The therapist agreed and suggested that Mrs. M initiate the rest and quiet-play period by taking John to his room and telling him that it is quiet-play time. After he remained quietly in his room for 5 minutes, she should go to the room and provide positive attention (by using attends and rewards) to him. The therapist told Mrs. M to initially provide positive attention to John for each 5-minute period that he stayed quietly in his room. She also was told that after 1 week she could lengthen the interval between positive attention statements to approximately 10 minutes. During subsequent weeks, she could continue to lengthen the time intervals between positive attention statements but was never to phase out her attention entirely for John resting or playing quietly during this hour of the day. During rest period, she was to ignore any of John's attempts to gain attention and matter-of-factly return him to his room if he left it. Mrs. M agreed to the intervention strategy. She and the therapist then role played the situation. With the therapist's help, the parent explained and demonstrated the new plan to John, who then participated in a brief practice session with his mother about the home plan.

The therapist then reviewed the importance of Mrs. M's attention to John. She was reminded to (1) make her attention to John contingent on his engaging in desirable "OK" behaviors and (2) ignore his undesirable "not OK" behavior. Subsequently, the therapist told Mrs. M to practice her use of attends and rewards with John. She was given the bug-in-the-ear, the therapist left the room, and for approximately 10 minutes Mrs. M and John engaged in activities chosen by John. During this time, the therapist prompted Mrs. M by way of the bug-in-the-ear regarding which positive attention statements (i.e., attends and rewards) she could use and when to use them. The therapist also praised Mrs. M for the use of positive attention statements that she gave without being prompted by the therapist. Following the parent–child interaction, the therapist praised Mrs. M for her performance. She was encouraged again to ignore "not OK" behavior and to use attends and rewards for "OK" behavior during the daily practice of the Child's Game at home, during normal activities with John, and during the rest period after lunch.

COMMONLY ENCOUNTERED PROBLEMS

Failure to Complete Homework Assignments or Attend Sessions

Not infrequently, a parent fails to complete a homework assignment or misses appointments. A single occurrence is not considered significant; however, repeated failure to complete the assignments or missed appointments should be a danger signal. Questions such as "What made it hard for you to attend the session/do this homework exercise?" and "What can you do to make it easier for you to attend the sessions/do this exercise?" can be effective ways to engage the parent in a discussion about these issues (Webster-Stratton & Herbert, 1994). The therapist should determine whether there are environmental factors preventing the completion of assignments and/or session attendance or if a lack of motivation on the parent's part is relevant. Examples of the former might include illness of the parent or other family members, marital stress, or transportation difficulties. In any case, the therapist should emphasize the importance of attending sessions and of completing the homework assignments. If motivational factors appear to be operating, then the therapist may wish to outline a set of contingencies for continued contact with the parent. For incomplete homework assignments, the therapist should inform the parent that progression through the program is being delayed and that completion of the homework assignments is necessary for progression to the next skill. Other contingencies might include a monetary deposit to be refunded upon completion of the program, charging the parent for missed sessions, or terminating contact if a predetermined number of assignments are not completed or sessions are missed. The use of a "parenting salary" (i.e., monetary payment for attendance or homework completion) can be an effective motivational strategy, especially with lower-SES clients (Fleischman, 1979; McMahon et al., 1996).

The Extremely Inappropriate Child

As discussed in Chapter 3, we believe it is important to teach positive parenting skills (attending and rewarding) before teaching a punishment procedure. However, we have had a very few cases in which the child was so out of control that it was impossible for the parent to practice and use the positive skills with the child until the disruptive behavior was addressed directly. In these few cases, we taught attending and rewarding to the parent, but did not have the parent practice the skills with the child in the clinic. Instead, we immediately taught TO to the parent, and then had the parent use TO and rewarding in practice sessions in the clinic and at home. After the child's extremely disruptive behavior decreased, we returned to teaching Phase I skills until the parent reached the behavioral criteria for these skills. We returned to the Phase II skills in the latter part of the program.

We rarely find it necessary to deviate from the typical sequence of the parent training program. Therefore, use of TO prior to achieving the criteria for positive parenting skills should be reserved for the most extreme cases.

Reinforcement as Bribery

Equating reinforcement with bribery is occasionally raised by a concerned parent early in Phase I as an objection to the use of reinforcement procedures. Because the HNC parent training program relies so heavily on social reinforcement (as opposed to material reinforcers such as food and money), this issue rarely arises. However, if a parent does express concern about "bribing" the child, it will be necessary for the therapist to clarify the difference between bribery and reinforcement.

A "bribe" is defined as something that is offered or given to someone to induce him or her to act dishonestly. In other words, bribery is a misuse of reinforcement, for we have stressed that the parent's positive attention skills are employed contingent upon appropriate behavior on the part of the child. The basic distinction between positive reinforcement and bribery, then, is the purpose of these procedures. Reinforcement should be given to teach the child various appropriate behaviors. Bribery would occur only if the parent were using reinforcement to corrupt the child's behavior (Krumboltz & Krumboltz, 1972). It is also helpful to explain that the parent's role is to socialize the child and that positive feedback teaches the child what is expected, not just by parents but by society in general.

The Flat-Affect Parent

Occasionally, a parent will meet the criteria for attends and rewards with respect to frequency, but the statements will be uttered in a flat tone of voice that is not reinforcing to the child. In this case, the therapist must help the parent to show appropriate affect while using these skills. This is not an easy task, as it is difficult to specify behaviorally exactly what proper affect is. Nevertheless, we have found that the most effective teaching procedure is the same one used to teach the other skills used in the program: brief discussion of the skill, modeling by the therapist, role playing by the parent with the therapist, and practice with the child. The modeling is particularly important, as it is easier to demonstrate flat affect and proper affect than it is to verbally describe them.

We have found that with flat-affect parents it is easiest to teach the attending skill first and then the use of proper affect. Trying to teach both at once is too complex for most of these parents. If this approach is not successful, then the flat affect may be a sign of other difficulties, such as depression or physical illness.

The Failure-to-Generalize Parent

A related but somewhat different issue is when parents have difficulty generalizing the parenting skills from the playroom context to the real world. This occurs primarily in the first phase of the program where the parent learns to use attends and rewards effectively in a play situation (i.e., the Child's Game) both in the clinic and at home, but not in daily interactions with the child.

The therapist's task with the parent who fails to generalize is to structure homework assignments such that the parent has to use the skills in everyday interactions with the child. This can be done by increasing the number of positive child behavior programs (above the three or so that are typically requested) that the parent is required to develop and implement following the teaching of the Phase I skills. In addition, our earlier suggestion that the parent check on the child periodically in order to obtain more opportunities to "catch the child being good" (and thus to use attends and rewards) can be structured so that the parent is asked to conduct such checks every 20 or 30 minutes and to keep a log of such contacts. By helping the parent use the skills in multiple daily interactions, the therapist is essentially programming generalization.

CHAPTER 7

Phase II: The Skills of Compliance Training

In this chapter, we first present a rationale and an overview of Phase II. We then describe the clear instructions sequence for enhancing child compliance to parental instructions. The various skills are described, followed by recommended homework assignments. We then discuss the use of standing rules, the application of the parenting skills to siblings and to situations outside the home, a sample Phase II session, and challenging problem situations and their solutions. The chapter concludes with a discussion of the final parent training session(s).

RATIONALE AND OVERVIEW OF PHASE II

As noted earlier, the program utilizes two major approaches to handling inappropriate (i.e., "not OK") child behavior. The second phase of the program is directly concerned with decreasing child noncompliance to parents' commands. We feel that the parenting skills learned in Phase I of the program, which are designed to increase appropriate (i.e., "OK") child behavior, are extremely effective in improving the parent's relationship with the child. However, there are times when a direct approach to dealing with child noncompliance is needed. It is important to emphasize that these new skills do not replace the differential attention skills from Phase I. Indeed, Phase II skills are effective only when used in conjunction with Phase I skills. The skills taught in the second phase of the program focus on parent behaviors to increase child compliance and decrease child noncompliance. Both antecedent (clear instructions) and consequent (rewarding compliance, applying a TO procedure for noncompliance) behaviors are included. These parenting skills are taught in the context of the Parent's Game. In contrast with the free-play activity of the Child's Game, in the Parent's Game the parent structures the activity by issuing commands and providing consequences for compliance and non-compliance. The Parent's Game is not practiced in the home setting, but only at the clinic. After the relevant skills are mastered in the clinic, they are employed in the home. In addition, parents also learn the use of standing rules.

Parent Introduction to Phase II

At the beginning of the session in which Phase II is to begin, the therapist brings back the two bar graphs from the assessment feedback session (Figure 5.2) and reminds the parent that the program utilizes two major approaches to handling "not OK" child behavior. So far, the program has focused on directly increasing "OK" child behavior through the use of positive attention such as attends and rewards, and reducing "not OK" child behaviors through ignoring. The therapist then summarizes the progress that the parent has made to date in increasing the proportion of "OK" behaviors, as compared to "not OK" behaviors.

The focus of Phase II, the therapist then tells the parent, is to directly address the "not OK" behavior of noncompliance to parental instructions and to increase the child's compliance. It is important to emphasize that the Phase II skills will not replace the differential attention skills from Phase I. Indeed, we believe that Phase II skills will be effective over the long term only when used *in combination with* Phase I skills.

The therapist gives Parent Handout 8: Introduction to Phase II (Appendix B) to the parent at the end of the session in which the rationale and overview of Phase II are presented.

THE CLEAR INSTRUCTIONS SEQUENCE

The primary Phase II parenting skills are taught as part of the clear instructions sequence. The clear instructions sequence is presented in Figure 7.1 as a flowchart and in Figure 7.2 as a series of three distinct paths. (Also see Parent Handouts 9–14 in Appendix B.) In all cases, the clear instructions sequence begins with the parent giving a clear instruction to the child. If the child complies to the initial clear instruction (Path A) or to a subsequent warning (Path B), then the parent provides positive attention and the sequence is ended. However, if the child does not comply to the warning, then a TO procedure is implemented (Path C). Each of the component skills and the individual paths of the flowchart are described in detail below.

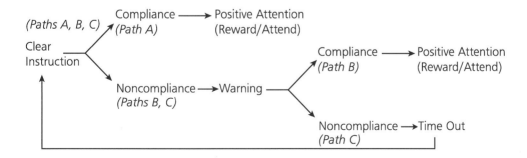

FIGURE 7.1. Flowchart of the clear instructions sequence.

- Issue a single clear instruction (e.g., "Please pick up your toys now").

Path A

```
Clear                Child              Reward/
Instruction    →     Complies    →      Attend
```

- If the child initiates compliance to the clear instruction within 5 seconds, provide positive attention (i.e., rewards, attends) (e.g., "Thank you so much for playing quietly—I really appreciate it when you do what I ask").

Path B

```
Clear                Child Does                       Child              Reward/
Instruction    →     Not Comply  →  Warning    →      Complies    →      Attend
```

- If the child does *not* initiate compliance to the clear instruction within 5 seconds, issue a warning: "If you do not [*state the behavior*], you will have to go to time out."
- If the child initiates compliance to the warning within 5 seconds, provide positive attention (i.e., rewards, attends).

Path C

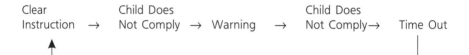

```
Clear                Child Does                       Child Does
Instruction    →     Not Comply  →  Warning    →      Not Comply→    Time Out
```

- If the child does *not* initiate compliance to the warning within 5 seconds, lead the child to the time-out chair without lecturing, scolding, or arguing.
- Tell the child: "Because you did not [*state the behavior*], you have to sit in the chair until I say you can get up."
- Ignore the child's shouting, protesting, and promises to comply.
- Leave child in time out for 3 minutes (including being quiet for the last 15 seconds).
- When the time is completed, remove the child from the chair and return to the situation that elicited noncompliance.
- Restate the original clear instruction.
- Implement the warning–time-out sequence again if noncompliance occurs.

FIGURE 7.2. Paths of the clear instructions sequence. Adapted by permission of the authors from McMahon, Slough, and the Conduct Problems Prevention Research Group (1994).

Clear Instructions

The focus of most parent training programs has been to modify the consequent events of child responding (Forehand, 1977). Antecedent events that might elicit inappropriate child behavior have been generally ignored. The analysis of such antecedent events is particularly relevant for child noncompliance. In this case, the antecedent event is the parental command. Our work in the laboratory (Roberts, McMahon, Forehand, & Humphreys, 1978), in the home (Williams & Forehand, 1984), and in treatment outcome studies (e.g., Peed et al., 1977) has demonstrated the clinical importance of parental command-giving behavior in influencing child compliance (see Chapter 10).

Introducing Clear Instructions

Several aspects of giving clear instructions initially are emphasized to the parent. First, the therapist stresses the importance of deciding ahead of time whether to give a command. Second, the therapist cautions the parent about giving commands in an indiscriminate manner (i.e., assuming an authoritarian style of interaction with the child; see "The Drill Sergeant" later in this chapter). Third, the parent is told not to give a command unless she or he is prepared to ensure that compliance follows it, regardless of how long that may take.

Some indications that a clear instruction is appropriate include situations when: (1) it is important to the parent that the child do something right away; (2) the parent is not willing to give the child a choice as to whether to do the behavior or not; and (3) the child is engaged in a behavior that might possibly harm people or property (McMahon et al., 1994). On the other hand, if the child's behavior is minor and is merely annoying, irritating, or attention seeking, then the differential attention skills from Phase I are the most appropriate response.

The therapist then tells the parent that the focus of training in clear instructions is to teach him or her to give clear, direct commands to the child. In this manner, the parent can have a powerful positive influence on the rate of child compliance. The therapist stresses the moral and ethical responsibility of giving clear instructions. If the child does not follow a parental command, the parent needs to be sure it is because the child *chose* to be noncompliant, not because of a failure to understand the instruction.

Examples of Unclear Instructions

A number of unclear instructions (beta commands) are then listed and described (see Figure 7.3). There are five general types of unclear instructions that can lower the rate of child compliance.[1]

---

[1] Our colleague Karen Wells has identified another type of unclear instruction, which she refers to as "repeated commands." In this situation, the child realizes that he or she can ignore the parent's commands until the parent has repeated the command a certain number of times (which varies from parent to parent). It is only when the "magic" number of repetitions has been reached that the parent decides to follow through, so the child delays responding until then.

Type	Examples
Chain commands	"Put your plate in the sink, rinse it off, put it in the dishwasher, and bring me the napkins."
Vague commands	"Be careful!" "Watch out!" "Act your age!" "Be a good boy (girl)!"
Question commands*	"Would you like to take out the trash?"
"Let's . . . " commands*	"Let's go clean up your room."
Commands *followed* by a rationale or other verbalization	"Please pick up the toys in here. (*Child: Why?*) Because your mother's boss is coming for dinner tonight, and we want the house to look nice. (*Child: But she won't come up here*)" Etc.

*These may be appropriate types of instructions in some situations. See text.

FIGURE 7.3. Types of unclear instructions.

1. *Chain commands.* These are a series of commands strung together, which may require the completion of several related or unrelated activities (e.g., "Pick up the blocks and put them in the box, then make your bed and put the dirty clothes in the hamper"). Especially with young children, chain commands may result in an information overload, with the result that the child fails to comply. Even where this is not an issue, however, chain commands preclude a clear definition of compliance unless the child complies to all parts of the chain.

2. *Vague commands.* These directives do not specify observable behaviors to be performed by the child and, as such, present an ambiguous situation for the child. Classic vague commands include "Be careful," "Watch out," and "Be a good boy." Although the parent probably often has specific behaviors in mind when issuing these commands (e.g., "Don't run into the street" or "Don't hit your brother"), the child has not acquired a long enough learning history to associate these vague directives with the specific behaviors. The result, at least from the parent's view, is noncompliance.

Parents who give vague commands may say something like "My child knows what I mean when I say 'Be a good boy.'" The therapist's response is to acknowledge that this may be true; however, it still provides the child with an opportunity to avoid complying by pleading ignorance as to what the parent really wanted the child to do.

3. *Question commands.* These are perhaps the most problematic type of command for parents. At issue here is the subtle distinction between a request and a command. A request implies that the child has the option of choosing whether to do as the parent has asked. Commands are directives in which the parent expects the child to follow through on the instruction. This is relatively straightforward. However, this distinction is blurred in adult–adult interactions. Most commands and requests to adults are phrased

in a question format (e.g., "Would you work this weekend?"). Parents then use the same type of phrasing with their children when they give a command. They are usually surprised that when they say to their 6-year-old "Would you like to take your bath now?" he or she says no. It is important to stress that requests themselves are not inappropriate. If the parent truly does mean to give the child the option of saying either yes or no to the request, then this type of statement is appropriate. Rather, it is when the parent expects compliance to a command but phrases it as a request that it becomes problematic.

4. *"Let's . . . " commands.* These are commands stated in such a fashion as to include the parent ("Let's pick up the toys"). If the parent intends to assist the child in the activity, then this is an appropriate form of instruction. However, parents often use this to trap the child into beginning an activity. The parent has no intention of becoming involved. The child feels tricked, and the typical result is an uncompleted task and another round of escalation in the coercive cycle.

5. *Commands* followed *by a rationale or other verbalizations.* A rationale for a parental command is not only appropriate but also desirable. However, analogous to the case of ignoring, the rationale should precede the command. For example, the parent might say, "We're having company tonight and I'd like the house to look nice. Please put away the toys in your room." In contrast, when the parent provides the rationale *following* the command, she or he is inadvertently obscuring the actual directive and increasing the likelihood that the child will forget the command. The net result is that the child is less likely to comply. In addition, some children will play the "why game" after commands as a way of avoiding the issue (e.g., "Why do I have to pick up my toys, Mommy? . . . But *why?*" and so on). It is not unusual for parents to get sidetracked when giving a rationale after a command and to completely forget the original command. In addition, parental participation in the "why game" serves to inadvertently reinforce the child's avoidance of complying to the parent's command by providing parental attention for the avoidance behavior.

After these unclear commands are described, the therapist then asks the parent if he or she engages in any of these. Most parents report using at least one type of unclear instruction with some frequency. We usually mention our own difficulties with particular types of unclear instructions. (One of the authors is well known for his mastery of question commands.)

Training in Clear Instructions

The major thrust of this segment of the program is to teach the parent to give clear instructions (alpha commands) to the child (see Figure 7.4). Giving clear instructions is done in the following steps.

1. *Get the child's attention.* The parent should first get the child's attention. Research with clinic-referred children indicates that they often simply ignore parental instructions (Dumas & Lechowicz, 1989). In order to get the child's attention effectively, there are several guidelines. The parent should be in relatively close proximity to the

- Get the child's attention.
  - Move close.
  - Say the child's name (maximum of two times).
  - Establish eye contact.
- State the instruction clearly.
  - Give one instruction at a time.
  - Use a firm voice.
  - Phrase as "do" command.
  - Use simple language.
  - Use gestures as appropriate.
  - Rationale (if given) *precedes* the clear instruction.
- Wait 5 seconds.
  - Count silently.
  - No verbalization to child.

FIGURE 7.4. How to give clear instructions.

child (certainly within the same room, and preferably within a few feet of the child) (e.g., Hudson & Blane, 1985). The parent should say the child's name and pause until eye contact is established. If the child pretends not to hear (what we like to call "selective deafness") or otherwise ignores the parent, then we instruct the parent to say the child's name a second time. If the child still does not respond verbally or with eye contact, then the parent assumes that the child is purposely ignoring. At that point, the parent proceeds with the clear instruction.

2. *State the instruction clearly.* The parent should give only one directive at a time. If there are several tasks that the parent wants completed, a separate clear instruction should be issued for each one. The parent's voice should be firm (but not angry) and slightly louder than usual. This is to provide a discriminative cue to the child that a clear instruction, as opposed to a request or other type of verbalization, will follow. The clear instruction should be phrased as a "do" command ("Please put the cars and trucks in the toybox") rather than a "stop" command ("Stop making a mess in here") if at all possible, since the former tells the child what behavior is expected (e.g., Jones, Sloane, & Roberts, 1992). ("Do" commands also make it easier for the parent to provide appropriate consequences.) The parent should say exactly what is meant without excessive verbalization, and the clear instruction should be phrased in language the child can understand. If appropriate, gestures may be used to explain the clear instruction (e.g., pointing to the cupboard in which the toy should be placed). As noted above, if a rationale or explanation concerning the parental command is given, it should occur *before* the clear instruction is stated.

3. *Wait 5 seconds.* The parent should not issue additional commands or any other verbalizations until the child *initiates* compliance or until 5 seconds have passed. The focus on initiation (rather than completion) allows the parent to begin reinforcing compliance immediately (see below). The parent should count *silently* from 1 to 5 and refrain from speaking to the child during this time. The adoption of a 5-second waiting period is not arbitrary—research (e.g., Wruble, Sheeber, Sorenson, Boggs, & Eyberg,

1991) suggests that, for children in this age range, the probability of initiated compliance is greatest within the first 5 seconds after the command and decreases significantly with the passage of each subsequent 5-second interval. (The following sections describe further steps to take if the child does or does not initiate compliance.)

The therapist then gives a number of unclear and clear instructions to the parent. After each instruction, the therapist asks the parent (1) whether it was a clear or unclear instruction and (2) why. For each unclear instruction, the therapist asks the parent to rephrase it as a clear instruction.

Goals for Clear Instructions: Behavioral Criteria

The behavioral criteria for successful completion of the clear instructions segment of Phase II are at least one 5-minute observation of the Parent's Game in which the parent gives (1) an average of two or more alpha commands (i.e., clear instructions) per minute and (2) no more than 25% of the number of total commands as beta commands. Training in clear instructions is limited to a maximum of two sessions.

Positive Attention for Child Compliance (Path A)

The next step in the clear instructions sequence is to provide consequences for the child. We introduce consequences for compliance first. If the child *initiates* compliance within 5 seconds after the command is given, the parent is instructed to employ the positive attention skills learned in Phase I (attends and rewards). This is portrayed as Path A in Figure 7.2—the parent gives a clear instruction, the child complies, and the parent provides positive attention (i.e., rewards and attends). Compliance to parental commands is definitely an "OK" behavior that the parent wants to increase! The focus on the initiation of compliance allows the parent to reinforce compliance frequently and immediately, thereby increasing the probability that the task will be completed as well. As noted earlier, attends are particularly useful in maintaining compliance to a task that takes some time to complete (e.g., picking up a number of toys). Labeled verbal rewards are most appropriate for the initiation and completion of compliance. Therefore, for a task that takes some time to complete, the therapist suggests that the parent:

- Give a labeled verbal reward as soon as the child initiates compliance.
- Use attends and rewards as the child continues to comply.
- Use a labeled verbal reward when compliance is completed.

An example of how a parent might mix praise and attends to maintain compliance to an extended task follows.

PARENT: Patrick, please put these wooden blocks into the box.

CHILD: (3 *seconds pass. Begins to put one or two blocks in the box.*)

PARENT: Great! You're picking up the blocks and putting them in the box.

CHILD: (*Puts additional blocks in the box.*)

PARENT: Now you've picked up some more blocks and there *they* go into the box. You're really working hard! (*Continues attending until the task is finished.*) Thank you so much for picking up all of these blocks—you did a wonderful job! I really appreciate it when you do what I ask.

As noted above, the clear instructions sequence that we employ consists of a series of alternative paths (Figures 7.1 and 7.2). We usually draw the sequence laid out in Path A of Figure 7.2 for the parent as we explain the procedure. This sequence is role played with the therapist and then practiced with the child. At this point, noncompliance is ignored.

The therapist gives Parent Handout 9: The Clear Instructions Sequence: Path A (Appendix B), to the parent at the end of the session in which clear instructions and Path A are introduced.

The Warning and Subsequent Child Compliance (Path B)

After the parent has successfully employed Path A with the child in both the clinic and at home, the therapist then describes Path B of the clear instructions sequence (Figure 7.2). As with Path A, it begins with the parent giving a clear instruction. However, the child does not begin to comply within 5 seconds, so the parent issues a warning. The warning is an "If . . . then" statement that specifies the desired behavior and the consequences for noncompliance (e.g., "If you don't pick up the toys, then you will have to sit in the chair"). The warning essentially functions as a second clear instruction. Inclusion of a warning has been shown to decrease the number of TOs necessary to gain child compliance (Roberts, 1982). The parent again allows 5 seconds for compliance to be initiated. If the child complies following the warning, the parent immediately praises and attends to the child. The path is then ended. The therapist cautions the parent against the temptation to add a critical statement to the positive attention after compliance to the warning (e.g., "Thanks for putting your coat away. So, why didn't you do it the *first* time I told you to?").

The therapist gives Parent Handout 11: The Clear Instructions Sequence: Path B (Appendix B), to the parent at the end of the session in which Path B is introduced.

The Time-Out (TO) Procedure (Path C)

If the child does not initiate compliance to a parental clear instruction within 5 seconds, or to the subsequent warning, then the parent is taught to use a TO procedure as a consequence for noncompliance. The TO procedure that we employ requires the child to sit on a chair facing a wall for 3 minutes (see Figure 7.5). The therapist introduces the procedure by saying that although punishment is not a preferred mode of interacting with a child, it is a necessary and appropriate action to take on some occasions. TO

- Chair TO
- Located in boring (but safe) area
- 3-minute duration plus 15-second quiet contingency
- Return to original clear instruction after TO
- Backups (if child refuses to go to TO or stay in TO) include:
  - Additional time in TO
  - Response cost (i.e., privilege removal)
  - TO room

FIGURE 7.5. Key elements of the time-out (TO) procedure.

means "time out from positive reinforcement." It is represented as a more extreme form of ignoring in which the child is removed from all sources of positive reinforcement (especially parental attention) for noncompliance. It is described as a relatively simple, guilt-free method of discipline that is an effective substitute for other methods of parental discipline, such as criticizing, hitting, and yelling. It allows the parent to avoid responding to the child in anger; therefore, the parent will be able to use punishment more consistently and less frequently.

"TO" has been used as a label for a variety of procedures, some of which are quite punitive (e.g., isolating a child for an indefinite period). It is also the case that most parents have been exposed to, or employed, something that has been referred to as TO. It is important that the therapist inquire as to whether the parent has used TO before, and if so, what the procedure involved (McMahon et al., 1994). The therapist should also inquire as to the parent's perception of the effectiveness of that particular form of TO.

Setting Up the Location

With assistance from the therapist, the parent should select an appropriate TO area in the home. The key to a successful location for TO is that it is boring! The parent is advised to place a chair in a corner of a hallway or an infrequently used room, such as a dining room. The chair should be far enough away from the wall so that the child cannot kick the wall. There should be no entertaining items, such as TV, radio, or toys, in the immediate vicinity. Likewise, the TO location should be safe—thus, bathrooms should generally not be used for TO because of the risk of the child having access to medications or other dangerous items. Closets also should not be used, as they are too confining, frightening for the child, and potentially dangerous.

Steps of the TO Procedure

In Path C, the child fails to initiate compliance within 5 seconds after the warning, so TO is implemented. By this time, the parent should realize that the child does not intend to obey the instruction, since the child has received both a clear instruction and a warning and has not complied to either one. The parent takes the child firmly by the hand, walks the child to the TO chair, and places the child on the chair facing toward a corner of the room. He or she then says, "Because you didn't _____, you have to sit in the chair until I say you can get up." This should be stated in a matter-of-fact voice that indicates that the parent is not pleased with the child's behavior. The parent should not provide a rationale or argue with the child while taking the child to TO or while the child is in TO. As in other situations, the time for explaining the TO procedure is when the child is behaving appropriately. (A modeling/explanation procedure for teaching the child about TO is described below.) Furthermore, the parent should completely ignore any temper tantrums, shouting, protesting, or promises to behave by the child on the way to TO or during TO.

The child should remain in TO for 3 minutes. Release from TO is contingent on 15 seconds of sitting quietly on the chair (Hobbs & Forehand, 1975). In this way, the parent avoids inadvertently reinforcing any acting-out behavior that might be occurring when the 3-minute mark is reached. Thus, 3 minutes is the minimum length of a TO interval. A kitchen timer may be helpful to both the parent and the child to keep track of the TO period. The timer should be visible to the child but out of reach. If the child is not sitting quietly when the timer rings at the end of the 3 minutes, the parent says, "You will have to stay in TO until you are quiet" (Schroeder & Gordon, 2002).

When the child has been quiet for the 15-second interval, the parent goes to the TO area, removes the child from the chair, and returns to the location and activity that elicited the noncompliant behavior. The parent then repeats the original clear instruction.

This return to the original situation and subsequent repetition of the clear instruction is *essential* to the success of the TO procedure. First of all, it prevents the child from using TO as a means of avoiding compliance. Some children would much rather sit in the corner for 3 minutes than take out the trash, clean up the kitchen, and the like. More importantly, this procedure ensures that the child learns the compliance behavior that is expected in that particular situation. The child also learns that once the parent gives a clear instruction, the child must follow through, whether it is before or after being placed in TO. When administered in this fashion, TO is truly a learning experience for the child.

Once the original clear instruction is repeated, then the entire sequence of events leading to TO potentially may be repeated as well. The usual case is that the child complies immediately after the clear instruction or after the warning. It is critical that the parent provide positive attention (via rewards and attends) for this compliance, even though the parent had to use TO to obtain compliance. The therapist should again remind the parent to avoid adding any critical statements (as was done at the end of Path B). Although there is the potential for the parent to enter an "endless loop" with the clear instructions sequence if the child *never* complied with clear instructions or warnings subsequent to the initial TO, our experience has been that it is unusual for the parent to have to repeat the entire clear instruction sequence after a TO.

After the TO procedure is explained and diagrammed, the therapist then walks the parent through all three paths of the clear instructions sequence. We include the first path of the clear instructions sequence (Path A of Figure 7.2), in which the child complies to the initial clear instruction, in this part of the session as a way of reminding the parent of *all* the possible scenarios that follow a clear instruction. The parent then practices each path of the clear instructions sequence with the therapist acting as the child. It is critical that the therapist comply to a certain number of the parent's clear instructions, so that the parent continues to practice providing positive attention for compliance.

The therapist usually gives Parent Handout 12: The Clear Instructions Sequence: Path C (Appendix B) to the parent at the end of the session in which Path C is introduced and practiced.

Challenges in the Use of the Clear Instructions Sequence

Our clear instructions sequence is a very exact, well-specified one. This is so that the parent will be encouraged to use the procedure in a consistent manner, which, it is hoped, will reduce any difficulties that may arise. Nevertheless, a number of potentially problematic situations can develop (see Figure 7.6). They are described below in the order in which we discuss them with the parent.

Tardy Compliance

In this situation, the child says "I will do it now" when the parent begins to take him or her to TO. It is critical that the parent follow through with TO at this point. If the parent does not, the child learns that he or she does not have to obey the clear instruction until TO is actually initiated, rather than complying to the initial clear instruction or warning.

Child behavior	Solutions
Tardy compliance	Follow through with TO.
Verbalizations in TO	Ignore.
Other misbehavior in TO	Ignore or use TO backups.
Refusal to *stay in* TO	Use TO backups.
Refusal to *go to* TO	Use TO backups.
Refusal to *leave* TO	Repeat original clear instruction or give child a clear instruction to leave TO. Continue with clear instructions sequence, including TO.
Compliance only to the warning	TO following noncompliance to the initial clear instruction.

FIGURE 7.6. Challenges in the use of the clear instructions sequence.

Verbalizations in TO

A situation that often accompanies the use of TO is the child using a variety of inappropriate verbalizations. They can range from whining, yelling, and crying to statements to the parent that "I am going to run away," "I hate you," "You are mean," or "You don't love me" to "I don't care" or "I like TO." The parent must ignore these types of comments, as they are another attempt to control the situation by the child. If the parent does not respond to these verbalizations, they will quickly disappear. On occasion (e.g., when these verbalizations are extending the length of TO significantly because of the child's failure to meet the 15-second quiet contingency), the parent may find it helpful to use the strategy for decreasing persistent "not OK" child behavior during ignoring that was described in Chapter 6 on pages 121–122. The parent makes a statement that is ostensibly directed to someone other than the child, but which serves as a reminder to the child about the contingencies that are in effect (e.g., "When Karen is quiet for a few seconds, then she will be able to leave TO").

Other Misbehavior in TO

Another situation is the child who continually "pushes limits" while in TO. This may be moving the chair backward away from the corner or kicking the wall. As with verbalizations during TO, these behaviors are usually attempts to get parental attention and thereby control the situation. Whenever possible, these behaviors should be ignored (i.e., if they do not pose a risk to the child, to others, or to property; see Chapter 6). However, if this is not the case, then the parent provides a single warning to the child, such as "If you [state the behavior] again, then I will [state one of the TO backups described below]." Only major behaviors that cannot be ignored should be treated in this manner. It is important that the parent ignore as many minor behaviors as possible since TO is intended to temporarily isolate the child from sources of positive attention and other types of reinforcement.

Refusal to Stay in TO

Once the entire clear instructions sequence has been described to the parent, the parent is then instructed on what to do if the child decides to leave TO while it is still in force. We define "leaving TO" as when the child's buttocks leave the TO chair, even for a second. We employ this admittedly arbitrary definition because some children attempt to manipulate the situation by gradually easing more and more of their body off of the TO chair, all the while maintaining that they are still in the chair. The decision rule allows the parent to adopt a standard and consistent definition of when the child is "out of TO."

If the child leaves the chair, he or she should be immediately returned to the chair. The first time this ever occurs, the parent gives the child a warning: "If you get off the chair again, then [specifies the backup to TO]." This warning is only presented once; that is, the first time the child ever leaves the chair. It is not repeated in subsequent TO periods. If the child gets off the chair again, the parent returns the child to the TO chair and administers the backup procedure (see below).

In the previous edition of this book (Forehand & McMahon, 1981), we described the use of a mild spanking procedure (two spanks on the child's bottom with an open hand) as the primary backup procedure if the child left TO while it was in force. Although that procedure was effective, we no longer employ it. Over the past 20 years, the use of physical punishment (even at the minimal level at which it was employed in the HNC program) has become increasingly less acceptable. In addition, research indicated that an alternative approach (see below) that did not involve physical discipline was comparable in effectiveness (Day & Roberts, 1983; Roberts, 1988; Roberts & Powers, 1990).

Based on our own experiences and those of others, we now present parents with one or more of the following alternatives as possible backup consequences for TO: (1) additional time, (2) a response-cost (privilege removal) procedure, and (3) a TO room. One backup involves the imposition of an additional 3 minutes to the initial 3-minute length of TO (i.e., 6 minutes total) ("Bryan, if you don't stay in the chair, you will get an extra 3 minutes of TO"). If a timer is used to mark the length of TO, it can be reset to 3 minutes when the child is returned to the chair (Schroeder & Gordon, 2002).

Response-cost procedures (i.e., privilege removal) can be employed instead of, or in addition to, the use of additional time as a TO backup. Especially with older children, we have found that many respond to removal of a privilege that is to occur at a slightly later time. For example, the parent might say to the child, "If you get out of the chair again, you may not watch television tonight." If this option is used, then the consequence should be in close temporal proximity (i.e., immediately or within a few hours), of moderate magnitude (no TV tonight, rather than no TV for the next 2 days), and, ideally, a logical consequence (e.g., television privileges are temporarily suspended because the child disobeyed the initial clear instruction because he or she did not want to miss any of a favorite cartoon show on TV) (Dreikurs, 1964).

Finally, a TO room can be an effective backup contingency (Day & Roberts, 1983; Roberts, 1988; Roberts & Powers, 1990). When used in this way, the parent might say, "If you get out of the chair again, then you will have to stay by yourself for a while." If the child does leave the TO chair, then the parent says, "Since you left the chair, you will have to stay by yourself for a while." The child is then put in a room that is closed either by a partition or a door. The parent holds the door shut as necessary. It is imperative that the room be well-lit, relatively spacious (i.e., *not* a closet), and absent of entertaining (e.g., radio, toys) or potentially dangerous (e.g., razors, medications) items. Because the parent is not able to observe the child during this period, it is essential that the room be boring as well as safe. After 1 minute, the child is taken back to the TO chair. The procedure is repeated as necessary.

In general, the first backup that we recommend that parents employ is adding 3 minutes to the original TO. If that proves ineffective over a number of TOs, then, for younger children (5 years and younger), we have the parent employ the TO room. For older children (6-8 years), the parent implements the response-cost procedure if the extra minutes backup is not effective, with the TO room as a third backup. However, the therapist can be flexible in the choice of initial and subsequent backups.

Refusal *to* Go to *TO*

Occasionally, a child may refuse to go to the TO chair. This is handled by using the same backup procedures employed when the child refuses to stay in TO.

Refusal *to* Leave *TO*

A related situation is the child who refuses to come out of TO when the TO period is over. We teach the parent either to repeat the original clear instruction (e.g., "Pick up the toys in the living room") or to give the child a clear instruction to leave the TO chair. In either case, if the child does not comply, then the parent continues with the clear instructions sequence, including another 3-minute TO if necessary.

Although this approach seems counterintuitive, the child's refusal to leave TO is essentially an attempt to control the situation by dictating when he or she will leave TO. Fortunately, most children quickly realize that their bid for control in this situation is not likely to succeed after an additional period of TO.

Compliance Only to the Warning

Some children may learn to comply to the warning rather than the initial parental clear instruction. These children realize that the parental clear instruction will be followed by a warning and that negative consequences will occur only for noncompliance to the warning. For these children, it may be necessary to have the parents employ TO immediately following noncompliance to the clear instruction. This strategy should be implemented only after several weeks of using TO, since this phenomenon may be only temporary.

The therapist usually gives Parent Handout 13: Challenges in the Use of the Clear Instructions Sequence (Appendix B) to the parent at the end of the session in which the challenges are introduced and practiced.

Teaching the Child about the Clear Instructions Sequence

Once the parent is proficient at implementing the procedures involved in one of the paths (e.g., Path A), then the teaching focus shifts to the child, where the same path is taught. Since the child has been in the room while the prior training has been occurring, he or she is likely to be somewhat familiar with the clear instructions sequence already. However, to ensure that this is the case, the therapist and parent provide formal instruction in the procedure for the child.

The steps parallel those employed in teaching the parent about the clear instructions sequence. The clear instructions sequence is explained step-by-step at a level appropriate to the child, beginning with Path A (see Figure 7.2). For example, the therapist might say:

> "Lisa, today you will get a chance to help your mom practice something new called 'clear instructions.' This means that when your mom has decided that she wants you to do something, she will first say your name. Then she will tell

you exactly what she wants you to do. If you do it right away (within 5 seconds), she will be really pleased and she will praise you. Do you know how long 5 seconds is? Let me show you. (*Therapist counts out loud.*) That's not very long, but it is plenty of time for you to get started. Let me show you what I mean."

The therapist and parent then demonstrate this path (with the therapist role playing the part of the child). The therapist asks the child "What should your mom do now?" at each step of the path.

A similar procedure is employed in explaining and demonstrating each of the remaining two paths of the clear instructions sequence to the child. Finally, all three paths are demonstrated to the child at the same time, with the therapist playing the part of the child and the parent administering the clear instructions and consequences. We have found that it works best for the therapist to comply to the first few clear instructions, then comply only to the warnings, and finally go to TO. After the TO, it is essential that the therapist return to the original situation and obey the clear instruction, and that the parent provide positive attention for compliance.

At each step, the therapist asks the child, "What's next?" If the child is correct, the child is praised and the actions are carried out. If the child answers incorrectly or does not know, the therapist again verbalizes the step and the parent carries it out.

When the therapist is role playing the child, the therapist should "talk to himself or herself" while in TO, saying things such as "I don't like this. . . . This is boring. . . . I *knew* I should have done what Mom said the first time." The TO should last the entire 3 minutes in the initial demonstration to the child, so that the child gets an accurate sense of its duration. The therapist should *not* be disruptive in TO when the child is being taught the basic TO procedure. However, the therapist can whine or complain a bit near the end of the 3-minute period so that the 15-second quiet contingency can be demonstrated. After the child has learned about the basic TO procedure, then the various challenges in the use of the clear instructions sequence described in Figure 7.6 are addressed.

With some children, the child can serve as a "coach" to the parent while the therapist acts as the child. In this manner, the child's understanding of the clear instructions procedure is assessed. With older children, the parent can implement the various alternatives of the clear instructions sequence with the child in a role play situation. The "pretend" nature of this practice is emphasized. The parent should never play the role of the child in this aspect of the training. Some children take this as a sign that parents can be told what to do and be put in TO. It is important that the gravity of the clear instructions sequence be stressed to the child. It is not a game and is not to be used with adults, siblings, or friends.

This instructional process has several positive benefits for both parent and child. It seems to facilitate the learning process for the child, thus resulting in less need for the parent to issue warnings, to use TO or backup contingencies, to repeat TO for noncompliance to the same clear instruction, and so forth. It also assuages a remaining qualm the parent often has concerning the use of clear instructions and especially TO: that the child does not understand, or will not accept, the procedure.

Goals for Consequences: Behavioral Criteria

The behavioral criteria for the successful completion of the consequences segment of Phase II are at least one 5-minute observation of the Parent's Game in which (1) a 75% child compliance ratio (child compliance/total parental commands plus warnings) is obtained and (2) a 60% rewards plus attends ratio (parental rewards plus attends issued within 5 seconds following child compliance to a parental command or warning) is obtained. Training in the consequences segment of Phase II is limited to no more than three sessions.

Homework Assignments

Practicing Clear Instructions and Reinforcing Compliance

Once the parent has begun to practice clear instructions in the clinic with the child, she or he should be asked to engage in this behavior at home as well. With respect to the home practice, the focus is initially on Path A of the clear instructions sequence (see Figure 7.2). The parent is advised to present the child with clear instructions to which the child is likely to comply. This is to provide the parent and child with some early successes in compliance training and to reduce the likelihood of noncompliance. The therapist should emphasize the importance of reinforcing compliance by using rewards and attends.

Because the parent has not been taught the remaining paths of the clear instructions sequence at this point, noncompliance can be a rather frustrating experience for the parent (for this reason, it is a good idea to initiate training in the remaining paths of the clear instructions sequence as quickly as possible after the completion of training in Path A of the clear instructions sequence). As a stopgap measure, the parent is instructed to ignore noncompliance or deal with it as it normally would be handled. The parent is given Parent Handout 10: Parent Record Sheet: Clear Instructions and Child Compliance (Appendix B) on which to record two clear instructions that he or she is to give to the child each day as well as the child's response and parental use of positive consequences (attends, rewards) for compliance.

To increase the likelihood of success, the therapist tells the parent to give clear instructions for tasks to which the parent is reasonably sure that the child will comply. In addition, the therapist enlists the child's assistance for the home practice:

> "Lisa, your mom is going to practice giving clear instructions to you over the next week. She needs your help to practice, so I'd really appreciate it if you do what your mom says when she tells you. That way, she'll get a chance to practice clear instructions *and* she'll be able to praise you when you do what she says."

The parent also lists unclear instructions that have been given, along with an alternative clear instruction that could have been given. A sample record sheet that has been partially completed is presented in Figure 7.7. In reviewing the record sheet for the

Parent Handout 10: Parent Record Sheet: Clear Instructions and Child Compliance

For the next week, give your child at least *two clear instructions* each day. Record each clear instruction below, whether or not your child complied, and the rewards and attends you gave for compliance.

Remember to make these easy instructions that you are reasonably sure that your child will comply to.

Date	Clear instruction	Did child comply?		Reward/attend for compliance
Tues 9/13	1. Lisa, pick up your toys now.	Yes	(No)	1.
	2. Come to dinner now.	(Yes)	No	2. Thank you for coming when I called you.
Wed 9/14	1. Please hand me Jane's toy now.	(Yes)	No	1.
	2. Lisa, come here right now.	Yes	(No)	2.
Thurs 9/15	1. Please come to dinner.	(Yes)	No	1. You came right away when I called you. Thank you.
	2. Please turn off the TV right now.	(Yes)	No	2. Thanks for doing what I told you right away!
	1.	Yes	No	1.
	2.	Yes	No	2.
	1.	Yes	No	1.
	2.	Yes	No	2.
	1.	Yes	No	1.
	2.	Yes	No	2.
	1.	Yes	No	1.
	2.	Yes	No	2.

List any unclear instructions you notice yourself giving during the week. Then change each unclear instruction to a clear instruction.

Unclear instructions	change to	*Clear instructions*
1. Lisa, would you pick up your toys?		1. Lisa, pick up your toys now.
2. Lisa, come to dinner now because we need to eat so we can go shopping.		2. Lisa, come to dinner now.
3.		3.
4.		4.
5.		5.

FIGURE 7.7. Sample Parent Handout 10: Parent Record Sheet: Clear Instructions and Child Compliance.

past 3 days, the therapist noted that the parent had issued two unclear instructions but, in both cases, had rephrased the instruction into a clear one. The parent indicated that she thought that she was beginning to "catch herself" whenever she was using unclear instructions. The therapist praised her and encouraged her to continue to pay close attention to the instructions that she gave her child. The therapist also pointed out to the parent that her child had complied to 60% of the clear instructions and that the parent had praised the child's compliance 75% of the time (i.e., three of four opportunities). The therapist and the parent discussed how clear instructions and praise for complying to the instructions are powerful ways to increase child compliance.

Time Out

Because the TO procedure is relatively more complex than the other parenting procedures taught in the program, we want to increase the likelihood that when TO is implemented in the home, it will be successful. The parent is not assigned to use TO at home until its proper use in the clinic setting has been demonstrated and the child generally remains in the chair during TO in clinic practice sessions. In fact, the therapist specifically asks the parent to refrain from using TO at home during this period.

Once the parent is proficient in employing TO in the clinic setting, the parent is encouraged to employ it at home. The therapist has the parent select a single situation in which noncompliance frequently occurs at home for the first potential use of TO. The parent is reminded to issue an appropriate clear instruction, reinforce compliance, and employ the TO procedure if necessary. The therapist asks the parent to record each administration of clear instructions and warnings, the child's response, and the use of parental consequences for compliance (rewards, attends) and noncompliance (TO) on Parent Handout 14: Parent Record Sheet: Clear Instructions Sequence (Appendix B). In addition, use of any backup procedures to TO is recorded as well.

A sample record sheet that has been partially completed is presented in Figure 7.8. In reviewing the record sheet with the parent, the therapist noted that for the past 4 days the child had complied to the original instruction twice, to the warning once, and to a restatement of the original instruction after a TO once. The therapist then noted that, with a single exception, the parent used labeled verbal rewards when the child complied to either clear instructions or to a warning. The therapist praised the parent for her successful use of the clear instructions sequence, including TO.

It is important to phone the parent in the interval between sessions after this assignment is made as a means of monitoring the use of TO and providing feedback and support when necessary. Depending upon the family, the phone calls may even occur on a daily basis. It is very important that the parent be successful in these early implementations of TO. If not successful, the parent may lose confidence in the procedure or in her or his parenting abilities, and the child may become more difficult to control. Once TO is used successfully in the one situation in the home, at the next session the parent is instructed to employ the TO procedure for all instances of noncompliance at home. The parent continues to monitor use of TO in the home on Parent Handout 14: Parent Record Sheet: Clear Instructions Sequence, which is brought to each session.

Parent Handout 14: Parent Record Sheet: Clear Instructions Sequence

Date	Time	Clear instruction/ warning	Child's response	Reward/attend for compliance	Time-out duration	Backup?
Sat 9/17	5:30 pm	Lisa, pick up your toys now!	Complied	Thanks!		
Sun 9/18	5:10 pm	Lisa, I want you to pick up your toys now.	No!			
	5:11 pm	If you don't pick up the toys, then you will have to go to TO.	Stared at me.		Yes 3 min	
	5:15 pm	Lisa, now pick up your toys.	Complied	Very nice job of picking up your toys.		
Mon 9/19	5:00 pm	Lisa, it is time to pick up your toys. Please pick them up.	Walked away			
	5:01 pm	If you don't pick up your toys, then you will have to go to TO.	Complied	Wow! I really like the way you put the doll in the box.		
Tu 9/20	4:55 pm	Please pick up the blocks now.	Complied	Great job of putting away all the toys!		

FIGURE 7.8. Sample Parent Handout 14: Parent Record Sheet: Clear Instructions Sequence.

Parents report that use of the clear instructions sequence seems to follow a relatively predictable pattern. When the procedure is first implemented at home, the parent may need to use TO a fair percentage of the time. There may even be a few instances of the child getting out of the chair before being permitted to leave. The child is testing the parent to see if the parent will be consistent in the use of TO. Once the child learns that TO can be expected to occur on a reliable basis following noncompliance, the next stage begins. During this period, there is an increase in the number of compliances to warnings but perhaps not to the initial clear instructions. The child is still testing the parent. When TO does occur, the child stays in the chair for the 3-minute period and then complies immediately to the subsequent repetition of the original clear instruction. Finally, the child settles into a developmentally appropriate routine. He or she complies to most clear instructions after they are stated initially and, if not, the child usually complies with the warning statement when it is given. Noncompliance still occurs but on a sporadic basis. The child has learned that he or she can expect consistent consequences for each act of compliance or noncompliance. Employing similar procedures, Roberts and Powers (1990) reported that refusal to stay in TO dropped significantly after the first week of implementation in the home and was essentially gone after 3 weeks.

EXTENDING PHASE II SKILLS: STANDING RULES[2]

Once the parent is successfully employing the clear instructions sequence (including TO as necessary) at home, then we teach the use of standing rules (see Figure 7.9). Standing rules are verbal "If . . . then" statements that specify (1) a particular prohibited child behavior or activity (e.g., "If you hit your brother . . . ") and (2) the consequence for breaking the rule (" . . . then you will have to go to TO"). Once stated, standing rules remain in effect permanently. Whenever the child breaks the rule, the consequence is implemented immediately.

Standing rules are a useful supplement to the clear instructions sequence. There are some situations in which the clear instructions sequence is cumbersome or even inappropriate (e.g., Jones et al., 1992). For example, a child is jumping on the couch. The parent gives a clear instruction (e.g., "Sit quietly on the couch") that terminates the activity, and the parent reinforces the compliance with positive attention. However, 30 seconds later the child is again jumping on the couch. Using the standard clear instructions sequence, the parent must give another clear instruction. As long as the child complies to the clear instruction or warning, this procedure might have to be repeated over and over. A standing rule of "If you jump on the furniture, you will have to go to TO" prevents this situation from occurring.

The therapist states that standing rules can be particularly useful for situations in which there is a danger to the child, someone else, or property (e.g., "You may not hit your sister"; "You may not leave the back yard"). There are two primary advantages to using standing rules in these types of situations. The first advantage is that the parent is able to provide a consequence for the inappropriate behavior immediately after its occurrence and is able to avoid situations in which the child manipulates the standard clear instructions sequence. The second advantage is that standing rules represent a developmentally more advanced type of parent–child interaction. The standing rule usually encompasses more general classes of behavior (e.g., no jumping on any piece of furniture) than the clear instructions sequence, and the rule is not stated every time. As such, it is especially appropriate for older children.

There are some potential disadvantages to the standing rules procedure as well. Because no clear instruction or warning is given to the child, the child's opportunity for complying to an immediate clear instruction or warning and for receiving positive attention for compliance is eliminated. Unlike the clear instructions sequence, there are no specific reminders to reinforce compliance that are built into the standing rules procedure. Thus, the parent may forget to provide positive attention for compliance to the rule. For these reasons, there should only be one or two standing rules in effect at any given time. In addition, we have found it helpful to have parents post the standing rule(s) in a prominent place, such as on the refrigerator. For children who are unable to read, the standing rule can be presented in the form of a picture. When a standing rule is first established, the therapist has parents provide positive attention to the child for

---

[2]Some of the information in this section is based on materials developed by our colleague Mark Roberts.

- "If . . . then" statement.
  - "If" specifies prohibited child activity.
  - "Then" specifies consequences for breaking the rule (i.e., TO).
- Once stated, continually in effect.
- TO implemented immediately when rule is broken.
- Parent rehearses standing rule with child at end of TO.
- Parent must *regularly* reinforce compliance to the rule.
- Maximum of two standing rules in effect at one time.

FIGURE 7.9. Standing rules. Partially adapted with permission from Mark W. Roberts, Idaho State University (1995).

complying to the rule several times per day for the first week or so. The therapist suggests that the parent put a sign next to the posted rule as a prompt (e.g., "Praise Doug for playing nicely with Karen").

Teaching the Parent about Standing Rules

The therapist first provides a description of standing rules to the parent, as well as the rationale for their use and relevant examples (see above). The parent is then asked to generate one or two "not OK" behaviors for which standing rules would be appropriate, as well as the rules themselves. The procedure for using a standing rule is the following:

- The parent considers whether the situation is best handled by a standing rule or by another parenting strategy such as the clear instructions sequence, positive attention alone, or differential attention. Standing rules should be used selectively and infrequently, as compared to the other strategies.
- The parent explains and demonstrates the standing rule to the child (see below), and it is posted in a prominent place (e.g., on the refrigerator).
- The parent reminds the child occasionally about the standing rule.
- The parent provides positive attention to the child on a regular basis for complying to the rule.
- If the child breaks the rule:
  - Using a firm voice, the parent says, "Since you [*state the rule violation*], you must go to TO."
  - The parent uses the standard TO procedure.
  - At the end of TO, the parent rehearses the rule with the child. Ask the child: "Why did you have to go to TO?" "What's wrong with [*state the misbehavior*]?" "What will happen if you forget again?" "What could you have done instead?" If the child answers incorrectly or refuses to answer, then the parent briefly and calmly provides the correct responses.
- The parent involves the child in an activity so that the parent can provide positive attention for appropriate behavior.

The rehearsal procedure with the child following completion of TO is very important. It is analogous to having the child return to the initial situation in the clear instructions sequence in that it provides the child with an opportunity to learn from the experience.

The therapist gives Parent Handout 15: Standing Rules (Appendix B) to the parent at the end of the session in which standing rules are introduced.

Teaching the Child about Standing Rules

Once the parent has decided to use a standing rule, the next step is to teach the rule to the child (see Figure 7.10). First, the child must *always* be told the rule in advance, at a time when he or she is behaving appropriately. Second, the parent provides a rationale for the standing rule. For example, if the standing rule is "If you hit your sister, then you will have to go to TO," then the parent might say, "I don't want you to hit her, because it might hurt her."

The third step is to rehearse the standing rule with the child. We first have the parent ask the child a series of questions: "What is it that you are to do?" "What will happen if you do [*the "not OK" behavior*]?" and "What could you do instead?" This last question is designed to get the child to generate more prosocial alternatives to the misbehavior. The next step is to demonstrate and role play enforcing the rule. If the rule is broken, the parent takes the child to the TO chair and says, "Since you [*state the rule violation*], you have to stay in TO until I say that you can get out." At the conclusion of TO, the parent practices the rehearsal procedures described above with the child.

During the Parent Training Session

After the therapist has presented and discussed the information about standing rules with the parent, the therapist and parent role play and practice the process of establishing and implementing a standing rule, as described above. The standing rule is then explained and demonstrated to the child using the process described in the preceding sec-

- Parent tells child the rule in advance.
- Parent provides rationale for the rule.
- Parent and child rehearse the rule.
  - Parent asks:
  - "What is it that you are not to do?"
  - "What will happen if you do [*the "not OK" behavior*]?"
  - "What could you do instead?"
- Parent demonstrates procedure and role plays with child.

FIGURE 7.10. Teaching the child about standing rules. Adapted with permission from Mark W. Roberts, Idaho State University (1995).

tion. Finally, the parent and child practice the standing rule in the session, with feedback from the therapist.

Homework

For homework, the therapist asks the parent to implement the one or two standing rules at home, with special emphasis on providing positive attention to the child for adherence to the rule. The parent is asked to complete Parent Handout 16: Parent Record Sheet: Standing Rules (Appendix B). A sample record sheet that has been completed is presented in Figure 7.11.

   After reviewing the record sheet from the past 4 days, the therapist praised the parent for praising the child for following the standing rule, and for using TO on the one occasion that the child broke the rule. The therapist also suggested that the parent should try to praise her child more frequently than two or three times per day during the first week or so that the standing rule was being implemented.

Parent Handout 16: Parent Record Sheet: Standing Rules

The standing rule that I will work on with my child is:

Do not hit the dog

Positive statements that I can make for following the standing rule are:

1. Thanks very much for patting the dog gently.

2. You are playing so nicely with the dog!

Date	Did my child follow the rule?		Number of times I praised my child for *following* the rule	Time out for *breaking* the rule?		Rehearse the rule after time out?	
Fri, 9/30	Yes	(No)	2	(Yes)	No	(Yes)	No
Sat, 10/1	(Yes)	No	3	Yes	No	Yes	No
Sun, 10/2	(Yes)	No	2	Yes	No	Yes	No
Mon, 10/3	(Yes)	No	3	Yes	No	Yes	No
	Yes	No		Yes	No	Yes	No
	Yes	No		Yes	No	Yes	No
	Yes	No		Yes	No	Yes	No

FIGURE 7.11. Sample Parent Handout 16: Parent Record Sheet: Standing Rules. Partially adapted by permission of the authors from McMahon, Slough, and the Conduct Problems Prevention Research Group (1994).

EXTENDING PHASE I AND PHASE II SKILLS

The Role of Siblings

Many parent–child conflicts occur in the context of interactions between the referred child and a sibling (see Chapter 1). Especially when the sibling is also 3–8 years of age, we usually ask the parent to bring both children to some of the parent training sessions. There are a number of reasons for adopting this strategy.

First, including the sibling in some of the sessions may relieve any pressure that the referred child may be experiencing as *the* problem in the family, and it lends credence to the therapist's assertion that the focus of intervention will be on the parent–child(ren) interactions. Second, we have found that, although only one of the children has been referred for treatment, a sibling often will display a very similar pattern of noncompliance and other inappropriate behavior (although perhaps at a lower intensity) (Snyder & Stoolmiller, 2002). Third, some of the referral problems may directly involve the sibling (e.g., excessive arguing, fighting). Fourth, generalization may be programmed more effectively, since the parent will need to deal with both children's behaviors in the home setting. By learning to handle these situations in the parent training sessions, the parent will be better equipped to deal with similar events at home.

Another advantage of having the sibling present during the parent training sessions is that it can facilitate the effectiveness of some of the parenting techniques. With respect to the Phase I skills of attends and rewards, the therapist has the parent practice the Child's Game with both children at the same time. The parent learns to switch her or his attention back and forth from one child to the other, as well as to use statements that include both children simultaneously (e.g., "You are both doing such a good job of coloring between the lines"). The therapist also teaches the parent to provide attends and rewards for cooperative play, sharing, and other "OK" sibling behaviors that the parent would like to increase. The therapist also suggests the use of ignoring for sibling behaviors such as minor teasing or tattling.

As noted in Chapter 6, the differential attention procedure can be even more effective when a sibling is present. For example, if one of the children is behaving inappropriately (e.g., whining) and the other sibling is not, then the parent ignores the first child and reinforces the sibling for an incompatible "OK" behavior at the same time (in this example, the parent might say, "I really like it when you talk in a regular voice"). This seems to facilitate the process in which the referred child (or sibling) learns the contingencies for various "OK" and "not OK" behaviors. As soon as the first child stops whining and begins to talk in a regular voice, the parent resumes interaction with that child as well.

Finally, the Phase II skill of TO (either through the clear instructions sequence or through a standing rule) is typically employed to deal with more intensive levels of sibling conflict, such as excessive teasing or physical aggression. In the latter case, we tell the parent that *both* sibs should be sent to TO. Trying to decide "who started it" is usually futile, and provides attention to both siblings for fighting, which inadvertently reinforces the behavior!

Depending on the situation, we usually have the parent bring the sibling only to the later sessions of Phase I and of Phase II. This is because the parent first needs to practice and learn the various skills individually with the referred child before attempting to practice the new skills in the parent training session with both children simultaneously. Subsequently, practice can take place with both children together. Having the parent attempt to practice a new skill right away with both children at the same time is usually too complex and confusing for the parent.

If both children cannot attend the sessions, all is not lost. As described in Chapter 10, even without directly teaching the parent to deal with an untreated sibling's problem behaviors, many parents are able to transfer their parenting skills to the sibling's behavior. The sibling responds by increasing his or her compliance to parental directions (Humphreys et al., 1978).

Even in families in which a sibling's behavior is not problematic, it is important to emphasize to the parent that the skills being taught are ones that improve interactions between the parent and all children. Therefore, the parent should apply the procedures to all children who are in the appropriate age range. In some of our cases in which this has not been explicitly stated, parents have asked, "Is it all right to use the techniques with my other children?"

Situations Outside the Home[3]

It is quite common for the parent to name at least one problematic situation with his or her child that occurs outside the home. The most frequently mentioned activities are riding in the car, going shopping or eating in restaurants, and visiting in others' homes. These public situations are often difficult for parents to handle constructively. The parent has less control of the situation than at home (and the child usually knows it). In addition, the parent may be concerned about criticism from others concerning the child's behavior and the parent's use of the parenting skills, or embarrassment about the child's reaction.

The therapist should have the parent defer implementation of the parenting skills in these situations until a satisfactory level of success has been achieved in employing the parenting procedures in the home. As noted above, the parent has less control of the environmental contingencies outside the home. Having problems employing the skills successfully at home almost guarantees that the parent's interventions in the car or at the grocery store will fail. However, by successfully employing parenting skills at home on a consistent basis, the parent increases the likelihood that these same procedures will be effective outside the home. It has been our experience that children respond rapidly and positively to these parenting skills in other settings once they are responding to them at home.

Although particular circumstances can vary tremendously, several guidelines for handling problems should be followed regardless of the setting (see Figure 7.12). The

---

[3]Some of the information in this section is based on materials developed by our colleague Mark Roberts.

key to successfully dealing with the child's behavior in situations outside the home is for the parent to plan ahead. The therapist encourages the parent to decide ahead of time how to handle the situation rather than having to react to it spontaneously. Prior to any excursion outside the home, the parent should explain to the child exactly what consequences will occur for "OK" and "not OK" behavior. This clearly delineates the rules to both the child and parent. The parent then employs brief "practice" sessions with the child in these settings. This is to assist the child in learning the desired behaviors and to increase the likelihood of a positive interaction between the parent and child. For example, if riding in the car is a problem, then a short ride through the neighborhood might be a first step, followed by subsequent rides of longer duration. If the child's behavior while shopping is problematic, then the parent takes the child to the grocery store for one or two items that the child likes (e.g., snacks, cereal).

The therapist emphasizes that the same skills taught in the parent training program for use at home can be employed to deal with difficulties outside the home. The parent is encouraged to look for opportunities to "catch your child being good." Attends and rewards should be used to reinforce "OK" child behaviors in these settings. A variety of examples of ways to increase the likelihood of "OK" behavior are listed in Parent Handout 17: Dealing with Situations Outside the Home (see Appendix B). For example, one tactic to facilitate longer car trips is for the parent to have a small set of toys (e.g., coloring books, cars and trucks) that are brought out only on these occasions. In this way, their novelty can be maintained for a longer time period. While shopping, involving the child in purchasing decisions is an excellent way to maintain good behavior and to begin consumer education at an early age. When visiting others, the parent should excuse himself or herself from the host to attend to the child on a frequent basis, in the same way that this is done during the parent training sessions (see Chapter 6).

Ignoring (in the context of differential attention), the clear instructions sequence, and standing rules can be employed to decrease "not OK" behaviors. If a command needs to be given, then the same clear instructions sequence should be employed. However, the actual TO procedure may vary according to the setting. The time limit for TO can be decreased from 3 minutes to 1 minute. We have found that this briefer TO is effective in these other settings. The therapist stresses that in no case should the child

- Plan ahead to increase likelihood of success.
  - Decide ahead of time how to handle situation.
  - Explain consequences for "OK" and "not OK" behavior to child.
- Set up brief "practice" sessions to guarantee child success.
- In the public setting:
  - Look for opportunities to "catch your child being good" (i.e., give positive attention for "OK" behaviors).
  - Use ignoring (in the context of differential attention), the clear instructions sequence, and standing rules as needed.

FIGURE 7.12. Dealing with situations outside the home. Partially adapted with permission from Mark W. Roberts, Idaho State University (1995).

ever be left alone while in TO in a public setting. Instead, the parent sits or stands near the child. The therapist notes that TO can be implemented in a variety of settings (see Parent Handout 17: Dealing with Situations Outside the Home for a list; Appendix B). For example, when in a store or restaurant, the parent may take the child out of the establishment and return to the car. The child is placed in the car for 1 minute. The parent stands next to the car (the parent must be sure that he or she has the car keys!), or the child is placed in the back seat and the parent sits in the front seat. Never leave the child in the car alone. Once the TO period is completed, the parent and child return to the store, where the parent reinforces the child's appropriate behavior (e.g., walking in the aisle, eating quietly). When driving in the car, the parent can simply pull over to the side of the road and ignore the child until the inappropriate behavior subsides. At the homes of others, the same procedures for establishing a TO area in the child's own home would apply. The parent should anticipate whether TO may need to be used when visiting others and, if so, explain to the host that a TO procedure may be necessary for inappropriate behavior and may have to be implemented during the visit.

Although the parenting skills are generally the same as those that the parent has been taught to employ at home, the public context of these problematic situations can impede the consistent use of the procedures. The therapist should empathize with the parent concerning the difficulty of using the procedures outside the home; however, at the same time the importance of consistently employing the parenting procedures in these situations must be stressed. In this way, the overall positive aspects of the parent–child interaction will be markedly enhanced.

During the session, the therapist asks the parent to identify a situation outside the home that is of concern. The therapist and parent discuss strategies for dealing with this situation, and then the therapist and parent role play the planned solution. The plan is then explained and demonstrated to the child. Finally, the parent and child practice the plan in the session, with feedback from the therapist. For homework, the therapist asks the parent to hold at least one "practice" session, followed by gradual implementation of the plan over the next couple of weeks.

SAMPLE SESSION

In prior Phase II sessions, Mrs. M learned how to deliver clear instructions and had been introduced to the consequences for compliance and noncompliance, including the use of TO. This session initially consisted of a 5-minute assessment observation of Mrs. M and John engaging in activities selected by the mother (the Parent's Game). During the observation, Mrs. M issued a total of 15 commands (13 alpha commands and 2 beta commands) and 2 warnings. Of the 13 alpha commands, John complied 11 times to the initial command and, for the remaining two commands, he complied to both warnings (for a 76% rate of compliance to total commands plus warnings). Finally, Mrs. M rewarded or attended to John 7 out of 11 times for complying to the initial command and rewarded him both times for complying to the warning (for a total of 69% contingent attention).

Following the observation, Mrs. M instructed John to play with toys by himself while she talked with the therapist. The therapist discussed Mrs. M's use of clear instructions (alpha commands) and rewards and attends for John's compliance during the preceding observation. The therapist noted to himself that Mrs. M and John had met the criteria for Phase II and praised Mrs. M for her performance. The therapist also pointed out to Mrs. M that John had complied to 76% of the clear instructions and warnings that she had issued. Mrs. M stated that she had noticed that John was complying much more frequently. At this point, Mrs. M went over to John and praised him for playing quietly and not interrupting while she and the therapist talked. When Mrs. M returned to her seat, the therapist praised her for attending to John's appropriate behavior.

The therapist then asked Mrs. M about her use of TO at home during the previous week. The homework assignment had been to use TO (if necessary) in one situation, which was for not picking up his toys when told to do so each night before dinner. Mrs. M had kept a record on Parent Handout 14: Parent Record Sheet: Clear Instructions Sequence of the number of instructions she issued, how often she had praised John for compliance, warnings that were issued for noncompliance, compliance to those warnings, and praise to John for complying to the warnings. The therapist and Mrs. M went over the record sheet. Mrs. M had used a high rate of rewards and attends to John for compliance to instructions to pick up his toys. Furthermore, she had had to warn John a total of eight times during the previous week following noncompliance to her instruction. Of those eight times, John complied six times. She had praised him all six times for complying. On the two occasions when John failed to comply when his mother issued the warning, Mrs. M reported using TO. On one occasion, John sat quietly for the required TO period and returned to the task of picking up toys. On the other occasion, John screamed loudly for 45 seconds and then left TO. Mrs. M reported that she returned John to TO and lengthened the period of time that he was required to stay in TO. Although he continued to scream for 2 minutes, John did not leave TO again. After John was quiet in TO, Mrs. M returned John to the task of picking up his toys. She reported that John did comply, but he appeared to be "upset." She reported that once the toys were picked up, John showed no further signs of "being upset" and did not have to go to TO during the remaining 2 days of the week prior to coming to the parent training session.

The therapist talked to Mrs. M about how she felt the use of TO had gone. She indicated that using TO was stressful for her because she "hated" confrontations with John. However, she also indicated that TO was effective and that it was less stressful than nagging or screaming at him, which is how she previously handled trying to get John to pick up his toys. Mrs. M indicated that she felt that she had effectively used TO for noncompliance to her instruction to pick up the toys, as well as rewards and attends for John's compliance.

Based on Mrs. M's meeting the criteria during the initial 5-minute observation and her report of appropriately using the clear instructions sequence for picking up toys and rewards for complying, the therapist decided Mrs. M was ready to use TO for noncompliance and other problem behaviors throughout the day. The therapist encouraged Mrs. M to use TO but cautioned her that it was only effective within the context of a positive home environment created by her rewards and attends for John's appropriate behavior. Mrs. M and the therapist then discussed other situations in which John was continuing to be noncompliant. These involved picking up toys before going to bed, coming when his mother called him to take a bath, and getting up when told to do so in the morning. They discussed the use of clear instructions, warnings, TO for noncompliance, and praise for compliance for these various situations. The therapist requested that Mrs. M keep a record for each of these situations during the coming week on the parent record sheet.

During the discussion between Mrs. M and the therapist that was just described, Mrs. M again left her chair to praise John. The therapist praised Mrs. M for continuing to attend to John's appropriate behavior. Furthermore, the therapist noted how effective it was to praise and attend to John playing quietly, as he had not interrupted them during their conversation.

The therapist next indicated that he thought it would be beneficial if Mrs. M and John spent the remainder of the session practicing the Parent's Game. Mrs. M was reminded of the importance of clear instructions, praise for compliance, and warnings and TO for noncompliance. The therapist told Mrs. M that she should initially tell John that they would briefly play the Child's Game and, when the therapist cued her, she then would inform him that they were to switch to the Parent's Game.

During the 5-minute Child's Game, Mrs. M issued 15 rewards, 5 attends, and 1 question. During the Parent's Game, 90% of her instructions were alpha commands, John complied to 89% of these, and she praised him for compliance 75% of the time. Mrs. M only gave one warning and John complied. Mrs. M praised him for this compliance.

Following the observation, the therapist met briefly with Mrs. M and asked her how she felt about the interaction. She indicated that she felt like she had done a good job, and the therapist enthusiastically confirmed this. The therapist reminded Mrs. M about her homework assignment, and an appointment was scheduled for the following week.

COMMONLY ENCOUNTERED PROBLEMS

The Drill Sergeant

The Drill Sergeant is a parent who gives numerous commands, expects 100% compliance, and believes children should "fall into line" with little explanation for why commands are issued and rules are in place. The therapist should note that issuing a large number of commands actually can be counterproductive, since the parent cannot follow through on all of the commands. In addition, the child probably will be overwhelmed and will often become even more noncompliant and oppositional. The therapist should point out that expecting 100% compliance is not only unrealistic but also is not desirable from a developmental perspective.

The Drill Sergeant frequently gives commands and rules that are unrealistic or developmentally inappropriate. For example, the parents of a 3-year-old child who was referred to us for treatment had a rule that the child was *never* to enter their bedroom. The parents had no rationale or explanation for why this rule should exist; not surprisingly, they reported considerable conflict with their child over the rule. Part of our intervention with this family focused on the need for logical rules and realistic expectations for a young child.

The beliefs of the Drill Sergeant likely will be evident early on. The Drill Sergeant sees little reason why a child should be attended to and rewarded for compliance. The parent believes that child compliance should occur "because I am the parent and in charge." This parent will either directly express reservations about attending because he or she sees it as unnecessary or will suggest reasons why attending will not work with his or her child. The therapist will likely need to spend significantly more time with this parent concerning both the overall approach of the parent training program (Chapter 5) and the Positive Reinforcement and Attention Rules that form the basis of Phase I (Chapter 6). The Drill Sergeant needs to understand the importance of creating a positive, nurturing environment through the use of attends and rewards in the context of the Child's Game. As we noted in Chapter 6, such an environment motivates the child to want to comply to parental commands. When parents are positive with their children, the child reciprocates and increases his or her compliance.

The Afraid-to-Confront Parent

In contrast to the Drill Sergeant, some parents learn and use the Phase I skills very well but do not wish to confront their child by issuing clear instructions and using TO following noncompliance. This parent issues few commands during the Parent's Game and accepts the child's every excuse for not complying. The parent may still be fearful of an intensive negative reaction from the child, despite the child's positive response to Phase I. Sometimes the parent may rationalize this behavior by stating that the parent values assertiveness over compliance.

In these cases, it is necessary to discuss the need to set firm and consistent limits for the child and to stress the developmental importance of the child's learning to follow directions from parents. Furthermore, in practice sessions with the child it may be necessary to give the parent clear instructions to issue to the child and to tell the parent exactly when and how to implement TO. Only with this type of structure will this parent ever learn to deal with the issue of exerting any control over the child.

This parent also tends to express concern over the Parent's Game as being unfair to the child. The parent may say that noncompliance to the commands used in the Parent's Game (e.g., "Put the red block on the green block") does not justify the use of TO. The therapist should acknowledge the artificiality of the Parent's Game while at the same time pointing out to the parent that the basic issue is one of noncompliance to the parent, regardless of the particular command. The therapist should also point out that the purpose of the Parent's Game is to provide the parent with an opportunity to learn how to elicit compliance and minimize noncompliance and for the child to learn the consequences for compliance and noncompliance as well. At the same time, the therapist should also agree that the parent would not likely issue a clear instruction or use TO in such a situation at home and should stress the importance of giving appropriate clear instructions in that setting.

The Compliant Child

A situation that occasionally arises is that a child who is noncompliant in the home (as determined by parent report, parent-recorded data, and home observations) is compliant in the parent training sessions. In fact, this is often the direct result of teaching the child about the various paths of the clear instructions sequence and practicing them within the sessions. As a consequence of the child's compliance in sessions, the therapist is unable to directly observe the parent practice actual implementation of the TO procedure with the child. In that situation, we may specifically ask the child whether he or she would be willing to role play being noncompliant so that his or her parent can get some practice with the TO procedure. This allows the therapist to prompt and instruct the parent in the actual use of TO with the child, albeit in a practice situation. The parent is then instructed to use the procedure at home. The therapist can receive detailed feedback from the parent over the phone or at the next parent training session concerning the effectiveness of the procedure. Modeling and role playing can then be utilized to assist the parent in working out implementation problems. If difficulties with TO continue to occur in the home, the therapist can make a home visit, observe the parent's use of TO, and assist the parent with the correct implementation of the procedure.

THE FINAL SESSION(S)

After the parent has met the behavioral criteria for Phase II, has been successfully employing the clear instructions sequence and standing rules in the home, and has been able to implement both Phase I and Phase II skills outside the home, then termination of the parent training program is appropriate. (In some cases, therapeutic contact may continue around other issues, such as parental depression or the marital relationship.) As in all interventions, the parent should be given a general idea as to when the program may be terminated well ahead of the expected termination date. The final session provides both the parent and the therapist with an opportunity to "wrap things up."

The parent is likely to have several procedural questions concerning particular situations that have arisen (or that she or he anticipates arising). By this time, the parent is equipped with the requisite knowledge and skills for handling most instances of problematic child behavior. Throughout the final stages of the program and especially in the final session, the therapist should encourage the parent to apply the skills already learned to these situations and should reinforce the parent for appropriate use of the skills. The therapist's task is more one of encouragement than instruction in the final session(s).

The therapist should emphasize that consistent use of the parenting procedures is the key to the ultimate success of the program. The child will engage in less limit testing and more appropriate behavior as he or she comes to realize that the parent provides predictable and consistent consequences for both appropriate and inappropriate behaviors. While the program is not a panacea, it will make family life a more enjoyable and profitable experience for all concerned. It does require that the parent continue to work at employing the newly acquired parenting skills. At the same time, the therapist also prepares parents for the reality of occasional relapses and mistakes in the future and stresses the parent's ability to self-correct, using the same approach and skills that the parent has been employing throughout the parent training program.

Finally, the parent also should be encouraged to contact the therapist if further questions or concerns arise. Depending upon the situation, at the last session the therapist may decide to schedule follow-up telephone calls or "booster session" clinic visits.

CHAPTER 8

======

Adjunctive Interventions

*I*n this chapter, we present four sets of adjunctive interventions that we have developed to enhance the effectiveness and generalization of our treatment effects. One procedure, developed
primarily by Karen Wells, involves employing a self-control program with parents who participate in the parent training program. The second procedure, devised primarily by the first author (RJM), consists of giving the parent an extensive knowledge of social learning principles
in addition to the parenting skills delineated in Chapters 6 and 7. The third adjunctive intervention, developed primarily by Douglas Griest, includes several components designed to address various family-related issues. The fourth set of procedures is focused on the development
of self-administered parent training materials. We describe a broad-based book for parents
written by the second author (RLF) and Nicholas Long and a more narrowly focused brochure for parents interested in improving their children's mealtime behavior. The empirical
evaluation of these adjunctive interventions is discussed in Chapter 10.

RATIONALE FOR ENHANCING PARENT TRAINING

As we indicated in Chapter 2, although parent training is regarded as the most effective
intervention for young children with conduct problems, there has been increasing recognition of the need to enhance basic parent training. Miller and Prinz (1990) delineated three approaches for accomplishing this. The first is to enhance the parenting
skills already taught in parent training programs by *adding* new interactional strategies.
The second approach involves broadening intervention to include a wider array of family influences, such as parent depression, marital adjustment, and parental expectations
of children. The third approach involves incorporating multiple systems—such as intervening in school as well as at home—into the therapeutic process.

Our view is that parent training is a necessary but not always sufficient intervention for dealing with child noncompliance and other conduct problems. When it is not
sufficient, one or more of the three approaches delineated by Miller and Prinz (1990)
may be necessary. In these next three chapters, we describe efforts (by ourselves and
others) to enhance the effectiveness and generalization of the HNC parent training program. In this chapter we delineate our efforts concerned with the first two approaches
presented by Miller and Prinz, namely, enhancing or strengthening parenting skills and

broadening intervention to address a wider variety of family influences. In Chapter 9 Karen Wells describes the adaptation of the parent training program to special populations. Finally, in Chapter 10 we consider parent training as a *preventive* intervention, which conceptually falls under the third approach described by Miller and Prinz.

USE OF A SELF-CONTROL PROGRAM WITH PARENTS

One strategy that may be particularly appropriate for enhancing changes in parenting behavior and, subsequently, child behavior is the use of self-control procedures. It has long been acknowledged that changes in child behavior may not provide sufficient reinforcement to maintain good parenting behavior (e.g., Conway & Bucher, 1976; Miller & Prinz, 1990). Similarly, after treatment particular individuals (e.g., helping agencies, spouses, neighbors, grandparents) may undermine continued change efforts by failing to reinforce or by punishing treatment-acquired parenting skills (Marholin, Siegel, & Phillips, 1976; Miller & Prinz, 1990). Self-control procedures may help circumvent these problems by teaching parents to provide themselves with antecedent and consequent events necessary to control their own behavior. In this way, parents are no longer totally dependent on the external environment to continue to reinforce treatment-acquired skills. The program described in this chapter was developed and experimentally tested by Wells, Griest, and Forehand (1980). The results of their study provide some evidence that self-control procedures can be of benefit to some parents in maintaining improvements in child behavior. As we noted earlier, the self-control procedures are not part of our parenting program, per se, but may be used as an adjunctive intervention to further facilitate child behavior change.

Our self-control training is designed to teach the parent self-monitoring and self-reinforcement skills. During the parent training sessions, the parent is given a multi-channel wrist behavior counter capable of recording two categories of behavior. After being taught each parenting skill, the parent learns to self-monitor by accurately counting the use of the skill. In Phase I, the parent is taught attending; subsequently, the parent is asked to self-monitor or count attends to the child on the wrist counter. The parent practices counting attends during a 10-minute role play situation with the therapist in which the therapist plays the role of the child. Subsequently, the parent counts the number of attends used with the child during a 10-minute practice session in which the therapist observes the parent and child interacting and also counts the occurrence of attends. Such practice sessions continue until the parent obtains at least 75% agreement with the therapist. Subsequently, the parent is taught the rewarding skills and then is taught to self-monitor these skills in the same way that self-monitoring was taught for attending. As with attending, the practice sessions continue until the parent obtains at least 75% agreement with the therapist.

In Phase II of the parent training program, the parent learns the clear instructions and TO skills (i.e., the clear instructions sequence) to a specified level of performance. Then the parent is taught to count the following parent–child interactive sequences: (1) clear instruction (parent behavior), comply (child behavior), reward/attend (parent behavior) (i.e., Path A of the clear instructions sequence), *or* clear instruction (parent behavior), noncomply (child behavior), warning (parent behavior), comply (child behavior), reward/attend (parent behavior) (i.e., Path B of the clear instructions sequence), on one behavior channel; and (2) clear instruction (parent behavior), noncomply (child behavior), warning (parent behavior), noncomply (child behavior), and TO (parent behavior) (i.e., Path C of the clear instructions sequence) on the second behavior channel. The therapist initially prompts accurate self-monitoring in a role play situation by informing the parent whenever one of these sequences occurs. Prompts are phased out as the parent begins to show proficiency in self-monitoring. Subsequently, the parent self-monitors during 10-minute practice periods with the child while the therapist observes the interaction and also counts occurrences of each of the two sequences. These practice sessions continue until the parent reaches 75% agreement with the therapist.

In the final session, the parent and therapist compose an individualized self-control program (including reinforcers) to be followed by the parent during the next 2-month period. First, a list of self-reinforcers is developed that includes material reinforcers (e.g., afternoon coffee break, special dessert) and high-probability behaviors (e.g., watching a favorite TV program, reading a favorite magazine) that can be applied daily, as well as three valued reinforcers (e.g., dinner out, shopping trip) that can be applied at 2- and 4-week intervals. Following this, the details of the program are outlined. Each day during the period that the program is in effect, the parent chooses a daily reinforcer from the list derived in the preceding session. Using a clock or timer for self-timing, the parent spends 15 minutes with the child in a potentially problematic situation (e.g., bath time, mealtime), reinforcing the child's appropriate behavior and providing consequences for child compliance and noncompliance. These behaviors are self-monitored using the wrist counter by recording each attending or rewarding response on one channel of the counter and interactive sequences in which TO occurs (i.e., Path C) on the second channel. Following each 15-minute "good parenting session," the parent self-administers the daily reinforcer only if (1) an average of at least four attends and/or rewards per minute was counted while the child was not in TO and (2) the parent reports that each occurrence of child noncompliance was handled appropriately (i.e., initially with a warning and then, if necessary, with TO). Although the parent is encouraged to employ treatment-acquired parenting skills as well as self-reinforcement throughout the day, these behaviors are self-monitored and recorded only during the daily 15-minute "good parenting sessions."

In order to motivate the occurrence of self-control behaviors (daily self-monitoring and self-reinforcement) and parenting sessions, each parent sets up a contract with the therapist after the details of the program have been explained. As part of the contract, the parent agrees to telephone in data from the daily 15-minute parenting sessions during the 2-month period according to a set schedule (i.e., initially daily, fading to approximately once per week). The number of attends and rewards is reported, as well as whether each act of child noncompliance was followed with TO.

The parent self-administers one of the three highly valued reinforcers after the first 2 weeks if the following criteria are met: phoned in data at least 75% of the required days and reached the criteria for daily self-reinforcement on at least 75% of these occasions. At the end of 4 weeks and 8 weeks, the same criteria are imposed for receiving a preselected valued reinforcer.

The parent receives brief instructions through the mail every 2 weeks, which (1) list daily reinforcers to be administered after parenting sessions, (2) inform the parent of the dates data are to be called in, and (3) inform the parent that the criteria for 2-, 4-, and 8-week self-reinforcement have or have not been reached as agreed upon with the therapist in the last treatment session. An example of a letter sent at the beginning of the first 2-week period after the last treatment session is presented in Figure 8.1.

The self-control program is effective in facilitating child behavior change (see Chapter 10). The program obviously involves a number of procedures, including the parent's learning to count his or her own use of parenting skills, instructions to practice and count the skills at home, setting up rewards for use of the skills, and telephoning data to an answering service. Which of these components, individually or in combination, are the effective ingredient(s) is unknown. For clinical purposes, a therapist may choose to incorporate one or more of the components of the self-control program into the treatment package. For example, having the parent discriminate each occurrence of a particular parenting skill used and recording it may be beneficial, particularly for the parent who has difficulty identifying the occurrence of a behavior or a chain of behaviors that constitute a skill. However, it is important to reiterate that the effectiveness of the individual components of the self-control program is not known.

TEACHING PARENTS SOCIAL LEARNING PRINCIPLES

Another procedure that has been suggested as a potential means of enhancing generalization is training parents in social learning principles in addition to behavioral parenting skills (Forehand & Atkeson, 1977). The reasons given for including formal training in social learning principles (O'Dell, Flynn, & Benlolo, 1977) have been that it is parsimonious in terms of time and effort (Patterson, Cobb, & Ray, 1973), parents need the theoretical framework supplied by such principles (Salzinger, Feldman, & Portnoy, 1970), and generalization is more likely to occur (Forehand & Atkeson, 1977; Miller & Prinz, 1990). Patterson and his colleagues have been the strongest advocates of training parents in social learning principles prior to beginning treatment. They have stated that such training should allow the subsequent performance of child management skills to "(a) accelerate more rapidly, (b) display greater generalization in that parents are able to innovate a number of their own programs for both the target child and siblings, and (c) be performed for a longer period following termination of the formal treatment program" (Patterson, Reid, Jones, & Conger, 1975, p. 53). Studies by McMahon, Forehand, and Griest (1981) and McMahon and colleagues (1984) analyzed the effectiveness of incorporating formal training in social learning principles into the parent training program on enhancing treatment outcome and generalization. They found that not only does the integration of formal training in social learning principles enhance treatment outcome, setting generality, and temporal generality with respect to behavioral and par-

Mrs. Jane Doe
892 Smith Street
Athens, Georgia 30601

Dear Mrs. Doe:

Listed below is a summary of the contract that we made in our last treatment session. These instructions apply on a *daily* basis for the next 2 weeks.

1. *Every day* choose one "daily reward" for yourself from the following list. The one you choose should be something that you really want to do or have that day.
   a. crocheting
   b. television
   c. reading a magazine or watching a video
   d. writing letters
   e. soaking in bathtub

2. Spend 15 minutes with Michael practicing the skills you learned (attending and rewarding compliance and appropriate behavior, using time out for noncompliance). *Time yourself with a clock.* Remember to *wear your behavior counter* and count attends and rewards on one channel and the number of times you use time out with Michael on the second channel.

3. If you give at least four attends and rewards each minute that Michael is not in time out (if he wasn't in time out at all, that would be a total of 60) *and* if you use time out every time Michael disobeys you after a warning, then give yourself your daily reward. *Remember*, if you do not spend the 15 minutes practicing or do not meet the criteria just presented, you should *not* give yourself your daily reward.

4. Call the voicemail number every day after your parenting session. State your name and provide the following information:
   a. Whether you had the 15-minute practice period with Michael.
   b. The number of attends and rewards you gave.
   c. Whether you used time out each time Michael disobeyed your warning.
   d. The number of times you used time out.
   e. If you met the criteria described above, name your daily reward and whether you gave it to yourself.

Thank you for your continued cooperation.

Sincerely,

Karen C. Wells, PhD

FIGURE 8.1. Sample letter sent to parent for first 2-week period.

ent perception measures, it also results in higher levels of parental satisfaction and/or maintenance of satisfaction with the parent training program (see Chapter 10).

In light of the potential benefits to be derived from this approach, we developed a variation of the HNC parent training program in which parents not only are taught the parenting skills but are given extensive background in the social learning principles on which the skills are based. It is important to note that the "basic" parent training program described in this book is based on, and utilizes, social learning principles. However, parental exposure to formal instruction in these principles is relatively limited (see Chapters 6 and 7). The social learning principles training component that is outlined in this chapter represents both a more systematic and more extensive presentation of the principles than is employed in the basic parent training program. These principles include the hypothesis that most social behavior is learned; the characteristics, rules, types, and schedules of reinforcement; shaping; reciprocity; negative reinforcement; extinction; and punishment. The principles are described to the extent that they are consonant with the general framework of the parent training program. Thus, in many cases, the additional material elaborates on issues that are already covered in the basic parent training program.

Instruction in social learning principles occurs via both didactic instruction by the therapist and brief reading assignments. The material for both types of instruction was selected from several behavioral parenting manuals. Specific reading assignments were drawn from the following sources: *Living with Children* (Patterson, 1976), *Families: Applications of Social Learning to Family Life* (Patterson, 1975), *Parents Are Teachers: A Child Management Program* (Becker, 1971, 1975), and *Parent Manual on Child Rearing* (Wittes & Radin, 1968). Since we developed the social learning principles adjunctive treatment a number of years ago, the reading assignments are from books published prior to 1980. Most of these books (Becker, 1971; Patterson, 1975, 1976) are still available from Research Press, P.O. Box 9127, Champaign, IL 61826; *www.researchpress.com*. More recently published books for parents that describe social learning-based parenting skills may also be consulted for appropriate reading assignments. Examples include *Parenting the Strong-Willed Child* (Forehand & Long, 2002), *Your Defiant Child* (Barkley & Benton, 1998), *The Incredible Years: A Trouble-Shooting Guide for Parents of Children Aged 3–8* (Webster-Stratton, 1992), and *Preventive Parenting with Love, Encouragement, and Limits: The Preschool Years* (Dishion & Patterson, 1996). Didactic instruction by the therapist is closely based on the material in the reading assignments, as well as drawn from other sources (Glogower & Sloop, 1976; Miller, 1975).

Instruction in specific social learning principles typically precedes training in the use of a particular technique. The reading assignments are distributed to the parent at the end of the session prior to the session in which the material is to be discussed. Relevant points from both sources are reiterated throughout the training as the skills are being applied. For example, the material concerning extinction is repeated and integrated into the teaching of the ignoring skill. To ensure that the parent is, in fact, learning these principles, he or she is required to meet specific criteria at three points in the parent training program: following the presentation of the rationale, following the presentation of the social learning principles appropriate for Phase I, and following the principles appropriate for Phase II. The criterion measurements are objective tests on which the parent is required to provide correct responses to at least 95% of the items. The parent is given three trials on which to do so. Based on a content analysis of the incorrectly answered items, the therapist provides further instruction in the relevant principles and then readministers the incorrectly answered items. The number of trials to criterion is noted by the therapist. It has been our experience that three trials are sufficient for all parents to meet the criterion; most parents do so in one or two trials. The Social Learning Criterion Tests are based on the didactic material and reading assignments. Specific items were drawn from previously published tests of social learning material and the reading assignments (Becker, 1971, 1975; Clement, as noted in Glogower & Sloop, 1976; Patterson et al., 1975) or were formulated by the first author (RJM). The Social Learning Criterion Tests and scoring keys are presented in Appendix C.

The reading assignments and didactic material for each of the major sections of the parent training program ("Rationale," "Phase I: Differential Attention," "Phase II: Compliance Training") are described below. The points at which this didactic material and the Social Learning Criterion Tests are introduced into the basic parent training program are noted by referring to the description of the assessment feedback session and the outline of the program presented in Chapter 5 (also see Figure 5.1). With respect to the reading assignments, the therapist should stress the importance of reading the assignments *before* coming to the next session, since these assignments form the basis of the upcoming didactic presentation. If the parent fails to complete the assignment, the therapist has the option of either postponing the session or having the parent read the assignment before the session begins.

Because of the additional reading assignments and didactic material, some minor changes in the usual sequencing and presentation of material are suggested. The most significant modification is that the rationale for the parent training program, which is typically presented in the assessment feedback session, would now be presented at the beginning of the first treatment session. This shift is necessary because, as currently configured, we present the rationale *prior* to the parent's decision to participate in the parent training program. A brief rationale for the parent training program can still be provided in the assessment feedback session, but the more elaborate version presented in this chapter would be presented to the parent at the beginning of the first treatment session. The therapist may choose to present both the rationale and the introduction to Phase I in the first session or split this information into two separate sessions.

Rationale

Reading Assignments

The initial reading assignments should be provided to the parent prior to the first treatment session. The assignments can be mailed, or the parent can pick them up from the clinic a day or two prior to the first treatment session. Both assignments provide an introduction to social learning. (Numbers in brackets refer to the order in which the assignments should be read.)

1. *Living with Children* (Patterson, 1976, pp. 3–5, items 1–7 [1]).
2. *Families: Applications of Social Learning to Family Life* (Patterson, 1975, pp. 5–7 [2]).

Didactic Material

The following material should be presented in Session 1 as an elaboration of the rationale usually given for the program (presented in Chapter 5, pp. 87–91, "Providing the Rationale" and in Figure 5.1, "Rationale of program" under "IV. Recommendations for intervention," p. 82).

I. Social learning. (This is an elaboration of "Behavior is learned and can be changed," Figure 5.1, p. 82.)
   A. Most behavior is learned (Wittes & Radin, 1968).
      1. People learn their behavior from other people.
      2. People teach, train, and change one another's behaviors.
      3. Parents and teachers teach, train, and change children.
      4. Adults teach, train, and change other adults (e.g., husbands teach wives and vice versa).
      5. Children teach, train, and change their parents!
   B. Social learning is concerned with how people teach people.
   C. It is important that you know how your behavior relates to and influences your child's behavior and how your child's behavior affects your behavior.
      1. People are often unaware of why they behave as they do.
      2. Both prosocial ("OK") and problem ("not OK") behaviors are learned.
   D. Most people, *except parents*, are usually trained for the jobs at which they work. Parents are just expected to know how to raise their children successfully.
      1. We think parents should have the opportunity to learn to use some of the methods that have been developed for teaching children.
      2. Parents can learn how to establish behaviors in their children that will bring them success in school and in life. You do not have to trust to fate or to your instincts to develop successful behaviors in your children.
   E. We will make use of social learning principles to help your child learn appropriate behaviors.
II. Potential negative effects of an overreliance on punishment. (This is an elaboration of "Decreasing noncompliance directly through punishment," p. 82.)
   A. Extensive punishment sets up escape/avoidance behaviors that may be more harmful than the behavior being punished (Wittes & Radin, 1968).
   B. Extensive punishment establishes emotional reactions, such as anxiety, for the child (Wittes & Radin, 1968).

C. Punishment may also make you feel guilty or upset if you punished because of anger or frustration.

D. Punishment will probably reduce noncompliance for a while, but we have found that the behavior is likely to reappear shortly after punishment occurs.

    1. Punishment does not eliminate your child's motivation for engaging in a behavior (so when an opportunity next presents itself, the "not OK" behavior will reoccur).

    2. For punishment to be effective, the behavior has to be punished every time. This is impossible (since you are not with your child every second), so the behavior actually gets stronger. (We will explain exactly how this occurs later in the program.)

E. Punishment loses its effectiveness with frequent and continued use, so more and more severe punishments are required.

F. If physical punishment is overused, you may provide a model of aggression for your child.

G. You become less effective as a parent for the following reasons:

    1. Your value as a positive influence on your child decreases, since you are always associated with punishment.

      a. Your child will avoid you.

      b. We also know that persons in the family who give out the most punishment typically receive the most punishment in return.

    2. Your control through punishment weakens as the punishment loses its effectiveness through too much use.

Social Learning Criterion

The Social Learning Criterion, Rationale Test (see Appendix C) should be administered after the rationale of the program (Chapter 5, "Providing the Rationale," pp. 87–91, and in Figure 5.1, "Rationale of program" under "IV. Recommendations for intervention," p. 82) has been presented in Session 1 (per the change noted above). The parent should be told that the purpose of the test is to make sure that the principles are understood before the program continues. The therapist should state that it is not a test, per se, but rather a way for him or her to determine which areas should receive the most attention.

Phase I

Reading Assignments

These materials should be distributed to the parent prior to the session in which the rationale and overview of Phase I are presented (Session 1, "II. Phase I," Chapter 5, p. 92). The reading materials discuss characteristics, rules, types, and schedules of positive reinforcement, reciprocity, and the "criticism trap."

1. *Parents Are Teachers: A Child Management Program* (Becker, 1971, pp. 35–41 [3]; 85–88 [7]; Unit 6 Review Sheet [8]). Assignment 8 is from Becker's (1975) *Review Tests for Parents Are Teachers.*
2. *Living with Children* (Patterson, 1976, pp. 25–26, items 1–6, p. 29 [5]; pp. 31–37, items 1, 3–6, 11–31 [6]).
3. *Parent Manual on Child Rearing* (Wittes & Radin, 1968, pp. 7–10 [4]).

Didactic Material

This should be presented at the beginning of Phase I (Session 1, "II. Phase I," Chapter 5, p. 92).

I. All behavior is maintained, changed, or shaped by the effects (consequences) of the behavior.
   A. These consequences either strengthen (reward or reinforce) or weaken the behavior.
   B. To strengthen a behavior, reinforce or reward it.
   C. A behavior can be weakened by no longer reinforcing it.
II. Based on the Positive Reinforcement Rule and the Attention Rule ("II.A.2. Explain two assumptions on which Phase I is based"), the following are critical to improving your child's behavior.
   A. Focus on strengthening a desirable ("OK") behavior that is likely to be rewarding to your child and that, at the same time, will compete with the undesirable ("not OK") behavior that you are weakening and which will eventually take its place (the child cannot do both behaviors at the same time).
   B. If you pay attention to your child when he or she is being good (i.e., compliant), then it is more likely that your child will engage in that behavior more frequently.
   C. At the same time, if you do not give your child attention (i.e., if your child is ignored) when he or she is engaging in "not OK" behavior, then these "not OK" behaviors are not as likely to occur in the future and will eventually stop.
      1. Extinction (ignoring) is the one method that eventually eliminates a behavior completely, since the child learns that there is absolutely no payoff for engaging in the behavior.
      2. For ignoring to be effective, the parent must ignore the behavior every time it occurs.
      3. *Therapist note:* When the parent first starts to ignore, there may be an initial burst of inappropriate behavior.
         a. This is normal, as the child is testing limits.
         b. The parent must be consistent.
   D. The opposite is also true.
      1. Paying attention to your child (watching, discussing, smiling, yelling, nagging, criticizing, etc.) when she or he is displaying "not OK" behavior will make that behavior more likely to occur in the future.

    a. We all frequently reward "not OK" behavior accidentally/unintentionally by occasionally "giving in" (paying attention to it), even though we "know better." This occasional reinforcement will cause the behavior to persist.

    b. Children do the same thing to us (they do not intend to reinforce us for scolding, but this happens when we scold since they stop the "not OK" behavior briefly).

    c. This situation is called the "criticism trap" (Becker, 1971, 1975), since the parent thinks criticism (negative attention such as scolding, nagging, etc.) is effective because the child stops the "not OK" behavior for a while. Thus, the parent uses criticism whenever possible. However, by paying attention to "not OK" behavior, this makes it more likely that the child will misbehave again.

    d. The end result is that home is not a very pleasant place, since the parent must always be ready with scolding, nagging, or criticizing.

  2. If you ignore (i.e., do not reinforce) your child when he or she is being good, you will get less "OK" behavior.

    a. Some old adages do *not* apply.

      (1) The child is "supposed to know" which behaviors are appropriate; therefore, he or she is expected to engage in those behaviors. But the only way the child knows whether to engage in a behavior is if that behavior has been reinforced in the past.

      (2) "Leave well enough alone" and "Let sleeping dogs lie" will only result in the "OK" behavior eventually disappearing.

    b. One adage does apply: "Catch your child being good" (Becker, 1971). Too often we tend to take "OK" behavior for granted.

  E. *Therapist note:* Use both positive and negative examples from the parent's and child's in-session behavior or from parent-report data to illustrate the role of parental attention in influencing the child's behavior.

  F. Once you realize how you are reinforcing your child, you can start to weaken "not OK" behavior and strengthen socially desirable "OK" behavior.

III. The following are characteristics of positive reinforcement. (This represents an elaboration of Session 4, "II.B. Learning to reward," presented on p. 94.) The ultimate goal of parental reinforcement is for the "OK" child behaviors that are reinforced to eventually become self-reinforcing to the child. In this way, your child will develop control over his or her own behavior.

  A. Be *specific*—tell your child exactly what behavior you are reinforcing (you will use attends and labeled rewards to do this).

  B. Reinforcement should follow *immediately* after "OK" behavior. If delayed, then it is possible that some other child behavior (which may be "OK" or "not OK") will be reinforced.

  C. Shaping (successive approximations) is useful when dealing with complex behaviors.

    1. When the child is learning a new behavior (particularly a complicated

one), he or she should be reinforced for each small step along the way that approximates the goal rather than as a prize at the very end.

2. If the task is too large, the child may have to wait too long for reinforcement.

3. Shaping sets the child up for success, since the child is being reinforced for trying and for improvements toward the goal.

4. Shaping can also establish work habits and responsibilities for later, since the child will learn to keep trying until he or she has mastered a task.

5. Shaping requires patience, since it is often easier in the short run for the parent to do a task for the child. However, in the long run, this may make the child dependent.

D. Reinforcement can be continuous (continuous reinforcement) or only occasional (intermittent reinforcement).

1. Continuous reinforcement is given every time the behavior occurs.

a. It is an excellent procedure for starting or strengthening a behavior.

b. Changes in behavior are more likely to occur if reinforcement is *consistent*. The behavior must be reinforced more than one time.

2. Intermittent reinforcement follows continuous reinforcement success.

a. It is given occasionally after the behavior occurs and in an unpredictable manner.

b. It is excellent for maintaining a behavior once the behavior is well established since it is very resistant to extinction.

c. Intermittent reinforcement applies to negative behaviors as well. If you *occasionally* pay attention to "not OK" behavior, then this behavior is strengthened and is stronger than if you reinforced it every time.

3. A short summary of positive reinforcement follows.

a. In the early stages of learning a task, reinforce every correct response.

b. As the behavior becomes stronger, require more and more correct responses before reinforcing (gradually shift to unpredictable intermittent reinforcement).

c. "To get it going, reward every time. To keep it going, reward intermittently" (Becker, 1971, p. 38).

E. Social reinforcers are in contrast to material reinforcers.

1. There are two general types of rewards, social and material (nonsocial).

a. Social reinforcers involve the parent's behavior (saying or doing something to the child).

b. Material reinforcers involve such things as money, tokens, privileges, candy, and the like.

2. Social reinforcers are more versatile than material reinforcers.

a. Social reinforcers are always available as immediate consequences of "OK" behavior, while this is not necessarily the case with material reinforcers.

b. Social reinforcers are useful for starting *and* critical for maintaining

"OK" behavior, while material reinforcers are not as effective in maintaining "OK" behavior.

   c. We have an endless supply of social reinforcers, but this is not the case with material reinforcers (e.g., money).

   d. Social reinforcers are what the child can expect to find in the real world as reinforcement for social behavior.

F. Appropriate reinforcers must be employed.

   1. It is very important that the reinforcer the parent uses is, in fact, reinforcing to the child.

   2. The reinforcer should also be of appropriate magnitude for the particular behavior.

      a. If the reinforcer is too large, the child will become tired of it quickly (satiation), and it will no longer serve as a reinforcer.

      b. If the reinforcer is too small, it will not motivate the child to change the behavior.

G. Reciprocity refers to the idea that, in terms of interactions among family members, "You get what you give" (Patterson, 1975, p. 20).

   1. It is not just children who are taught by reinforcement. Children influence parents' behavior as well.

      a. The criticism trap is one example.

      b. Children also influence adult behavior by positive reinforcement.

   2. Everyone (adults as well as children) has to receive at least a minimal amount of social reinforcement. If you do not, you will probably become depressed.

      a. Many parents are in this situation since they may get little or no social reinforcement from their child or spouse (they may be divorced, spouse may be too busy with job, etc.).

      b. If a parent is not getting much social reinforcement, that parent is not likely to *give* it to a child or spouse.

   3. The following points are made in summary of the idea of reciprocity.

      a. The person in the family who gives the most reinforcement/punishment receives the most reinforcement/punishment.

      b. To receive a positive input from another family member, you have to give one first.

      c. If you give a negative input to another family member, then you should expect one in return. Unfortunately, this is much more likely to be reciprocated than a positive input (Miller, 1975).

Social Learning Criterion

The Social Learning Criterion, Phase I Test should be administered at the conclusion of the preceding didactic material. The test and scoring key are in Appendix C.

Phase II

Reading Assignments

The materials are distributed at the end of the last complete session of Phase I. The reading assignments discuss the potential negative effects of punishment, how to use effective punishment, and indications for its use.

1. *Parent Manual on Child Rearing* (Wittes & Radin, 1968, pp. 15–18 [9]).
2. *Parents Are Teachers: A Child Management Program* (Becker, 1971, pp. 121–128 [10]).

Didactic Material

"I. Clear instructions and shaping" is presented in Phase II during training in how to give clear instructions (Session 6, "V.C.2. State the instruction clearly," p. 97). The remaining didactic material is presented when introducing Path C to the parent (Session 8, "VI. Introduce Path C," p. 100).

I. Clear instructions and shaping
   A. If the behavior you desire is relatively complex, break it down into the smaller units or steps necessary to achieve that behavior. Remember, we talked about shaping (successive approximations) by reinforcement? The same applies here.
   B. Examples at home include the following:
      1. Rather than say "Pick up all the toys," say "Put the three blocks in the box" or "Put the cars in the box" and the like.
      2. Rather than say "Make your bed," say "Pull the sheet up first," "Now pull the blanket up," and so forth.
II. Effective punishment
   A. Punishment is an event that occurs following a behavior; it weakens the future rate of the behavior (Becker, 1971, p. 121). It involves the presentation of negative consequences or the withdrawal of reinforcers.
   B. As noted earlier, punishment is not the preferred mode of interacting with the child. Briefly review the potential negative effects of punishment (see Becker, 1971, pp. 126–127).
   C. Use of punishment per se is not immoral. There are times that punishment *is* necessary and is the most appropriate action to take.
      1. Punishment is appropriate in an emergency to save the child from danger (e.g., in careless crossing of the street) (Wittes & Radin, 1968).
      2. When the inappropriate behavior is so frequent that there is not any "OK" behavior to reinforce, punishment may be necessary.
      3. When reinforcement will not be effective because it is less pleasurable for the child than the "not OK" behavior in which he or she is engaging, punishment may be needed (Wittes & Radin, 1968).

    D. Generally, however, punishment should be used as little as possible.

    E. Most of the rules regarding effective punishment are similar to those for reinforcement. Effective punishment (Becker, 1971, p. 127) is characterized by the following conditions:

       1. Is given immediately.

       2. Relies on taking away reinforcers and provides a clear-cut method for earning them back.

       3. Includes a verbal warning signal. This eventually serves as a cue and helps the child develop internal controls so that external controls like punishment are needed much less often.

       4. Is carried out in a calm, matter-of-fact way.

       5. Is given along with much reinforcement of behaviors incompatible with the punished behavior.

       6. Is consistent. The procedure is carried out the same way each time, and reinforcement is not given for the punished behavior. Remember, if you are not consistent, you may end up making the behavior worse.

  III. The punishment procedure we recommend and which you will learn here is called TO, which is short for "time out from positive reinforcement."

Social Learning Criterion

The Social Learning Criterion, Phase II Test should be administered at the conclusion of the preceding didactic material. The test and scoring key are presented in Appendix C.

PARENT ENHANCEMENT THERAPY

As noted in Chapter 1, there is evidence that various family-related issues, such as the parent's perception of a child's behavior, the parent's personal adjustment and marital satisfaction, and the parent's extrafamilial relationships, are associated with child behavior problems. In some cases, these family-related issues may inhibit the effectiveness of behavioral parent training programs (Chapter 5). Griest and colleagues (1982) added a Parent Enhancement Therapy (PET) adjunct to the HNC parent training program to determine whether it would enhance treatment outcome and generalization. This adjunct contained interventions designed to address four different areas: parents' perceptions of the child's behavior, parents' personal adjustment, marital adjustment, and parents' extrafamilial relationships. The premise of this adjunctive intervention was that every parent plays a tripartite role that consists of being a parent, a spouse, and an individual, and that the three roles are integrally interrelated. Training consisted of didactic presentations, modeling, role playing, and homework assignments. Components of the PET package were presented prior to, during, and after the standard parent training program. The sequence of components is presented in Table 8.1.

**TABLE 8.1. Sequence of Parent Enhancement
Therapy Components**

<u>Prior to Phase I</u>
- Parental perceptions/expectations about their child's behavior
  - Increase awareness of positive child behavior
  - Develop realistic expectations about the child
- Parent's personal adjustment
  - Cognitive restructuring for depressive symptoms

<u>Between Phase I and Phase II</u>
- Parent's marital adjustment
  - Spouse–partner communication

<u>After Completion of Parent Training</u>
- Parent's marital adjustment (cont.)
  - Spouse–partner problem solving
  - Increasing pleasant activities
- Parent's extrafamilial relationships
  - Identification of sources of positive support outside the family
  - Increasing positive support outside the family

Included in the enhancement therapy were several modules to assist parents in developing realistic expectations about their children. The first module had parents list positive and negative aspects of their child. The purpose of this exercise was to help parents realize that their child, although noncompliant, had positive, as well as the typically identified negative, aspects to his or her behavior. A second module had parents list current expectations for their child. Parents then were asked to consider each expectation in terms of whether it was realistic or unrealistic. Information in the module outlined how parents could have unrealistically high expectations for a child, which would frustrate the child because of constant failure. On the other hand, it was pointed out that parental expectations could be too low, which could lead to the child not learning age-appropriate behaviors. Parents also were given handouts concerning problem behaviors that are developmentally normal at particular ages (e.g., enuresis at 1½ years of age, temper tantrums at age 2) and a chart of developmental norms for children at different ages.

With respect to the parents' personal adjustment, we included a module on cognitive restructuring for depressive symptoms. Parents were given information about how negative thoughts usually intercede between an event and emotion. Various types of negative thoughts (e.g., catastrophizing, overgeneralizing, personalizing) were delineated, and it was shown how these can relate to depressive symptoms. Procedures for combating negative thoughts (e.g., debating with one's self and offering a new explanation) were presented.

The PET adjunct also included a component focusing on marital adjustment. This component consisted of three modules on the enhancement of communication, problem-solving skills, and pleasant activities engaged in by spouses. Improvement of communication skills involved accurately tracking what your partner is saying, emphasizing with and reflecting what your partner is saying, and verbally praising your partner. Problem-solving skills included defining the problem, discussing one problem at a time, making sure both spouses understand the problem, brainstorming solutions, and reaching a solution. Pleasant activities involved the two spouses spending time together several times each week in an activity enjoyed by both of them.

The final component of the PET adjunct involved assisting parents in reducing stress and enhancing positive interactions outside the home for themselves and, specifically, for their parenting behavior. The therapist helped parents identify people with whom they had primarily positive interactions. The importance of increasing interactions with these individuals was stressed. Parents were also told ways to enlist the support of friends and the extended family in parenting (e.g., to enlist a friend's help in dealing with the child, to explain parenting principles the parent has learned).

TOWARD THE DEVELOPMENT OF A SELF-ADMINISTERED VERSION OF THE HNC PARENT TRAINING PROGRAM

For the past 30 years there has been an abundance of parent training interventions that can be totally or partially self-administered and that require little, if any, professional consultation (McMahon & Forehand, 1980, 1981; Taylor & Biglan, 1998). These programs are usually in the form of written materials (i.e., books, brochures), although videotapes, audiotapes, and computer software are becoming increasingly popular (e.g., MacKenzie & Hilgedick, 1999; Webster-Stratton, 1990a). The primary advantage of self-administered materials is that they enable therapists to extend their services to a greater number of individuals with minimal increments in professional time. Self-administered materials can be an important component of a multilevel system of intervention, either as stand-alone interventions or as a component of a more intensive intervention (Sanders & Dadds, 1993).

In this section, we describe both a narrowly focused brochure for dealing with a specific child behavior problem (i.e., inappropriate mealtime behavior) and a broad-based book for parents that presents and expands upon the HNC parent training program.

Improving Children's Mealtime Behavior

It may be beneficial to develop self-administered materials for specific problems and settings within the home. Also, by delivering parent training materials directly to the home, the issue of setting generality (i.e., from the clinic to the home) is eliminated.

Early on, we developed and evaluated a written brochure to teach parents to improve their children's mealtime behavior (McMahon & Forehand, 1978). The purpose of such an intervention was to serve as a prototype for dealing with situations in which a full parenting program may not be necessary, because the child's noncompliant behavior is limited to specific situations. If parents can read and effectively implement the intervention, then therapist contact will not be necessary (McMahon & Forehand, 1980, 1981). The importance of mealtime as an opportunity for the child to learn social, interactional, and cultural values has long been stressed (Dreyer & Dreyer, 1973; Finney, 1986). However, preschool-aged children often engage in high levels of problematic behavior at mealtime, including noncompliance, messy table behavior, leaving the table, and excessive demands for attention (Beautrais, Fergusson, & Shannon, 1982; Sanders, Patel, Le Grice, & Shepherd, 1993). Furthermore, coercive parent behaviors are associated with such problem mealtime behaviors (Sanders et al., 1993).

The brochure describing the program for mealtime behaviors is presented in Appendix D. A slight variation of this program was demonstrated by McMahon and Forehand (1978) to be effective with nonreferred children when used alone (i.e., with no therapist–client contact) (see Chapter 10). The program can be used as a supplement to the parent training program or can be used independently of the program in situations where the assessment procedures (see Chapter 4) indicate no problems in parent–child interactions except in this particular circumscribed situation.

Based on the approach that we employed for developing the mealtime brochure, our colleague Nicholas Long has developed similar brochures for numerous other behavior problems displayed by preschool children (e.g., tantrums, bedtime, dressing). (They are available at *www.parenting-ed.org*, in the "Parenting Handouts" section.) Similar materials have been developed and evaluated by Sloane and his colleagues (e.g., Gmeinder & Kratochwill, 1998; Sloane, Endo, Hawkes, & Jenson, 1990).

A Broad-Based Book for Parents of Young Children

The second author (RLF) and Nicholas Long have written a book titled *Parenting the Strong-Willed Child: The Clinically Proven Five-Week Program for Parents of Two- to Six-Year-Olds* (Forehand & Long, 1996, 2002). This book, which is intended for parents, consists of four sections. The first section explains the factors that cause or contribute to children's noncompliant behavior, as well as the differential diagnosis of ADHD and noncompliant behavior. The second section describes an adaptation of the HNC parent training program. The five primary skills (attends, rewards, ignoring, clear instructions, and TO) are presented to parents in the context of a self-administered program that is designed to be conducted over a 5-week period. Similar to the clinical version of the program, there is extensive emphasis on parental practice of the skills with the child on a daily basis and demonstrated mastery of a parenting skill before moving on to the next skill. The third section of the book focuses on ways in which parents can develop a more positive family atmosphere. The goal is to enhance and maintain the positive behavior changes that have occurred as a function of the 5-week parenting skills program. Topics include how to make interactions in the home more positive, improve communication skills, enhance children's self-esteem, develop greater patience in dealing with children, and help children deal with peer-related problems. In the fourth section, strategies for managing specific behavior problems (e.g., temper tantrums, bedtime and sleep problems, aggression, dressing problems, and sibling rivalry) are discussed.

As of this writing, the effectiveness of the Forehand and Long (2002) book as a self-administered intervention has not been evaluated. However, ongoing research is examining the effects of a parent group intervention based on the book (see Chapter 10). In addition, a pilot study described in Chapter 10 suggests that a self-guided written booklet explaining the HNC parenting skills may be effective in reducing the parent-reported intensity of oppositional behavior displayed by children with ADHD (Long, Rickart, & Ashcraft, 1993).

CHAPTER 9

Adaptations for Specific Populations

KAREN C. WELLS

In this chapter, the focus is on adaptations of the basic parent training program for special populations. The populations include children with ADHD, children who are abused and neglected, children with developmental disabilities, children with enuresis or encopresis, and children in inpatient settings. Adaptations to the program related to adherence to medical regimens are also presented.

Since its original development by Hanf and modification and evaluation by Forehand and his colleagues, the HNC parent training program has been adapted by a number of clinical researchers and applied in part or in whole to a variety of special child populations. It is the purpose of this chapter to present an overview of the literature on those special populations and the adaptations to the original HNC program that have been mandated by the unique characteristics and needs of those populations. Because the most systematic body of clinical adaptation and research with special populations has involved children with ADHD, this chapter will focus most heavily on that population. However, adaptations for other special populations (i.e., abused and neglected children, children with developmental disabilities, children with enuresis or encopresis, children in inpatient settings) and situations (i.e., adherence to medical regimens) will be discussed as well.

Karen C. Wells, PhD, is an Associate Professor of Medical Psychology in the Departments of Psychiatry and Behavioral Sciences and Psychology–Social and Health Sciences at Duke University, Durham, NC.

ATTENTION-DEFICIT/HYPERACTIVITY DISORDER

ADHD is a heterogeneous behavioral disorder of uncertain etiology (Conners & Erhardt, 1998). As its sobriquet suggests, ADHD is characterized by "inattention and/or hyperactivity–impulsivity that is more frequent and severe than is typically observed in individuals at a comparable level of development" (American Psychiatric Association, 2000). In the current version of the DSM, there are three subtypes of the disorder: primarily inattentive, primarily hyperactive–impulsive, and combined. The inattentive subtype refers to children who primarily display distractible and inattentive behavior resulting in maladaptation. The hyperactive–impulsive subtype refers to children who primarily display fidgety, hyperactive, and impulsive motor behaviors resulting in maladaptation. The combined subtype represents children who display impairments in both arenas.

The disorder typically begins in early childhood and lasts into adulthood in a substantial subset of cases. It frequently leads to social and academic impairments (Klein & Mannuzza, 1991). One-third of adults diagnosed in childhood continue to exhibit the full set of symptoms, albeit in somewhat altered form, and as many as 60% continue to have at least one significant impairing symptom (Weiss & Hechtman, 1994).

Prevalence rates for ADHD in children are roughly 5–7% in community samples and substantially higher in clinic samples. Rates of physician office diagnosis of ADHD have doubled from 1993 to 1997, probably reflecting an increase in educationally based referrals after the disorder became recognized as eligible under the category of "Other Health Impaired" under section 504 of the Individuals with Disabilities Act (Conners & Erhardt, 1998).

As noted in Chapter 1, ADHD is frequently associated with the disruptive behavior disorders of ODD and CD. For example, up to 40% of children and 65% of adolescents with ADHD also display ODD, and up to 30% of children and 50% of adolescents with ADHD also display CD. Individuals with ADHD may also display anxiety, depressive, tic, or learning disorders, either as comorbid disorders or as secondary consequences of the primary disturbances of impulse, attention, and motor control. Some authors believe that these patterns of comorbidity may reflect stable ADHD subgroupings, with correlated differences in natural history, risk factors, and response to treatment (March, Wells, & Conners, 1995).

Rationale for Treatment with Parent Training

Treatment with stimulant medication (e.g., methylphenidate, dextroamphetamine, pemoline) is by far the most common treatment for ADHD. In a meta review-of-reviews, Swanson (1993) found several thousand published studies supporting the efficacy of stimulant medication in ADHD. Nevertheless, medication does not always ameliorate associated problems such as oppositional defiant behavior, other aggressive behavior, poor peer relations, deficient problem-solving skills, or academic underachievement, nor does it sufficiently "normalize" the behavior of children with ADHD. Likewise, despite the results of large group outcome studies, some children are not helped by stimulant medications or have unacceptable side effects that prevent their use for the particular child. Some parents object to the use of medication and reject this treatment. Finally, even for children who are effectively treated with stimulant medication during the school day, parents must manage these children in the afternoon, evenings, weekends, and/or summers when they may not take medication. Therefore, the search has continued for other primary or adjunctive treatments for the child with ADHD (Wells, 1987; Wells et al., 2000).

The extension of parent training to populations with ADHD began in the early 1980s. This extension seems to be based on several areas of research. Many studies have documented the disturbed and conflictual nature of parent–child interactions in families with a child with ADHD. These studies have shown that, especially in high-demand, task-oriented situations, children with ADHD are less compliant to their parents' instructions, sustain their compliance for shorter time periods, are less likely to remain on task, and display more "negative" behavior than their normal same-age counterparts. In what Johnston (1996b) has labeled a "negative–reactive" response pattern, mothers and fathers of children with ADHD display more directive, commanding behavior; more disapproval; fewer contingent rewards for prosocial and compliant behaviors; and more general negative behavior than the parents of normal children (Barkley, Karlsson, & Pollard, 1985; Befera & Barkley, 1985; Cunningham & Barkley, 1979; Mash & Johnston, 1982; Tallmadge & Barkley, 1983).

While disrupted parent–child interaction probably does not cause ADHD, it may play a primary role in the development, escalation, and maintenance of the oppositional and aggressive behavior that is characteristic of ODD and CD and that often accompanies ADHD. Furthermore Barkley (1998b) has suggested that the high rates of noncompliance displayed by children with ADHD are indicative of a deficit in rule-governed behavior that may be manifested by appearing not to listen, to fail to initiate and follow through on instructions, and to be poor at adhering to task directions. These findings suggest that intervening in parent–child interactions of children with ADHD is important.

In addition, research has shown that family dysfunction and the co-occurrence of conduct problem behavior are among the most robust predictors for poor adult outcomes for individuals with ADHD diagnosed in childhood (Fischer, Barkley, Fletcher, & Smallish, 1993; Taylor, Sandberg, Thorley, & Giles, 1991). Since parent training attempts to change family processes that are directly associated with child conduct problems, it theoretically may be associated with reduction in long-term risk for these individuals (although this has not yet been demonstrated empirically).

ADAPTATIONS OF PARENT TRAINING FOR ADHD

Although a number of clinical researchers have employed parent training with families of children with ADHD, the investigators most associated with adapting this particular parent training program for this population are Russell Barkley (e.g., Anastopoulos, Smith, & Wien, 1998; Barkley, 1998a) and Wells and colleagues (1996). Barkley developed an intervention involving 11 steps, whereas the latter group of investigators developed an extended, 27-session parent training program, based on the program described in this volume, for the Multimodal Treatment Study for ADHD (MTA). The MTA is a large, multisite study of multimodal treatment for ADHD (including parent training) and the largest treatment trial ever funded by the National Institute of Mental Health (Arnold et al., 1997; Richters et al., 1995).

As noted in Chapter 2, Barkley and Forehand both trained with Constance Hanf at the Oregon Health Sciences University and learned the basic parent training program from her. Although Forehand and his colleagues conducted the basic research on the empirical validity of the program with noncompliant children, Barkley, because of his general interest in the field of ADHD, initially adapted the program to the ADHD population. The MTA parent training program (Wells et al., 1996, 2000) incorporated many of Barkley's adaptations, but embellished and extended his basic program, as will be described later.

Barkley's Adaptation

The fundamental parent training program for ADHD, as described by Barkley (Anastopoulos et al., 1998; Barkley, 1998a), involves 11 steps (see Table 9.1) that are administered over the course of 8–12 sessions (although more sessions may be necessary depending on the speed with which parents can learn and incorporate steps). Adaptations to the basic parent training program include: (1) a review of information on ADHD; (2) a focus on the child's independent play as a target behavior; (3) teaching parents to become sensitive to the limits that their child's short attention span can place on compliance to task-related instructions; (4) teaching parents to repeat an instruction so the parent is sure the child attended to it; (5) setting up a home token system; and (6) setting up a home-based reinforcement system for behavior at school.

TABLE 9.1. Barkley's Training Program for Parents of Children with ADHD

Session	Content
1	Review of information on ADHD
2	Causes of oppositional defiant behavior
3	Developing and enhancing parental attention
4	Attending to child compliance and independent play
5	Establishing a home token economy
6	Implementing time out for noncompliance
7	Extending time out to additional noncompliant behaviors
8	Managing noncompliance in public places
9	Improving child school behavior from home: The Daily School Behavior Report Card
10	Managing future misconduct
11	One-month review/booster session

Note. From Barkley (1998a). Copyright 1998 by The Guilford Press. Reprinted by permission.

MTA *Parent Training Program*

The parent training intervention (Wells et al., 1996, 2000) used in the MTA study of multimodal treatment for ADHD (Arnold et al., 1997; Richters et al., 1995) is a 27-session treatment that incorporates adaptations of the 8–12 session basic parent training program described in this volume and by Barkley (Anastopoulos et al., 1998; Barkley, 1998a), but extends well beyond the basic program (see Table 9.2).

TABLE 9.2. MTA Group Parent Training Program for Children with ADHD

Session	Content
	Intensive Treatment Phase
1	Structured Clinical Interview, Review of ADHD, and Introduction to Treatment
2	Setting Up School/Home Daily Report Card
3	Overview of Social Learning and Behavior Management Principles and Review of Daily Report Card
4	Attending and "Special Playtime"
5	Rewarding and Ignoring Skills in "Special Playtime" and "Catch Your Child Being Good"
6	Using Positive Skills and Premack Principle to Increase Targets: "Catch Your Child Being Good" and Independent Play
7	Giving Effective Commands to Children, Establishing Behavior Rules, and Attending and Rewarding Compliance to Instructions
8	Time-Out Procedure
9	Home Token Economy 1
10	Home Token Economy 2
11	Response Cost
12	Planned Activities Training and Setting Generalization
13	Stress, Anger, and Mood Management 1
14	Stress, Anger, and Mood Management 2
15	Peer Programming in Home and School
16	Preparing for the New School Year
17	Parent Skills for Academic/School Support at Home
	Compliance, Generalization, and Integration Phase
18	Review of Attending, Rewarding, and Ignoring Skills; Review of "Special Playtime"
19	Review of Commands, House Rules, and Time Out
20	Review of Home Token Economy and Response Cost
21	Review of Academic Support/Homework Programs at Home
22	Planning for the Second Summer
23	Review of the First Scripted Parent–Teacher Meeting
24	Review of the Second Scripted Parent–Teacher Meeting
25	Review of the Third Scripted Parent–Teacher Meeting
26	A Final Review of the Scripted Parent–Teacher Meetings
27	Preparing Parents to Coordinate Work with the Schools and Problem Solving School Issues

Note. From Wells et al. (2000). Copyright 2000 by Kluwer Academic Publishers. Reprinted by permission.

Adaptations to the TO procedure and dealing with situations outside the home will be presented as examples of adaptations of the basic parent training program. First, due to the attentional deficits and motor fidgetiness of children with ADHD, a manageable duration of TO is utilized that does not exceed the capacity of the child. The rule of thumb is a half-minute for every year of age of the child (e.g., 2½ minutes for a 5-year-old). Second, due to motor fidgetiness, parents are encouraged to ignore minor motor movements of the child while he or she is in the TO chair and to implement the protocol for escape from TO only after the child has walked beyond an imaginary or real boundary that surrounds the chair (e.g., masking tape on the floor that encircles the TO chair). A motorically "driven" child with ADHD may not be able to contain himself or herself while sitting in the chair for several minutes; therefore, standing or moving around beside the chair within the boundary is tolerated.

For many children with ADHD, difficulties with behavior control also extend to difficulty with affect control and regulation. Because of this, children with ADHD will frequently engage in more severe, disruptive, and long-lasting tantrums while in TO than do children with oppositional behavior alone. This eventuality should be predicted by the therapist and extensively role played ahead of time with the parents. The extreme importance of ignoring even these highly aversive and disruptive tantrums while the child is in TO is especially stressed with these parents. Methods for dealing with impulsive, destructive behaviors that may take place while the child is in TO also should be discussed in advance. For example, children who impulsively kick the walls, leaving scuffmarks, should be ignored, if possible, at the moment. The TO procedure should be followed through to completion. Then, an overcorrection procedure can be implemented such that children must obtain a cloth, sponge, and cleaning materials and wash and rewash the wall, making restitution for the destructive behavior. We have also had older children with ADHD spend their own money, earned in the token system, to purchase the cleaning materials or paint necessary to repair the damage. In this way, consequences are brought to bear for the child's impulsive behaviors.

For the child with ADHD, controlling his or her behavior in unfamiliar situations outside of home is especially difficult, as these situations may be filled with highly salient distracters. Therefore, parents are encouraged to use shorter intervals for reinforcement (i.e., the child can earn a point on the index card and praise after every 10 minutes of good behavior on the outing) and to preestablish a highly valued backup reward that is delivered immediately upon completion of the outing if enough points have been earned. Alternatively, points earned on an outing can be added to the home token system as soon as the family returns home. Whereas children with mild behavior problems can usually be managed with social contingencies alone, children with ADHD usually need a very tight reinforcement and behavior control system to manage their behavior in these difficult situations outside of home.

While incorporating all of the basic principles and strategies already described, the MTA parent training program was designed more intensively and comprehensively to address multiple settings and domains of child and family functioning in ADHD. First, great emphasis is placed on intervention in the school setting, where many, if not most, ADHD children display considerable difficulties related to attention deficits and disruptive behavior, even in the absence of specific learning disabilities (Conners & Erhardt, 1998; Wells et al., 2000). In this program, many sessions are devoted to discussing, modeling, and role playing with parents, both in therapy sessions as well as in visits to the school, advocacy, and teacher consultation skills. In parent training sessions, parents are taught skills for entering the school system and requesting a meeting with the teacher and all other school personnel involved with the child (e.g., principal, resource teacher, school psychologist, preceding year's teacher) at the beginning of the school year. In the meeting, the parents' goal is communicating with those personnel about the child's ADHD diagnosis, any relevant comorbid diagnoses (e.g., learning disability, ODD), and what behaviors can be expected in the classroom based on the preceding year's classroom performance. If the child is taking medication, this is explained to the school personnel, and their cooperation is elicited in administering the medication on the appropriate schedule if needed. The parent is then taught how to request that the teacher(s) implement the home-based reinforcement system and how to lead the teacher(s) through the steps involved in setting up and implementing such a system. It is our experience that parents who have successfully created and administered a home token economy system with their child are in the best position to consult with the school about setting up the home-based reinforcement system. Such parents have personal experience with the fine details that are necessary to make such a system operate effectively and can answer the teachers' questions from the stance of an experienced "expert."

Much discussion and role playing of these school consultation and advocacy skills takes place in parent training sessions early in the program. In addition, the therapist accompanies the parent to the first school meeting to provide in vivo modeling for the parent of the skills required in setting up and conducting such a school meeting and advocating in an assertive manner for the child. In parent training sessions toward the end of the program, the parent and therapist rehearse "scripts" for the parent to use in meetings with the teacher. These meetings are designed to monitor and fine-tune the home-based reinforcement system and other behavioral programs that have been in effect for the child and for the parent and teacher to work together in modifying the school interventions as needed. Parents go to the school and conduct the meeting with the teacher independently and then come back to sessions to review with the therapist how the meeting went.

We emphasize to parents that it will probably be necessary to conduct such school meetings every school year from now on, and to be constant advocates for their child in the school setting. To underscore this point, we audiotape the final parent training session, in which all of the school advocacy skills are reviewed, and then suggest that parents keep and listen to the audiotape at the beginning of each new school year to remind themselves of what needs to be done with the school (Wells et al., 2000). This is especially important as children make the transition from elementary school to middle school, where there will be an entirely new staff that has no history with the child.

Other innovations in the MTA parent training program involve training parents in cognitive strategies for changing maladaptive cognitions and attributions frequently related to parenting a child with ADHD (e.g., "My child is 'bad' "; "My child behaves like this on purpose just to annoy me"; "I must be a very incompetent parent"), and stress management strategies, including calming "self-talk" and relaxation skills, to use in disciplinary encounters with the child that traditionally have evoked anger and loss of control. These interventions were included to address findings from empirical research as well as frequent clinical observations that parents of children with ADHD experience anger and irritability, more parenting stress, and a decreased sense of parenting competence than other parents (Fischer, 1990; Mash & Johnston, 1990).

Empirical Evaluation of Parent Training for ADHD

There are a number of studies in the literature investigating the parent training program or an adaptation of the program described in this volume, either alone or compared with other treatments for children or adolescents with primary symptoms or diagnoses of ADHD (e.g., Anastopoulos, Shelton, DuPaul, & Guevremont, 1993; Barkley, Guevremont, Anastopoulos, & Fletcher, 1992; Barkley et al., 2000; Erhardt & Baker, 1990; Horn, Ialongo, Greenberg, Packard, & Smith-Winberry, 1990; Pisterman et al., 1989, 1992a, 1992b; Pollard, Ward, & Barkley, 1983). In addition, several other systematic research programs have included other variations of parent training as one component of an overall clinical behavior therapy (e.g., Dubey, O'Leary, & Kaufman, 1983; Pelham et al., 1988) or a comprehensive psychosocial treatment program (Wells et al., 2000) for children with ADHD.

The controlled evaluations of parent training as a single intervention generally show that it produces reductions in some measures of ADHD symptomatology based on parent report and in behavioral measures of noncompliance and other disruptive behaviors such as tantrums. In addition, Pisterman and colleagues (1992a) reported positive effects on parenting stress and sense of competence that were independent of parent and child behavior. Nevertheless, the literature on parent training as a single intervention for ADHD is not extensive, nor is it experimentally rigorous.

The evaluation of parent training in combination with stimulant medication shows little evidence for the superiority of combined treatment relative to stimulant medication alone on child outcomes. For example, in a study of the additive effects of methylphenidate and a combined parent training and self-control therapy program, Horn and colleagues (Horn et al., 1991; Ialongo et al., 1993) found no evidence for the superiority of the combined treatments. However, there were no assessments of parent or child behaviors in the home, and there was no assessment of parent stress. Importantly, only 20% of the sample displayed comorbid disruptive behavior disorders (CD or ODD), limiting the ability to detect effects on noncompliant and aggressive behavior in this sample.

When parent training is one component of a more comprehensive, multimodal, clinical behavior therapy program, there is clear evidence that the intervention is more effective than control conditions (for reviews, see Hinshaw et al., 1998; Wells et al., 2000). In addition, when stimulant medication is combined with multimodal behavior therapy (including parent training as one component), there is evidence for superiority of the combination treatment over single modality treatment (either stimulant medication alone or clinical behavior therapy alone) when multiple child outcome measures

are combined into one overall measure (Conners, 2001). However, none of these studies has as yet assessed long-term effects of parent training, multimodal behavior therapy,
or medication treatment for children with ADHD. (The MTA study will follow children treated with multimodal behavior therapy, including parent training, into their
high school years; however, this follow-up study of the original 7- to 9-year-old sample is
ongoing, and results are not yet available.) It may be that the most important impact of
parent training, which improves family processes and reduces child oppositional and aggressive behavior, will be in reversing the poor long-term outcomes of these children,
since family dysfunction and child aggression are robust predictors of poor outcome in
ADHD.

CHILD ABUSE AND NEGLECT

Another major area of clinical concern for which the basic parent training program has
been adapted and extended is child abuse and neglect. As noted in Chapter 2, behavioral parent training programs (including the HNC parent training program) have
been identified as "supported and accepted treatments" for intrafamilial child abuse
(Saunders et al., 2001). In a recent review, Ammerman and Galvin (1998, p. 46) noted
that many of the parent training programs that have been developed for maltreating
parents have been adapted from the HNC parent training program. For example, Wolfe
and his colleagues (e.g., Wolfe, Edwards, Manion, & Koverola, 1988) adapted the HNC
parent training program for a sample of parents under supervision from a child protective services agency. They also included a number of additional components, including
individual treatment for the abused children and the abusing parents, to accommodate
the multiple areas of need for these parents and their abused children. Similarly, Lutzker
and colleagues adapted the HNC parent training program and incorporated it into their
"ecobehavioral" multicomponent approach to the treatment and prevention of child
abuse and neglect (Project 12-Ways; Lutzker, 1984; Lutzker, Campbell, Newman, &
Harrold, 1989). (See also Urquiza & McNeil, 1996, for a discussion of the potential
application of PCIT [e.g., Eyberg & Boggs, 1998] to intervention with abusing parents.)

   The use of parent training, along with other treatments, is based on empirical work
documenting that abusive parents display a high level and degree of conflictual, coercive behavior with their children, coercive chains culminating in abuse, and a low level
of positive engagement with their children (e.g., Oldershaw, Walters, & Shaw, 1986;
Schindler & Arkowitz, 1986). As noted in Chapter 1, their children demonstrate lower
levels of compliance than do nonabused children (although infants and toddlers may
display so-called compulsive compliance; Crittenden & DiLalla, 1988). Wolfe and
Sandler (1981) concluded that "an abusive act by a parent toward a child often represents the parent's inability to deal effectively with the child's behavior due to a lack of
appropriate child management skills" (p. 323). For these reasons, parent training has
been investigated as one treatment component in these families. However, because abusive parents often display many other psychosocial difficulties including poverty, marital
conflict, and personality and psychological dysfunction (Azar & Wolfe, 1998; Wolfe,

1999), parent training is one component of a multicomponent treatment approach. Because description of a total therapeutic approach for child abuse is beyond the scope of this chapter, the reader is referred to Azar and Wolfe (1998) for descriptions of comprehensive treatment of child abuse and neglect, including parent- and child-focused treatments. However, modifications to the basic parent training program for this population will be described below.

One of the first modifications to the basic parent training program is the context of its implementation. With this population, intervention has often occurred directly in the homes of abusive parents by highly trained upper-level graduate students or professionals (e.g., Lutzker, 1984). Because there is danger of abusive parents misusing parenting instructions, it is deemed important for the therapist to train parents in the home environment in which the skills are displayed and to have an opportunity to observe and prompt new parenting skills in the natural environment. Abusive parents also may receive home visits or telephone calls between the formal skills-teaching sessions to support them in their practice and to directly prompt the newly learned techniques. In the Wolfe and colleagues (1988) study, mothers viewed videotaped sessions and critiqued their own behavior. This procedure seemed to encourage parental interest in their children and in their own performance, and was found to be rewarding and informative to the participants. In addition, Wolfe and colleagues taught parents in vivo desensitization with their child present (following preparatory instructions and rehearsal). In this manner, mothers had an opportunity to practice relaxation, diversion, and similar coping responses in the presence of realistic child behavior. Similarly, Project 12-Ways also includes a stress-reduction component (Campbell, O'Brien, Bickett, & Lutzker, 1983; Lutzker, 1984).

Wolfe also advocates the use of written contracts with abusive parents regarding giving up physical forms of punishment. According to Azar and Wolfe (1998), this is the most basic and difficult issue in undertaking parent training with maltreating parents. Because positive control strategies take some time to produce results, a contract to refrain from physical punishment and to use some nonphysical form of punishment may be discussed much earlier in the program than usual. If a nonphysical form of punishment, such as TO, is taught early in the program, the contract includes a statement that the parent will continue in the program long enough to learn the positive strategies for behavior control that are usually taught first with nonabusive families.

Another point of emphasis in parent training with this population is the risk that ignoring poses for these parents. Because ignoring mild disruptive child behavior may result in an increase in the child's aversive behavior before a reduction occurs (i.e., extinction burst phenomenon), abusive parents must not only be warned that this might take place, but cognitive and physiological coping strategies should be provided to parents to get them through this stressful period. As noted earlier, Wolfe and colleagues (1988) taught parents relaxation and other coping strategies and had parents practice these *in vivo* when the child displayed aversive behaviors.

Finally, my own clinical experience working with neglectful parents is that they, in particular, profit from a focus on the Child's Game component of the HNC parent training program (see Chapter 6). Neglectful parents are frequently very disengaged from their children and from their role as parent. The Child's Game, with its emphasis on giving the parents skills for attending to and interacting with their child in a relaxed and positive way, is often a first step back to reengagement with the child. However, parents often feel very uncomfortable and awkward when first practicing the Child's Game in parent training sessions and, consequently, may give up easily on homework practice. It is very important to provide a great deal of therapist support to the parent while modeling and role playing the Child's Game in these sessions. The therapist should give frequent prompts and praise to the parent, either via the bug-in-the-ear or by sitting close to the parent on the floor as the parent is practicing with the child. After practicing, the therapist should debrief the parent regarding feelings experienced while doing the practice. Parents frequently will report initial feelings of discomfort, and the therapist must normalize these feelings and support the parent through them.

In a study investigating the use of parent training in families where there is actual child abuse or risk for child abuse, Wolfe and his colleagues showed improvements in parenting skills and decreases in child behavior problems for maltreating and neglectful parents who receive parent training (Wolfe et al., 1988). In this study with a sample of parents and children under supervision by a child protective services agency, an adaptation of the HNC parent training program was compared to standard social service agency contact, with generally superior results for the groups receiving parent training (Wolfe et al., 1988). Support for the parent training component in Project 12-Ways has been provided in single-subject studies with neglecting parents (e.g., Campbell et al., 1983; Dachman, Halasz, Bickett, & Lutzker, 1984). Findings from these studies, in conjunction with those of other investigators (see Azar & Wolfe, 1998), provide strong support for the inclusion of behavioral parent training in comprehensive programs of treatment for families displaying child abuse and neglect.

DEVELOPMENTAL DISABILITIES

Parent training has been applied frequently with parents of children who display developmental disabilities. In fact, one of Hanf's original studies was with children described as "severely handicapped" (Hanf & Kling, 1973). The term "developmental disabilities," as it has been used in the parent training literature, includes children with mental retardation, autism, and speech and language disorders. In addition to their primary intellectual, social, and/or language deficits, such children often display deficits in self-help skills and attention, unresponsiveness to environmental cues, low frustration tolerance, perseverative or self-stimulatory behaviors, as well as high levels of noncompliant behavior.

The noncompliant behavior of children with developmental disabilities is often of primary concern early in treatment programs, since high levels of noncompliance make it difficult to teach these children in other areas. For example, it is difficult to teach a child with mental retardation to dress himself or herself independently if he or she cannot or will not follow a direction to "put your arm through your shirt sleeve." Likewise, a child with speech or language delays must be able to follow directions before speech training can be effective. For this reason, noncompliant and oppositional behavior has been an important behavioral target in programs for children with developmental disabilities and may be a prerequisite for self-help skills training and language training programs. As noted in Chapter 1, parents of children with mental retardation consider noncompliance to be the most pressing issue in dealing with their children (Tavormina et al., 1976).

Just as with other populations, modifications to basic parent training procedures for children with developmental disabilities arise from the unique needs and abilities of these children. At the outset of treatment, it is important to challenge a frequently held belief among parents of youngsters with developmental disabilities—that their child's noncompliant and other misbehavior is a fixed attribute resulting from the developmental disability rather than behavior that can be altered. Breiner (1989) recommends that this attitude must be elicited and challenged early in parent training to counter the reluctance that parents may display toward active intervention with their child.

There are several adaptations of the clear instructions component of the HNC parent training program for children with developmental disabilities. Because many of these children show attentional deficits (or, in the case of children with autism, extremes of social avoidance), it is important to gain the attention of the child with developmental disabilities in a very concrete way before giving an instruction. Parents are taught to obtain eye contact with the child and say "Look at me" prior to issuing a command. Furthermore, parents are taught to give very short instructions with a minimum of excessive verbiage. Along these same lines, Sanders and Plant (1989) emphasized that the level of verbal explanations to the child must be simplified compared to the basic parent training program (see Chapters 6 and 7). Breiner (1989) also recommends ending each instruction with the word "now." The word "now" becomes a cue to the child that a consequence will definitely follow if the child does not comply with the instruction. (Concomitantly, parents' use of the cue word "now" over time also becomes a self-prompt to the parent to follow through with a consequence.) Among other specific recommendations given by Breiner (1989) and Breiner and Beck (1984) is the use of physical prompts or cueing to get behavior started once a command has been given. For example, after obtaining the child's attention and giving a specific instruction, the parent may gently guide the child's hands to begin compliance with the task.

Ducharme (e.g., 1996; Ducharme, Popynick, Pontes, & Steele, 1996) has developed an "errorless compliance training" procedure that has shown great promise in increasing compliance to parental instructions by young children with developmental disabilities. This procedure involves the initial use of parental instructions to which there is a high probability of compliance, followed by the gradual introduction of instructions to which the probability of compliance is less likely. The hierarchy of commands is determined through both a parent-completed checklist and observation of parent–child interaction. Parents also receive training in how to give clear instructions (the components of which are very similar to those described in Chapter 7) and to provide positive attention for compliance (see Chapter 7). The errorless compliance training procedure has been shown to result in increased compliance to all parental commands, with the effects generalizing to untrained instructions and maintained for up to 15 months after treatment (e.g., Ducharme et al., 1996).

In working with parents of children with developmental disabilities, more emphasis is placed on tangible reinforcers in association with attends and rewards than on verbal reinforcement alone. For example, with children who are profoundly retarded or autistic, food reinforcers may be coupled with attends and rewards to increase the salience of reinforcement and to further enhance the reinforcing value of the parent.

Another modification to the basic parent training program for families with youngsters with developmental disabilities derives from the fact that these children may learn at slower rates and require more structured learning situations than other children (e.g., Lovaas & Newsom, 1976). More reinforcement trials will, therefore, be needed in order to teach these children new skills. This is stated explicitly by the therapist to the parents, especially those who may have a nondisabled older child and are accustomed to steeper learning curves. Parents are encouraged to set aside particular times of the day to work with their disabled child on language skills, self-help skills, or general compliance and to provide multiple reinforcement trials during these specific planned activities. The use of shaping is especially emphasized with parents while working with children with developmental disabilities on specific skills and tasks. Skills and tasks (e.g., brushing one's teeth, making up one's bed) may be broken down into even more elemental steps than those used with nondelayed youngsters, and parents are supported in persisting with their children in daily skills practice sessions over weeks if necessary until the skill is learned.

For children with language delays and behavior problems, attends can also play a role in language acquisition in addition to their value as a social reinforcer (Cunningham, 1989; McElreath & Eisenstadt, 1994). Cunningham also recommends that questions that are directly related to the child's play and conversation be actively encouraged, as questions help to elicit verbal responses and sustain conversation. (As noted in Chapter 6, questions are typically discouraged in the Child's Game.)

A final issue in parent training for families with children with developmental disabilities has to do with generalization of intervention effects. Many studies have shown that these children do not adequately generalize skills and behaviors learned in one setting to other settings; nor do their parents adequately generalize the use of parenting skills from one child behavior or situation to other behaviors or situations (e.g., Cushing, Adams, & Rincover, 1983; Koegel, Rincover, & Egel, 1982). Although generalization cannot be assumed with any child or parent population, parent training for families with children with developmental disabilities should focus particular attention on generalization. For example, parents learn parenting techniques for multiple target behaviors and in multiple situations (Sanders & Plant, 1989). Learning behavioral principles in addition to specific techniques may result in greater generalization than technique training alone (Koegel, Russo, & Rincover, 1977) (as is the case for parents of children with conduct problems; McMahon, Forehand, & Griest, 1981; see Chapter 8).

The literature on the empirical evaluation of parent training with families with children with developmental disabilities is reviewed in detail in Breiner (1989), Breiner and Beck (1984), Handen (1998), and Newsom (1998). These reviews indicate that parent training produces significantly greater improvements in child compliance, reductions in child aggression and other child target behaviors, and improved behavior rating scale scores as compared with control conditions (e.g., Eyberg & Matarazzo, 1980; Mash, Lazere, Terdal, & Garner, 1973; Mash & Terdal, 1973; Tavormina, 1975). These studies strongly suggest that parent training is an important component of intervention with these children and produces greater changes in relevant target behaviors than nonspecific control treatments (e.g., discussion groups). Including parents in a comprehensive approach can improve the intervention and generalization effects obtained in work with children who are developmentally disabled.

The HNC parent training program has also been employed with children with developmental disabilities on a limited basis (see Chapter 10). Two studies (Breiner & Forehand, 1982; Forehand et al., 1974) provide some preliminary support for the program's success with children who have developmental and physical limitations (i.e., developmental disabilities, deafness).

A few small-scale studies suggest that adaptations of the basic parent training program have potential for use with *parents* with developmental disabilities. For example, Peterson, Robinson, and Littman (1983) taught some of the positive attention skills of Phase I (using the PCIT approach; e.g., Eyberg & Boggs, 1998) to six parents with developmental disabilities. They found that these parents increased attending and praise statements and decreased their use of commands in the context of the Child's Game; however, only the lower frequency of commands was maintained after treatment. In another study, Lloyd, Case, Ducharme, and Feldman (1988) taught three mothers with developmental disabilities to effectively use components of the clear instructions sequence (clear instructions, praise for compliance, TO for noncompliance) to increase their children's compliance.

OTHER POPULATIONS

Enuresis and Encopresis[1]

During the assessment of children referred for noncompliance and other behavior problems, it is not uncommon to find that the child is also enuretic (or, less frequently, encopretic). Conversely, children referred for a presenting problem of enuresis or encopresis may display oppositional behavior as a co-occurring problem (Mellon & Stern, 1998). In either situation, it is frequently necessary to treat the child's oppositional/noncompliant behavior first, using the parent training program, before focusing treatment specifically on the elimination problem.[2]

This strategy is followed for several reasons. First, most behavioral programs for treatment of enuresis and encopresis require a great deal of parent–child interaction around toileting and a parent who is able to elicit cooperation from the child, if the program is to be successful. For example, the treatment program designed by Houts and colleagues (Mellon & Houts, 1998) for enuresis requires that, when bedwetting occurs, the parent have the child get out of bed, turn off the urine alarm, and remake the bed. In addition, during waking hours, the parent must conduct a retention control procedure with the child in which the child is instructed to postpone urination for increasingly

[1]This section is adapted from Forehand and McMahon (1981, pp. 110–111).

[2]Appropriate medical assessment to identify potential physical causes for enuresis and encopresis should be conducted prior to the decision to implement a psychosocial intervention.

longer periods after drinking a large glass of water. These procedures (called Full Spectrum Home Treatment), although very effective, can be unpleasant for both the parent and child. If the child is noncompliant, then these training procedures are likely to become the focus of a new source of conflict and oppositional resistance between parent and child. Implementing the procedures in the middle of the night is aversive enough for parents. Trying to implement them with a noncompliant child may be more than the parent is willing to deal with, and the program may fail for that reason. Likewise, if the child is cooperative initially with the procedures but the parent fails to provide positive social reinforcement for appropriate toileting and compliance with procedures, then the program is again likely to fail. Interventions for encopresis require similar levels of cooperation from both the child and parents (see Mellon & Stern, 1998). Second, even if the treatment for enuresis or encopresis is successful, children who are extremely noncompliant may be more likely to relapse (e.g., Dische, Yule, Corbett, & Hand, 1983).

In any case, the HNC parent training program provides the parent with the requisite skills to elicit compliance and cooperation from the child in following the treatment procedures for enuresis or encopresis. In our experience, implementation of the HNC parent training program for noncompliance has sometimes resulted in resolution of the enuresis or encopresis without directly targeting these problems. From a theoretical point of view, this probably happens when enuresis or encopresis has functioned more as oppositional behavior (noncompliance with self-care rules) rather than as the result of a toileting skills deficit or nighttime anxiety about toileting. By changing parent–child interactions related to general oppositional behavior, enuresis and encopresis may change as part of the oppositional response class.

Inpatient Child Populations

Children whose emotional distress or behavioral disturbance has reached a level to require inpatient psychiatric hospitalization are a population requiring special management. During the course of daily experience on an inpatient unit, the child briefly interacts with several professionals, including the attending psychiatrist, psychologist, and nurses who administer the specific psychiatric treatments (formal therapy or medications). However, the persons with whom patients often have the greatest frequency of interaction and who are confronted with the greatest behavior management challenges are the front-line staff members who are typically paraprofessional aides or technicians. These individuals often find themselves in a "parental" role vis-à-vis the child as they attempt to move the child through the daily schedule, and are confronted with managing the same kinds of extremely oppositional, highly disruptive, and out-of-control emotions and behaviors that may have necessitated inpatient hospitalization in the first place. In my role as the chief inpatient psychologist for a children's psychiatric inpatient unit several years ago, I found that the HNC parent training program served as an excellent foundation for training front-line staff members in appropriate methods and skills for interacting with and managing hospitalized children.

In adapting the procedures to the inpatient setting, staff members are taught the basic skills of attending, rewarding, and ignoring just as they are described in this volume. My experience was that the procedures were well received by the children, even those as old as 12 years. Once staff members learned the skills, they were then asked to use them as they were supervising the children to whom they were assigned through the daily schedule. For example, if a staff member was assigned to monitor a young child through the morning routine of dressing, making up the bed, brushing teeth, and so on, the staff member would attend and reward as the child performed these self-care behaviors. Likewise, staff members assigned to socially isolated children would prompt children to play games with adults or other children and then attend and reward as the child played. Each morning in rounds, when each child was discussed, the staff would designate one or two prosocial behaviors relevant for each child that all staff members would monitor, and then apply attending and rewarding whenever they "caught the child being good." The prosocial behaviors were written into the medical chart and became an official component of the care plan for that child. For other children, especially those with a history of emotional neglect or abuse, one or more daily sessions of the Child's Game, in which a staff member interacted one-on-one with the child providing a high frequency of positive attending and rewarding, were specifically prescribed. These sessions provided for the beginning of establishment of trust with a staff member and became a way of modeling for parents or other family members to whom the child would ultimately be discharged a new way of interacting positively with the child.

The training in use of clear instructions is especially important with staff members on an inpatient psychiatric unit. I have seen staff members who fall on both ends of the "commanding" continuum (see Chapter 7). Some staff members can become overly authoritarian and rigid, functioning like drill sergeants, barking orders at children. At the other extreme are staff members who are too timid to confront highly disruptive children with assertive directions. In the training component about giving clear instructions, staff members model and role play how to give assertive directions to children in a calm, respectful, but firm tone of voice, using the procedures described in Chapter 7.

The application of TO as a consequence for noncompliant and highly disruptive behavior is the component of the HNC parent training program requiring the greatest adaptation for inpatient populations. Because this tends to be a population of children displaying excessive levels of disruptive behavior and emotion dysregulation, we found it necessary to have a three-staged approach to implementation of TO. The initial steps of the TO procedure are followed as described in Chapter 7. That is, the child is given a warning for initial noncompliance to an instruction or violation of pre-established unit rules and then taken to a TO corner on the unit after noncompliance with the warning. However, because hospitalized children frequently became highly disruptive in the corner or refused to stay in the corner, a second step was then implemented in which children were escorted to the "seclusion room" for a more restricted, open-door TO. If they came out of the open seclusion room once, they were escorted back with the warning that if they came out again, the door would be locked. This warning was then implemented if the child came out of the room a second time. As soon as the child stopped tantrumming in the locked seclusion room, the steps of TO were implemented in reverse order. First, the door was opened with a statement to stay in the open room for 5 more minutes. If the child was able to comply, after 5 minutes he or she was escorted to the corner TO and told to stay there for 5 minutes. Thereafter, the TO ended and the child was allowed back into the community environment of the unit. Finally, it was the responsibility of the staff member who implemented the TO to observe the child over the next 30 minutes and catch the child in some prosocial behavior that could be attended to and praised. If the original instigating event was noncompliance to a staff member's instruction, then the child was taken back to the original situation and given the instruction again.

Throughout this TO process, it was emphasized to the child that his or her goal was to work on self-control of behavior and emotions. The child was encouraged to employ self-control strategies learned in individual therapy sessions (e.g., relaxation, cognitive control strategies). By exerting self-control, he or she could avoid the escalation to more restrictive stages of TO. However, if self-control failed, the immediate implementation of gradually more restrictive steps let the child know that the adults would provide appropriate external controls and assured the other children on the unit that the adults would not allow the unit environment to become dangerous or out of control.

The incorporation of "locked TO" into this three-stage TO sequence must adhere to all state regulations regarding the use of locked seclusion in restrictive, therapeutic environments for children. For example, in some states, any time a child is placed in locked seclusion, a physician must be consulted about the situation within a short period of time, and a specific order approving the locked seclusion must be placed in the medical chart. Children must be monitored frequently while in locked seclusion (on our unit, every 5 minutes while the child was in seclusion, a staff member visually observed the child through a window on the seclusion room door to monitor the child's status and ensure his or her safety). Professionals in charge of the milieu program on inpatient units must thoroughly familiarize themselves with state regulations and incorporate training in these regulations into staff training programs.

In addition to providing a viable and effective model for training front-line staff members in appropriate, effective, and consistent methods for interacting with children on the inpatient unit, a second advantage of the HNC parent training program is that it also can be used for training parents of hospitalized children. Because children experience and become familiar with the "parenting" strategies being implemented by staff members, it smoothes the way for parents who simultaneously participate in individual or group parent training sessions and learn the same strategies. Furthermore, as parents learn the strategies, they can watch the unit staff using the strategies with the child on the unit during visits, and eventually implement the strategies themselves on the unit with backup and support from the unit staff. This shaping procedure facilitates the generalization of intervention effects from the unit to home, promoting a smoother and often earlier transition to discharge and outpatient follow-up.

ADHERENCE TO MEDICAL REGIMENS

It is quite common for children with both acute (e.g., ear infections) and chronic (e.g., asthma, diabetes) medical illnesses to display difficulties of noncompliance with their medically prescribed regimens of care (Huszti & Olson, 1999; Manne, 1998). Noncompliance may be circumscribed to the arena of adherence to the medical regimen or may be one component of more general oppositional behavior. In either case, the model of parent training for treatment of noncompliance outlined in this volume can be a very useful approach in the overall treatment plan for the child. As was discussed with enuresis and encopresis, it is frequently useful to employ the HNC parent training program for treatment of general noncompliance prior to a specific focus on medical noncompliance. As the child learns to become less oppositional and more cooperative and compliant with routine parent instructions and rules, generalization of this effect to medical compliance may occur. Even if generalization to medical compliance does not occur "spontaneously," child acceptance of the techniques (e.g., TO) targeted toward medical noncompliance will be greater if the child has already experienced the techniques directed toward other target behaviors. Greater child acceptance will help parents in their ability to follow through with consequences when needed.

When applying parent training to children with chronic medical illnesses, special adaptations and intensive support to parents may be required, especially when health-threatening symptoms occur during the application of parenting techniques. For example, one parent with whom I worked was very reluctant to apply any consequences for negative behavior to her son with asthma, for fear that he would become upset and have an asthma attack. Over the years, the child had developed serious oppositional behavior and was also noncompliant with his care regimen. He experienced frequent hospital admissions to the emergency room in respiratory distress because of this, and was referred to the psychology service by his physicians.

The parent training program was implemented, and the first half of the program was accepted well by the parent and child with no adaptations. However, when the procedure for implementing TO was taught to the mother and child, the child threatened to have an asthma attack and the mother said that she would not implement the procedure. We, therefore, arranged to have the psychologist implement the procedure with the child in a hospital room, with the child's physician in the room to monitor the child, while the mother watched from behind a one-way mirror. The child again threatened to have an asthma attack while sitting in the corner, but the psychologist and physician persisted with the procedure while monitoring the child. The mother became anxious behind the one-way mirror, but was reassured when her child did not experience severe respiratory distress. Thereafter, a shaping program was instituted in which the physician was no longer in the room, but was available by pager, while the psychologist implemented the procedure and the mother watched. Finally, the mother implemented the procedure with support from the psychologist. Once the mother had established parental control over the child's noncompliance, she began successfully to apply her parenting skills to the child's refusal to take medication, with the result that the child's medical noncompliance improved considerably.

This case illustrates several issues that can arise in implementing parent training with children with medical illnesses. First, because of parental anxiety about the child's medical status, parents often become reluctant to expect developmentally appropriate behavior from the child and to provide firm consequences for noncompliance with age-appropriate instructions and rules, even those associated with the child's medical care.

In parent training, parents must be helped to understand what the child is capable of, and supported in adjusting their expectations for their child. Furthermore, because anxiety may inhibit parents from following through with consequences, they may require a great deal of reassurance and support to implement consequences for the first time. The modeling and shaping program illustrated in this case, in effect, constituted a desensitization program for the parent in which her anxiety about applying consequences to her child was gradually diminished. The case also illustrated the importance of a close, cooperative effort among all the members of the treatment team in implementing an intervention plan for a medically ill child. Without a clear statement by the physician to the mother that treatment of the child's oppositional behavior was critical to the child's care, and without the physician's support and presence in the initial steps of this program, it is unlikely that the mother would have been able to follow through. The case illustrates that psychologists and other parent trainers must establish good working relationships with pediatricians and other medical care providers in working with this population of children.

FINAL THOUGHTS

Since the publication of the first edition of this volume in 1981, many clinicians and researchers have applied the HNC parent training program to diverse populations of children. As described in this chapter, the basic program has largely remained intact, although adaptations have been developed to fit the needs and abilities of special child and parent populations. This process has been an exemplar of clinical science at its best; that is, an established clinical program has been retained in its essential elements but refined by clinical researchers responding to what is known about the special characteristics of particular populations and then evaluated empirically with those populations. This process expands the horizons of empirical clinical psychology and brings effective interventions to a wider population of children and families in need.

By adapting and expanding the HNC parent training program to special populations, clinical researchers also have moved the program out of the laboratory, where the first demonstrations of efficacy occurred, and into the real world of clinical populations and settings where demonstrations of effectiveness are now taking place. For many clinical populations, parent training is now considered to be an essential component of treatment for some (e.g., ADHD; Pelham, Wheeler, & Chronis, 1998) and a treatment of choice for others (e.g., conduct problems; Brestan & Eyberg, 1998). Several major research projects that are evaluating the effectiveness of parent training combined with other psychosocial interventions show promise of improving the outcomes achieved with more traditional forms of child treatment (Arnold et al., 1997; Conduct Problems Prevention Research Group, 1992, 2000; Richters et al., 1995). Parent training in its basic and adapted forms is rapidly becoming a fundamental treatment in clinical child psychology and psychiatry.

CHAPTER 10

Review of Treatment Research and Current Directions

The preceding chapters presented how to assess and treat child noncompliance and related conduct problem behaviors. In this chapter, we describe research that we have conducted in order to provide an empirical basis for our procedures. We view this chapter as "must reading," since a therapist implementing the program should know the data on which the intervention procedures are based. The chapter concludes with an overview of some of our current efforts in the area of prevention.

In the first part of this chapter, we describe seven types of research pertaining to the effectiveness of our parent training program. First, various components of the program have been examined individually in a series of laboratory investigations to specify the variables in the parent training package that are effective in modifying child noncompliance. Second, we examined the immediate outcome of using the program with noncompliant children in several investigations. Third, we assessed the generalization of treatment effects across settings, time, siblings, and behavior, as well as the social validity and positive side effects of these generalized changes. Fourth, we examined several procedures for enhancing generalization. Fifth, we have examined the use of self-administered interventions based on the HNC program in three investigations. Sixth, we describe two studies that have compared the parent training program with other interventions. Finally, our recent research has focused on prevention, and we describe two of those efforts in the final section of the chapter.

LABORATORY INVESTIGATIONS

A first step in our research program was to specify the parameters and variables in the parent training program that are effective in modifying noncompliance. In essence, we wanted to demonstrate that the variables or skills in the program were related to child noncompliance and to identify parameters of the variables that were most effective in changing this behavior. We chose to conduct these studies in a laboratory setting. Use of such a setting has allowed the control of extraneous variables that may systematically or unsystematically affect child compliance in the home. Furthermore, more closely supervised introduction and withdrawal of treatment conditions has been possible. These studies were conducted with nonreferred, at-risk, or clinic-referred children.

All of the studies described in this section were conducted in laboratory settings equipped with observation windows and adjoining observation rooms. Children who participated in these investigations were 3–7 years old. In all cases, the experimenter used a bug-in-the-ear radio signaling device to cue the parent how to respond to the child. The studies, the majority of which were conducted by the authors, are summarized in Table 10.1. In addition, selected studies conducted by our colleague Mark Roberts concerning TO and the clear instructions sequence are included.

The results of these studies lead to the following conclusions. First, it is important to label verbal praise given to children, supporting the efficacy of teaching parents the use of labeled verbal rewards in the first phase of the parent training program. Second, teaching parents to use attends and rewards in the context of the Child's Game can lead to increases in compliance and decreases in noncompliance and inappropriate behavior. Third, as the number of parental instructions increases, child compliance decreases. This lends support to the first component of the parent training program, in which parents are initially taught to reduce the number of instructions to their children. Fourth, teaching parents how to issue clear instructions increases child compliance, and the combination of teaching parents how to issue clear instructions and use TO further enhances child compliance. Fifth, the TO studies suggest that the most effective and efficient TO condition is one in which the parent removes the child from all sources of reinforcement rather than just ignoring the child, uses a TO duration longer than 1 minute (but for ethical reasons under 5 minutes), releases the child from TO when the child is being quiet, and utilizes a physical barrier (removal to a TO room) when the child leaves the TO chair. A verbalized reason for TO is optional, as it neither adds to nor subtracts from the effectiveness of TO in suppressing child noncompliance. We do teach the parent to use a verbalized reason, since most parents feel more comfortable in utilizing the TO procedure with their child when this is done. Sixth, utilizing the clear instructions sequence (i.e., positive attention for compliance, a warning for noncompliance, and TO for noncompliance to the warning) not only increases compliance but decreases child negative verbalizations (e.g., "No, you're mean!"). Finally, a series of three studies by the first author (RJM) and his colleagues indicates that the effects of various parenting skills taught in the parent training program (i.e., ignoring, TO, contingent positive attention) can be enhanced by having the parent include a verbal rationale or a rationale plus modeling procedure when initially introducing each skill to the child. As described in Chapters 3, 6, and 7, we place a great deal of emphasis on teaching the child about the various parenting skills *before* they are implemented.

TABLE 10.1. Laboratory Investigations

Study	Component of program examined	Experimental question examined	Findings
Bernhardt & Forehand (1975)	Verbal rewards	Are labeled verbal rewards more effective than unlabeled verbal rewards?	Yes
Kotler & McMahon (2003)	Attends and rewards	Does training in attends and rewards lead to improvements in compliance and noncompliance?	Yes
Forehand & Scarboro (1975)	Instructions	Is number of instructions related to child compliance?	More instructions associated with less compliance.
Roberts, McMahon, Forehand, & Humphreys (1978)	Clear instructions and TO	Does clear instruction training enhance compliance, and does clear instruction training plus TO further enhance it?	Yes
Scarboro & Forehand (1975)	TO and ignoring	Is TO more effective than ignoring?	Both equally effective, but ignoring required more administrations, suggesting TO more efficient.
Gardner, Forehand, & Roberts (1976)	TO	Does inclusion of verbalized reason for TO change effectiveness of TO?	No
Hobbs, Forehand, & Murray (1978)	TO	Is 4-minute TO more effective than briefer (1-minute or 10-second) TO?	Yes
Bean & Roberts (1981); Hobbs & Forehand (1975)	TO	Is contingent release from TO more effective than noncontingent release?	Yes
Day & Roberts (1983); Roberts (1988); Roberts & Powers (1990)	TO	What is an effective backup for leaving TO?	Physical barrier (TO room) or spank; physical barrier associated with less disruptive behavior in TO.
Roberts (1982)	Clear instructions	Does use of a warning enhance TO?	Yes
Roberts & Hatzenbuehler (1981)	Clear instructions sequence	Do consequences for compliance and noncompliance increase compliance and decrease negative child verbalizations?	Yes

(continued)

TABLE 10.1. *(continued)*

Study	Component of program examined	Experimental question examined	Findings
Davies, McMahon, Flessati, & Tiedemann (1984)	Ignoring	When parent introduces ignoring to child, is effect of ignoring enhanced by parents including a verbal rationale or verbal rationale plus modeling?	Yes
McMahon, Davies, & Tiedemann (1983)	TO	When parent introduces TO to child, is effect of TO enhanced by parents including a verbal rationale or verbal rationale plus modeling?	Yes
McMahon, Tiedemann, & Davies (1987)	Contingent positive attention	When parent introduces contingent positive attention to child, is its effect enhanced by including a verbal rationale or verbal rationale plus modeling?	Yes

IMMEDIATE OUTCOME STUDIES

The laboratory investigations present data clearly indicating the importance of parental use of positive attention, ignoring, clear instructions, and TO in modifying child non-compliance and other inappropriate behavior, as well as in the use of rationales and modeling in introducing the procedure to the child. In addition to the examination of the various components of the parent training program in the laboratory setting, several early studies were conducted in which the effectiveness of the entire parent training program was evaluated. Each of these studies limited behavioral assessment of treatment outcome to the clinic laboratory setting. These studies are detailed in Table 10.2.

Forehand and King (1974) successfully used the parent training program to treat eight preschool noncompliant children and their mothers. In the Child's Game (free-play situation), mothers significantly increased their use of rewards and significantly decreased their use of commands and questions from baseline to posttreatment. In the Parent's Game (parental control situation), maternal rewards again increased significantly from baseline to posttreatment, as did child compliance. These results suggest that both parent and child behaviors changed in the desired and predicted direction with treatment.

Forehand and King (1977) subsequently used the parent training program in the treatment of 11 preschool children and their mothers. Parent perception measures and observational data on mother–child interaction in the clinic indicated that after treatment the mothers perceived their children as significantly better adjusted and, as in Forehand and King (1974), parent and child behaviors changed. Improvements in maternal perception of the child and the maternal and child behaviors were maintained at a 3-month follow-up. Relative to a nonclinic "normal" sample of 11 mother–child pairs,

TABLE 10.2. Outcome-Related Investigations

Study	Sample size	Comparison/control group	Outcome data	Follow-up	Focus	Miscellaneous
			Immediate outcome			
Forehand & King (1974)	8	—	CO	—	Clinic outcome	
Forehand & King (1977)	22	NON	CO, Q	3 mo	Clinic outcome	
Breiner & Forehand (1982)	10	ATT	HO, PR, Q	—	Developmentally disabled sample	
Forehand, Cheney, & Yoder (1974)	1	—	CO, Q	3 mo	Case study with developmentally disabled child	
			Generalization/social validity			
Peed, Roberts, & Forehand (1977)	12	WLC	CO, HO, Q	—	Home generalization	
Forehand, Griest, & Wells (1979)	20	—	HO, PR, Q	—	Home generalization	Relationship of multiple outcome measures
Rogers, Forehand, Griest, Wells, & McMahon (1981)	31	—	HO, Q	—	Home generalization	SES
McMahon, Forehand, & Tiedemann (1985)	55	Different age groups	HO, Q	2 mo	Home generalization	Child age
Breiner & Forehand (1981)	32	NON	HO, SO	—	School generalization	
Forehand, Sturgis, et al. (1979)—Study 2	16	NON	HO, SO, Q	—	School generalization	
Forehand, Breiner, McMahon, & Davies (1981)	16	—	HO, SO	—	Prediction of change in school behavior	
Forehand, Sturgis, et al. (1979)—Study 1	11	—	HO, Q	6 and 12 mo	Temporal generalization	
Baum & Forehand (1981)	34	—	HO, Q	1–4.5 yr	Temporal generalization, social validity	
Forehand, Rogers, McMahon, Wells, & Griest (1981)	18	—	HO, Q	8 mo	Temporal generalization	

(continued)

TABLE 10.2. *(continued)*

Study	Sample size	Comparison/control group	Outcome data	Follow-up	Focus	Miscellaneous
Forehand, Steffe, Furey, & Walley (1983)	34	—	Q	11–86 mo (3.6 yr)	Temporal generalization	
Forehand & Long (1988)	42	NON	CO, Q (P,T,C)	4.5–10.5 yr (7.5 yr)	Temporal generalization, social validity	
Long, Forehand, Wierson, & Morgan (1994)	52	NON	Q (P,C)	14 yr	Temporal generalization	
Humphreys, Forehand, McMahon, & Roberts (1978)	8	—	HO	—	Sibling generalization	
Wells, Forehand, & Griest (1980)	24	NON	HO	—	Behavioral generalization	
Forehand, Wells, & Griest (1980)	30	NON	HO, Q	2 and 15 mo[a]	Social validity, positive side effects	
Cross Calvert & McMahon (1987)	90 mothers	PTA, PR, PRM	Q	—	Social validity	Nonreferred sample
McMahon, Johnson, & Robbins (2003)	96 students, 57 mothers	TAD, WI, TAD + WI	Q	—	Social validity	Nonreferred samples
McMahon, Tiedemann, Forehand, & Griest (1984)	20	TA, SL	Q	2 mo	Social validity	
			Positive side effects			
Brody & Forehand (1985)	24	MD, non-MD	HO, Q	—	Marital satisfaction	
Forehand, Griest, Wells, & McMahon (1982)	27	High, medium, low marital satisfaction	HO, Q	2 mo	Marital satisfaction	
Roberts, Joe, & Rowe-Hallbert (1992)—Study 3	39	—	Q	—	Parenting locus of control	

			Enhancement of generalization			
Wells, Griest, & Forehand (1980)	16	PTA, PT + SC	HO, PR	2 mo	Maternal self-control adjunct	
McMahon, Forehand, & Griest (1981)	20	TA, SL	HO, Q	2 mo	Social learning principles adjunct	
Griest et al. (1982)	32	PTA, PET, NON	HO, Q	2 mo	PET adjunct	
		Self-administered interventions				
McMahon & Forehand (1978)	3	Multiple baseline across subjects	HO	6 wk	Self-administered	Mealtime behavior
McMahon & Lehman (2003)	40	TAD, WI, TAD + WI, NTC	CO, Q	—	Self-administered/clear instructions	Nonreferred sample
Long, Rickart, & Ashcraft (1993)	32	WI + meds, meds	Q (P,T)	—	Self-administered	Children with ADHD
		Comparisons with other interventions				
Wells & Egan (1988)	19	PTA, SFT	CO, Q	—	Comparative	
Baum, Reyna McGlone, & Ollendick (1986)	34	PT + CSC, PT + C – ATT, STEP + C – ATT	CO, Q (P,C)	6–8 mo	Comparative	
		Prediction of dropout/follow-up participation				
McMahon, Forehand, Griest, & Wells (1981)	48	—	HO, Q	—	Dropout	
Furey & Basili (1988)	53	—	HO, Q	—	Dropout	
Griest, Forehand, & Wells (1981)	16	—	HO, Q	8 mo	Participation in follow-up	

Note. Sample size is total. *Control/comparison group*: NON, nonreferred; ATT, attention control; WLC, waiting-list control; PTA, parent training alone; PRM, parent training plus verbal rationale and modeling; TAD, therapist administered; WI, written instructions; TAD + WI, therapist administration plus written instructions; TA, technique alone; SL, social learning principles adjunct; MD, maritally distressed; non-MD, non-maritally distressed; PTA, parent training alone; PT + SC, parent training plus maternal self-control adjunct; PET, parent training plus Parent Enhancement Therapy; NTC, no-training control; SFT, systems family therapy; PT + CSC, parent training plus child self-control; PT + C – ATT, parent training plus child attention control; STEP + C – ATT, Systematic Training for Effective Parenting plus child attention control. *Outcome data*: CO, clinic observation; HO, home observation; PR, parent-recorded data; Q = questionnaire; P, parent report; T, teacher report; C, child report.
[a] Consumer satisfaction/social acceptability data only at 15-month follow-up.

the treated children were less compliant prior to treatment and more compliant after treatment. Furthermore, prior to treatment mothers of the clinic children perceived their children as less well adjusted than mothers of the nonclinic children perceived their children. However, following treatment, the two groups of parents did not differ significantly in their perceptions of their children.

As noted in Chapter 9, two studies (Breiner & Forehand, 1982; Forehand et al., 1974) have examined the immediate effects of the parent training program with children with disabilities (i.e., developmental disabilities, deafness). A pilot study by Breiner and Forehand (1982) with children with developmental and language disabilities showed significantly greater changes in parent behaviors and attitudes and in parent satisfaction with parent training, as compared to an attention-control treatment. In addition, a case study by Forehand and colleagues (1974) reported positive intervention effects with a deaf child.

OUTCOME STUDIES EXAMINING GENERALIZATION AND SOCIAL VALIDITY

Although the earlier outcome studies suggested the immediate effectiveness of the parent training program in improving parent–child interactions in a clinic setting, lack of experimental control and failure to assess parent and child behavior outside the clinic setting limited the conclusions regarding the effectiveness of the program. Of primary importance, then, was the need to assess the generalization of these treatment effects across settings (from clinic to home and school), time (after termination of treatment), behaviors (from treated to untreated behaviors), and siblings (from treated to untreated children). It also was important to determine whether the treatment effects were socially valid and whether there were any side effects of the parent training program on other aspects of family functioning. See Table 10.2 for a description of these studies.

Generalization to the Home Setting

In order to evaluate the effectiveness of the parent training program in comparison to a nonintervention control group and to investigate the generality of treatment changes from the clinic to the home, Peed and colleagues (1977) compared six mother–child pairs who received treatment by way of the parent training program to six mother–child pairs in a waiting-list control group. In the clinic setting, parent and child behaviors changed for the treatment group as in the Forehand and King (1974, 1977) studies. Of primary importance, the treatment effects generalized to the home setting: significant increases from the pretreatment to posttreatment occurred for child compliance and for maternal rewards, attends, and contingent attention to compliance. Maternal use of beta commands decreased significantly. The control group did not change significantly from the pretreatment to postwaiting period in either the clinic or home, providing support for the notion that the treatment program rather than the passage of time was responsible for the mother and child behavior change in the treatment group.

When parent perception measures were examined, mothers in both groups perceived their children as better adjusted at posttreatment than at pretreatment, indicating that the changes in perceptions of the mothers in the treatment group did not result from treatment per se. This finding suggests that a parent perception measure alone may not be an adequate criterion upon which to base judgments concerning the effectiveness of parent training programs.

In an analysis of the relationship among multiple outcome measures, Forehand and colleagues (1979) reported that both observational data collected by independent observers and parent-recorded data indicated generalization of treatment effects to the home setting. However, for a given participant, the degree of change across the different types of outcome measures (parent questionnaire data were also collected) was not uniform.

Two investigations examined the extent to which family SES (Rogers, Forehand, Griest, Wells, & McMahon, 1981) or child age (McMahon et al., 1985) might relate to generalization of treatment outcome to the home setting. Neither of these variables related to behavior change in the home, suggesting that the parenting program is equally effective across SES levels and across children within the 3- to 8-year-old range.

Generalization to the School Setting

The effect of the parent training program on child behavior in the school was of concern because Johnson, Bolstad, and Lobitz (1976) reported data suggesting that children may increase their inappropriate behavior in school when inappropriate home behavior is treated by parent training programs. In order to determine whether such a "behavioral contrast" effect existed, or whether setting generality (a decrease in inappropriate school behavior when noncompliance and other inappropriate behavior decreased in the home) occurred with our parent training program, two different investigations have been conducted.

In both studies (Breiner & Forehand, 1981; Forehand, Sturgis, et al., 1979), child behavior was assessed not only in the home but at preschool or school before and after parent training. Furthermore, randomly selected children served as controls in the school setting. In the home assessments, children whose parents received parent training increased their compliance; however, relative to the control children, they did not systematically change either their compliance or inappropriate behavior (e.g., tantrums, demanding attention) in preschool or school. Thus, treatment-induced changes in child behavior in the home were not associated with systematic behavior change in the school, either in terms of setting generalization or a behavioral contrast effect (McMahon & Davies, 1980). However, it is important to note that more recent investigations using other Hanf-based parent training programs have reported generalization to the school (e.g., McNeil et al., 1991; Webster-Stratton, 1998). Based on the existing inconsistent data, assessment of school behavior when conducting parent training is important in order to ascertain whether intervention in the school setting is warranted (see Chapters 4 and 5).

Further analyses of the data from the Breiner and Forehand (1981) study indicated that it may be possible to predict changes in the school behavior of these children on the basis of pretreatment levels of compliance and inappropriate behavior at school in combination with the amount of change in home behavior from pretreatment to posttreatment (Forehand, Breiner, McMahon, & Davies, 1981). This combination accounted for 55% and 70% of the variance in predicting changes in school compliance and inappropriate behavior, respectively.

Temporal Generalization (Maintenance)

At this point, our data indicated that the parenting program was immediately effective in changing parent and child behavior in both the clinic and home. However, the maintenance of these effects (i.e., temporal generality) was unknown. Several subsequent studies examined the temporal generality of the parent training program (Baum & Forehand, 1981; Forehand & Long, 1988; Forehand, Rogers, McMahon, Wells, & Griest, 1981; Forehand, Steffe, Furey, & Walley, 1983; Forehand, Sturgis, et al., 1979; Long, Forehand, Wierson, & Morgan, 1994). These studies have included the following characteristics: (1) ranged from 6 months to 14 years in length of follow-up; (2) included between 10 and 34 children; (3) utilized behavioral observations (most studies), parent perception questionnaires, teacher report (one study), and, when children reached adolescence, youth-report measures; and (4) often included a community sample to serve as a normative group comparison.

These investigations indicated that the HNC program has a high degree of temporal generalization. Improvements in both child and parent behaviors and parental perceptions of the children generally were maintained at follow-up assessments up to 14 years after treatment termination. The apparent exception to this pattern of maintenance has been the finding that, while such positive parent behaviors as attends plus rewards and contingent attention occur more frequently at follow-up than prior to treatment, they decrease from posttreatment levels. However, these decreases in positive attention are programmed into the parent training program, since parents are told that the initial frequent use of positive attention can be gradually decreased, but not eliminated, as the children's negative behaviors decrease. Finally, when compared to the normative sample on parent, teacher, and child report at follow-up, differences rarely emerged. This suggests that the program is associated with "normalization" of children.

Sibling Generalization

Humphreys and colleagues (1978) examined the generalization of treatment effects from one sibling to another. During pretreatment and posttreatment home observations, the interactions of each mother and clinic-referred child and of the mother and a sibling of the clinic-referred child were observed in the home. During treatment, the therapist did not discuss the application of the parenting techniques to the untreated sibling. From pretreatment to posttreatment, the mothers significantly increased their use of positive attention contingent on compliance, rewards, and attends, and decreased their use of beta commands toward the *untreated* children. In addition, the untreated children increased their compliance. These results suggest that mothers can generalize their skills for dealing with noncompliance to other children in the family without the aid of direct programming by the therapist and that the untreated children respond by increasing their compliance to maternal commands.

Behavioral Generalization

One study has examined behavioral generalization of the parent training program, that is, the relationship between a treated child behavior (noncompliance) and untreated child behaviors (other inappropriate behavior, including tantrums, aggression, crying, etc.). Wells, Forehand, and Griest (1980) treated 12 noncompliant clinic-referred children and their mothers. Observations of child behavior were collected from these families and from a nonclinic normative comparison group of 12 mother–child pairs. The clinic-referred children significantly increased their compliance from pretreatment to posttreatment, whereas the children in the nonclinic group did not change significantly on these measures. Of importance for behavioral generalization, untreated child inappropriate behavior decreased significantly from pretreatment to posttreatment for the clinic, but not the nonclinic, group. The clinic-referred group displayed significantly more inappropriate behavior than the nonclinic group at pretreatment but not at posttreatment. These results provide evidence that generality from treated to untreated child behavior occurs with the HNC program, and suggest that the successful treatment of noncompliance is sufficient in many cases to reduce other inappropriate behaviors that are not treated.

Social Validity

Based on Kazdin (1977) and Wolf (1978), Forehand and colleagues (1980) examined the social validity of the parent training program by using four procedures: (1) social comparison (i.e., do referred children differ from a normative sample before treatment but not after treatment?); (2) subjective evaluation (i.e., do maternal perceptions of child behavior change with treatment?); (3) social acceptability of treatment (i.e., are the treatment procedures appropriate for the referral problem?); and (4) consumer satisfaction (i.e., is the parent satisfied with treatment?). Fifteen clinic-referred children and their mothers and 15 nonclinic children and their mothers served as participants. Behavioral observations in the home setting were conducted at pretreatment, posttreatment, and at a 2-month follow-up for the clinic-referred group and at comparable times for the nonclinic group. Parental questionnaires regarding the adjustment of their children also were completed before and after the treatment period and at the 2-month follow-up. At 15 months after treatment, measures of consumer satisfaction and social acceptability of treatment were collected from parents in the clinic-referred group. Only mothers in the clinic-referred group completed the parenting program.

    The social comparison method of assessing social validity indicated that children in the clinic (treatment) group were less compliant and more inappropriate prior to treatment, but not after treatment or at follow-up, than were children in the nonclinic group. Furthermore, children in the clinic group demonstrated an increase in compliance and a decrease in inappropriate behavior from pretreatment to posttreatment.

With respect to the subjective evaluation procedure, mothers in the treatment group reported significant improvement in their children's adjustment from pretreatment to posttreatment; however, they still perceived their children as less well adjusted than nonclinic mothers perceived their children at posttreatment. At the follow-up assessment, the two groups of mothers did not differ in their perceptions of their children's adjustment, suggesting that changes in maternal perceptions may follow rather than accompany changes in child behavior.

On the measure of social acceptability of treatment and consumer satisfaction collected 15 months after treatment termination, mothers in the treatment group indicated that they viewed the treatment procedures as appropriate for dealing with their children's behavior problems. Furthermore, they reported that they viewed their children more positively and as improved as a result of treatment, felt confident in managing their children, viewed the therapists as being very helpful, and frequently used the skills taught in the program. Thus, all four procedures suggested that the program is socially valid.

Two additional studies have examined the treatment acceptability of the HNC parent training program and its components. In a study by Cross Calvert and McMahon (1987), 90 nonreferred mothers of 3- to 8-year-old children evaluated treatment acceptability (based on a written description) of the individual parenting skills (i.e., attends, rewards, ignoring, clear instructions, and TO), three methods of introducing each skill (rationale, rationale plus modeling, no introduction), and the program as a whole. The mothers rated all aspects of the HNC program and the program as a whole very positively. Strategies to increase appropriate child behavior (attends, rewards, clear instructions) were rated as more acceptable than strategies used to reduce inappropriate child behavior (ignoring, TO). Presenting a rationale was rated as the most acceptable method of introducing the new parenting strategies to the child (see Davies et al., 1984; McMahon, Davies, & Tiedemann, 1983; McMahon, Tiedemann, & Davies, 1987).

The second investigation examined the acceptability (based on a written description) of three different modes of administration of the HNC parent training program: (1) the "standard" therapist administration, (2) self-administration in the form of a written manual, and (3) therapist administration plus the manual (McMahon, Johnson, & Robbins, 2003). Two studies were conducted, differing only in terms of sample composition: 96 undergraduate students in the first study and 57 nonreferred mothers of 3- to 8-year-olds in the second study. Findings were comparable across the two studies and replicated the findings of Cross Calvert and McMahon (1987) concerning the greater acceptability of parenting strategies to increase appropriate child behavior (attends, rewards, clear instructions) than those strategies used to reduce inappropriate child behavior (ignoring, TO). Administration of the parent training program in the form of written instructions, whether alone or in combination with therapist administration, was evaluated as comparable in acceptability, usefulness, and difficulty to the standard therapist administration of the parent training program.

Three additional investigations have utilized consumer satisfaction indexes of social validity. The studies were conducted at postassessment and follow-up intervals ranging from 2 months to 7½ years (Baum & Forehand, 1981; Forehand & Long, 1988; McMahon et al., 1984). Mothers at these assessments expressed a high level of satisfaction with the HNC program and with the therapists. They reported that they continued use of the parenting skills and that they found them useful and easy to implement. The mothers also reported that their children's behavior had improved at the end of the treatment program and at follow-up and that they would return to the clinic again if behavior problems appeared.

In the most thorough assessment of consumer satisfaction with the HNC parent training program, McMahon and colleagues (1984) also made comparisons of both perceived usefulness and difficulty among the various teaching methods and parenting skills. The various teaching methods employed by the therapists were rated as quite useful and as relatively easy to follow. The more performance-oriented teaching methods in the clinic (e.g., therapist demonstration, practice with the child in the clinic) tended to be rated as more useful and sometimes as less difficult than the more didactic modes of instruction (e.g., lecture, written materials). With respect to relative satisfaction with the various parenting skills, rewards was generally the most useful and least difficult parenting skill, while ignoring was rated as one of the least useful and most difficult parenting skills. Alpha commands (i.e., clear instructions) and TO tended to be seen as less difficult and more useful at the follow-up than at posttreatment.

The overall results of these studies strongly suggest that the HNC parenting program is a socially valid one. Furthermore, this social validity endures well after treatment termination.

Positive Side Effects

In addition to the work in generalization of treatment and social validity, we also have examined several side effects of the HNC parent training program. In the Forehand and colleagues (1980) study reported in the preceding section, evidence was found for positive side effects on maternal psychological adjustment; specifically, ratings of depressive symptomatology for the mothers of clinic-referred children improved significantly from pretreatment to posttreatment. Furthermore, while their depressive symptoms differed significantly from those of mothers of nonclinic children at pretreatment, the two groups did not differ significantly at posttreatment and at a 2-month follow-up.

In two investigations we have found evidence of a short-term positive "side effect" of the parent training program with respect to marital satisfaction (Brody & Forehand, 1985; Forehand, Griest, Wells, & McMahon, 1982): mothers with low levels of marital satisfaction prior to treatment improved significantly on this dimension after completing the parent training program. However, the gains were not maintained at a 2-month follow-up (Forehand et al., 1982). Mothers with medium or high levels of marital satisfaction did not report any change in marital satisfaction. Thus, this positive side effect was temporary and was limited to mothers with low levels of marital satisfaction. We have not examined whether marital conflict (e.g., as assessed by the OPS; Porter & O'Leary, 1980), as opposed to marital satisfaction, is affected by participation in the HNC parent training program.

Finally, other investigators using the HNC parenting program also have found positive side effects. Specifically, in a study by Roberts, Joe, and Rowe-Hallbert (1992), parents who completed the parent training program (supplemented with additional strategies for a number of specific child misbehaviors) reported a more internal locus of control concerning their parenting at posttreatment.

ENHANCEMENT OF GENERALIZATION

Once the basic treatment outcome and generalization of the parenting program were established, our investigations shifted to ways in which we might enhance treatment generalization. We have focused on developing adjunctive interventions that can be added to or combined with the basic parent training program (i.e., a constructive treatment strategy; Kazdin, 2002). In this section, we describe three investigations of different adjunctive interventions designed to enhance generalization: (1) maternal self-control procedures (Wells, Griest, & Forehand, 1980); (2) incorporation of formal training in social learning principles into the basic parenting program (McMahon, Forehand, & Griest, 1981); and (3) the efficacy of a multimodal family treatment approach (Parent Enhancement Therapy) (Griest et al., 1982) for improving the overall level of family functioning. These three interventions were developed as adjuncts to the basic parent training program because they address important factors that can adversely affect parenting. Our goal in these investigations was to examine the incremental effectiveness of incorporating these additional treatment components into the HNC program. The adjunctive interventions are described in Chapter 8, and the details of the studies are presented in Table 10.2.

Self-Control Training

Wells, Griest, and Forehand (1980) assigned 16 mothers and their clinic-referred noncompliant children either to parent training alone or parent training plus self-control. All mother–child pairs participated in the parenting program. Mothers in the combination group also learned to self-monitor their use of their new parenting skills and to reinforce themselves for the use of these skills during a 2-month follow-up period. Each mother and the therapist composed an individualized self-control program immediately after the posttreatment assessment. A list of self-reinforcers was compiled, and the mother entered into a contract with the therapist in which she agreed to practice the parenting skills with her child on a daily basis. Following each 15-minute "good parenting session," the mother administered one of these daily reinforcers to herself if she had provided positive attention to her child's appropriate behavior and provided the appropriate consequence (TO) for child noncompliance. The mother also was encouraged to employ her treatment-acquired parenting skills as well as self-reinforcement strategies throughout the day.

Of primary interest in terms of outcome were analyses of differences between the two groups at follow-up as a function of the self-control contract followed by half of the mothers. Children in the group receiving parent training plus self-control were significantly more compliant and less inappropriate than the children in the group receiving parent training alone. Unexpectedly, no differences were obtained between groups on the observational measures of parent behavior (rewards plus attends, beta commands, contingent attention). It should be noted that two mothers in the self-control group did not actively participate in the self-control program. Thus, while the results of this study provide some evidence that self-control procedures may be of benefit to some mothers in the enhancement of temporal generality, the failure to find concomitant improvements in parent behaviors in this group and the failure of two of the mothers to participate actively in the self-control program suggest that research is needed to determine which parents might benefit from such self-control training.

Training in Social Learning Principles

McMahon, Forehand, and Griest (1981) analyzed the effectiveness of incorporating formal training in social learning principles into the HNC program on enhancing treatment outcome and generalization. Twenty mother–child pairs who were referred for treatment of the child's behavior problems were assigned to one of two groups. The technique-alone (TA) parent training group received behavioral skill training via the treatment program. Therapists did not include any reference to, or explanations of, social learning principles in their interactions with these parents. The social learning (SL) parent training group received the same behavioral skills training. In addition, mothers in this group were given specific didactic instruction and brief reading assignments in various social learning principles that were relevant to the parent training program, such as characteristics of positive and negative reinforcement, shaping, extinction, and punishment. Instruction in these principles was integrated into the program such that instruction preceded training of a particular technique, but relevant points were repeated throughout the program as the skills were being applied. Families were assessed at pretreatment, posttreatment, and 2-month follow-up through home observations and parent-report measures.

At posttreatment and follow-up, not surprisingly, mothers in the SL group demonstrated a superior knowledge of social learning principles. The mothers in the SL group emitted a higher frequency of attends plus rewards and higher percentages of contingent attention than did TA mothers at either posttreatment and/or follow-up. Children in the SL group were significantly more compliant to maternal commands than were children in the TA group at the follow-up. Mothers in the SL group generally viewed their children in a more positive light than did mothers in the TA group at both posttreatment and follow-up. Mothers in both groups expressed a high level of overall satisfaction with their treatment program at both posttreatment and follow-up. Mothers in the SL group tended to be more satisfied with their program at posttreatment than were TA mothers.

In a more extensive analysis of the consumer satisfaction data collected in the McMahon, Forehand, and Griest (1981) study, McMahon and colleagues (1984) found that mothers in the TA group reported practice with the children in the clinic and therapist demonstration to be more difficult at both posttreatment and follow-up than did mothers in the SL group. At the follow-up, there were several additional differences between the two groups. One type of homework assignment, attends, and the overall group of parenting skills were judged significantly less useful at follow-up than at posttreatment for the TA group. The mothers in the SL group maintained their ratings on these measures from posttreatment to follow-up. In addition, the SL group rated the overall group of parenting skills as significantly more useful than did the TA group at follow-up. Taken in combination with the findings of McMahon, Forehand, and Griest, these results indicate that the integration of formal training in social learning principles enhances treatment outcome, setting generality, and temporal generality and is associated with higher levels of parental satisfaction and/or maintenance of satisfaction with the parent training program.

Parent Enhancement Therapy

The most comprehensive adjunctive therapy that we have examined is a multimodal treatment package designed to enhance general family functioning (Griest et al., 1982). As noted in Chapters 1, 2, and 5, as well as below, there is compelling evidence that various family-related issues, such as a parent's perception of a child's behavior, the parent's personal and marital adjustment, and the parent's extrafamilial relationships, are associated with child conduct problems. Furthermore, these family-related issues may inhibit the effectiveness of behavioral parent training programs.

Several of our investigations have been concerned with the interactions among maternal perceptions of the children, maternal personal adjustment, maternal marital status and satisfaction, and parent and child behavior (see Forehand, Furey, & McMahon, 1984, for a review). This research indicated that the negative perceptions of the mothers of clinic-referred children are influenced by a combination of the children's behavior and the mothers' own level of personal adjustment (e.g., depressive symptoms) (Griest et al., 1979, 1980). In fact, one of our investigations has suggested that there are at least two identifiable subgroups of mothers of clinic-referred children: mothers with a deficit in parenting skills per se (and whose children are more deviant than are nonclinic children) and mothers who are experiencing personal adjustment problems but whose children are no more deviant than are nonclinic children (Rickard et al., 1981).

Not only is there an association between level of maternal personal maladjustment and her negative perceptions of her children, as reported by Griest and colleagues (1979, 1980), but also with failure to complete the parenting program (Furey & Basili, 1988; McMahon, Forehand, Griest, & Wells, 1981), to participate in follow-up assessments (Griest, Forehand, & Wells, 1981), and to maintain improved perception of child adjustment at a 2-month follow-up (Furey & Basili, 1988) (see Table 10.2). Marital satisfaction is also implicated in maternal interactions with clinic-referred children (Bond & McMahon, 1984; Rickard, Forehand, Atkeson, & Lopez, 1982): low marital satisfaction was associated with increased depressive and anxious symptoms and more negative maternal perceptions of child adjustment. All of these investigations suggest the importance of considering family-related issues when conducting parent training.

The Griest and colleagues (1982) investigation determined whether including several additional treatment modules related to the broader family issues described above resulted in enhanced treatment outcome and generalization beyond the positive effects reported in some of our earlier investigations. A total of 17 mothers and their clinic-referred noncompliant children were assigned either to parent training alone or to parent training plus PET; 15 additional mothers and their nonclinic children served as a quasi-control group. All clinic-referred mother–child dyads were treated individually by way of the parent training program. In addition, mothers receiving parent training plus PET also received treatment related to the following areas: parents' perception of the children's behavior; marital adjustment; parents' personal adjustment; and parents' extrafamilial relationships. Treatment consisted of didactic presentations, modeling, role playing, and homework assignments. Components of the PET package were presented prior to, during, and after the basic parent training program.

Home observations at pretreatment, posttreatment, and a 2-month follow-up indicated that parent training plus PET was more effective than was parent training alone in changing inappropriate child behavior at posttreatment, as well as in maintaining child compliance, inappropriate child behavior, parental rewards, and parental contingent attention at the follow-up. The quasi-control group did not change over the three assessment periods, suggesting that the behaviors measured were generally stable over the three assessment periods. The parents' perception of the usefulness of the PET was also examined after treatment and at a 2-month follow-up. On a scale ranging from "extremely harmful" to "extremely helpful," the parent training plus PET group rated the additional treatment as "helpful."

The results of this study indicate that the maintenance of treatment effects of parent training can be enhanced by combining this approach with a treatment package that focuses on parental perception of child behavior, parental personal and marital adjustment, and the parents' extrafamilial relationships. It is important to note that the treated parent–child pairs in the present study were not selected because they demonstrated difficulties in one or more of the four areas targeted for treatment in the enhancement therapy. Therefore, the extent to which the present findings can be generalized to families with severe difficulties in one or more of these areas is uncertain. The limited treatment delivered in the PET package may not be sufficient with such families. In such cases, more intensive adjuncts (see Table 5.1) may be indicated.

SELF-ADMINISTERED INTERVENTIONS

The use of self-administered interventions based on the HNC program has been examined in three quite different ways (see Table 10.2). Also, as noted earlier in this chapter, McMahon and colleagues (2003) reported that administration of the HNC parent training program in written form (alone or in combination with therapist administration) has been evaluated as comparable in acceptability, usefulness, and difficulty to the standard therapist administration of the HNC program.

A Brochure for Dealing with Inappropriate Mealtime Behavior

As noted in Chapter 8, we developed and evaluated a written brochure to teach parents to improve their children's mealtime behavior (McMahon & Forehand, 1978) that served as a prototype for dealing with situations in which the child's noncompliant behavior is limited to specific situations. As mealtime problem behaviors are frequently reported by parents of preschool children (e.g., Sanders et al., 1993), we chose these problem behaviors to test the effectiveness of an abbreviated self-administered intervention.

Three preschool-aged children and their mothers participated in the study. All were from middle-class families. Observations were conducted in the home by independent observers during mealtime. A multiple-baseline design across subjects was employed to assess the effects of the treatment brochure. Prior to baseline observations, each mother specified the mealtime behaviors she wished to modify in the Mealtime Behavior Checklist (see Appendix D). Following the final baseline observation, the experimenter delivered the brochure to the mother. The brochure described the procedures of rewards and TO by presenting a short rationale for each technique, along with step-by-step instructions for their implementation, and examples of their use at mealtime (see Appendix D for the brochure). There was no therapist–client contact other than an initial interview to describe the project and the delivery of the brochure to the mothers after baseline, and there was no feedback given to the mothers at any point in the study. After baseline, observations continued in the home during mealtime for 7–16 days. Approximately 6 weeks following the final observation, five additional follow-up observations were carried out to assess maintenance.

Inappropriate mealtime behavior decreased substantially, ranging from 50% to 80%, for the children following introduction of the treatment brochure. Furthermore, the changes were maintained for all three children at the follow-up observations. Maternal behavior also changed following introduction of the brochure: all mothers substantially increased both rewards to their children's appropriate mealtime behavior and suitable responses to inappropriate mealtime behavior, as compared to baseline levels of response. At the 6-week follow-up, successful handling of inappropriate mealtime behavior maintained or continued to improve. Rewards for appropriate mealtime behavior did decline at the follow-up; however, this decline was expected, as mothers were instructed in the brochure to thin out the schedule of reinforcement gradually.

This study indicates that written instructions alone can effectively prompt mothers to modify their nonreferred children's inappropriate mealtime behavior in the home setting, and that these changes are maintained for at least 6 weeks.

Written Instructions for Path A of the Clear Instructions Sequence

McMahon and Lehman (2003) recently examined the effectiveness of written instructions in enhancing the therapist administration of the parenting program. Because this was a preliminary study, a nonreferred sample was employed, and only a single component of the parent training program was evaluated. Specifically, parents were trained to give clear instructions to their children and to follow child compliance with positive attention (i.e., Path A of the clear instructions sequence; see Figure 7.2). (The written instructions are available upon request from the first author [RJM]). Forty mothers and their 3- to 6-year-old children were assigned to one of four conditions: (1) "standard" therapist-administered parent training; (2) written instructions only; (3) a combination of therapist-administered training and written instructions; or (4) no-training control group. This design allowed the examination of not only the effectiveness of written instructions in enhancing the therapist-administered intervention but also the effectiveness of written instructions alone. The analyses generally indicated that the combination of therapist-administered and written instructions was the most effective intervention. Mothers and children in this condition engaged in a higher proportion of the clear instructions–child compliance–contingent attention sequence (i.e., Path A) than mothers in either the written instructions or control conditions. The mothers in this condition also gave a higher level of contingent attention than did the control group mothers, and they tended to be more knowledgeable and satisfied with the intervention than mothers in the other intervention conditions. Thus, the findings of this study suggest the value of written instructions as an adjunct to the standard administration of the parent training program by a therapist. The handouts we utilize in the program (see Appendix B) serve as our written instructions.

A Self-Administered Booklet for Parents of Oppositional Children with ADHD

Finally, Long and colleagues (1993) conducted a pilot study to examine the effects of a self-administered booklet explaining the skills in the HNC program to parents of children with ADHD and high levels of oppositional behavior. The study involved 32 families who were randomly assigned to the intervention condition (booklet plus medication) or the comparison group (medication only). Parent ratings collected 2 months after distribution of the booklet indicated that the intensity of oppositional behavior problems was less for children whose parents had received the booklet than for children in the comparison condition. There was also a trend for the children in the intervention group to have fewer behavior problems. Teachers, who were blind to the purposes of the study, also rated the intensity of behavior problems of the children in the intervention condition to be less than the children in the comparison condition.

   Taken together, these studies suggest the potential value of employing self-administered written materials in the HNC parent training program.

COMPARISONS WITH OTHER INTERVENTIONS

Two independent replications have compared the effects of the HNC parent training program with other interventions for children with conduct problems (see Table 10.2). Wells and Egan (1988) randomly assigned 19 children (aged 3–8 years) who had been diagnosed with ODD to either the HNC parent training program or to systems family therapy (Haley, 1976; Minuchin, 1974). They found that, at the end of treatment, the parents in the parent training condition displayed higher levels of positive attention (attends plus rewards) and contingent attention in clinic observations. Furthermore, the children in the parent training condition displayed higher levels of compliance to instructions than children in the systems family therapy condition. The two treatment groups did not differ on parental self-report measures of personal (depression, anxiety) or marital adjustment.

Baum and colleagues (1986) compared the effectiveness of the HNC parent training program (with or without a child self-control adjunct) to a parent discussion group based on the Systematic Training for Effective Parenting (STEP) program (Dinkmeyer & McKay, 1976). (The parent training alone and STEP conditions also included a child attention control.) Children ranged in age from 6 to 10 years. For parents and children receiving the parenting program, improvements occurred in the observed parent and child behaviors at posttreatment and at a 6- to 8-month follow-up. No change in behavior occurred with the STEP intervention.

These two studies provide substantial support for the effectiveness of the parent training program. By comparing the program to other interventions, Wells and Egan (1988) and Baum and colleagues (1986) demonstrated that the parenting skills taught are necessary to achieve changes in parent and child behavior and are more effective than other approaches.

CURRENT DIRECTIONS: MOVING TOWARD PREVENTION

Parent training interventions that occur with preschool- and early school-age children can be viewed as preventative in nature in that they attempt not only to alleviate current child conduct problems but to also decrease the likelihood that children will develop the more serious conduct problems that are characteristic of later stages in the early starter pathway of conduct problems (see Chapter 1). In fact, our long-term data suggest that this may be the case with the HNC parent training program (Forehand & Long, 1988; Long et al., 1994). Another reason to intervene early through preventative efforts is that parent training programs have a better track record in treating conduct problems manifested in the preschool- and early elementary school-age periods than during adolescence (McMahon & Wells, 1998).

Given these factors, it becomes relatively easy to argue for a focus on targeted prevention, in which family-based interventions occur early on in the developmental progression of conduct problems. Much of our effort in recent years has focused on research that is preventative in nature. In this section we describe two ongoing prevention efforts: (1) parent education groups utilizing a book based on our parenting program and (2) a large-scale preventive intervention, Fast Track, that has incorporated major components of the HNC parenting training program. The first effort is a modified version of the HNC parent training program in which intervention occurs with groups of parents who have at-risk children demonstrating preclinical levels of noncompliance. The second effort is a prevention program for at-risk children in which the teaching of parenting skills is one of several intervention components. For many children, more than parenting skills may be needed; Fast Track is an excellent example of a comprehensive program. Finally, an important aspect of both of these preventive interventions is the inclusion of significant numbers of ethnic minority families.

Parent Education Groups

As noted in Chapter 8, the book *Parenting the Strong-Willed Child: The Clinically Proven Five-Week Program for Parents of Two- to Six-Year Olds* (Forehand & Long, 2002) has been utilized successfully as the core of a six-session parent education group. In each of the first five 2-hour sessions, one of the skills in the HNC parenting program is taught, along with selected material from the first or third sections of the book concerning causal and contributing factors to the development of noncompliance and the development of a more positive family atmosphere. The final 2-hour session integrates the parenting skills and uses them to address specific child behavior problems that occur (i.e., the fourth section of the book). The leader's guide (Long & Forehand, 2000b) is available from Nicholas Long (*LongNicholas@exchange.uams.edu*).

The parent education group intervention, which has been evaluated in pilot work with 54 parents, is associated with significant decreases in parent reports of child problem behavior (Long & Forehand, 2000a, 2002a). Currently under way is a large-scale, grant-supported independent evaluation of the parent education group intervention by Mark Edwards, a psychologist at the University of Arkansas for Medical Sciences. This project is being conducted with some 150 families of at-risk Head Start children, approximately 75% of whom are ethnic minority. In addition to an evaluation of the parent education group format intervention, this project is evaluating the parenting program as administered by therapists to individual families.

The Fast Track Project

Fast Track is a multisite collaborative study that is investigating the effectiveness of a comprehensive intervention designed to prevent the development of serious conduct problems in a large at-risk sample of young school-aged children (Conduct Problems Prevention Research Group, 1992, 2000). The project is being conducted at four sites in the United States that represent urban, semi-urban, and rural communities. The first author (RJM) is the principal investigator at one of the sites and was in charge of developing the parenting intervention. The high-risk sample consists of 891 children who have been identified by both parents and teachers as displaying high levels of conduct problem behaviors during kindergarten. An additional 387 children constitute a representative normative sample from the same schools as the high-risk children. Adequate representation of girls (31%) and minorities (53%, most of whom are African American) ensures that it will be possible to examine both the developmental course and the effects of the intervention with various subgroups of children. The children are followed on an annual basis from kindergarten through high school and beyond. Assessments include interviews with the children, parents, and teachers; observations of parent–child interactions and child interactions in the classroom and on the playground; peer sociometric interviews; and review of archival records.

Half of the children in the high-risk sample are participating in an intensive and long-term intervention designed to address the developmental issues involved in the early starter pathway of conduct problems. The intervention begins in the first grade and continues through the tenth grade. However, there are two periods of most intensive intervention: school entry (first and second grade) and the transition into middle school (fifth and sixth grades). The intervention at school entry targets proximal changes in six domains: (1) disruptive behaviors in the home; (2) disruptive and off-task behaviors in the school; (3) social-cognitive skills pertaining to affect regulation and social problem-solving skills; (4) peer relations; (5) academic skills; and (6) the family–school relationship. Integrated intervention components include parent training, home visiting, social skills training, academic tutoring, and a universal teacher-administered intervention designed to increase social and emotional competence in the classroom. The family-based components of the intervention during first and second grades are described below. (See Bierman, Greenberg, & the Conduct Problems Prevention Research Group, 1996, for detailed descriptions of the other intervention components.) The intervention at the entry into middle school in grades 5 and 6 (and through grade 10) includes interventions with increasing emphasis on parent/adult monitoring and positive involvement, peer affiliation and peer influence, academic achievement and orientation to school, and social cognition and identity development (Conduct Problems Prevention Research Group, 2000).

Three family-based components occur during the elementary school phase of the Fast Track intervention: (1) a parenting skills group; (2) a parent–child relationship enhancement group; and (3) a home-visiting program (see McMahon et al., 1996, for more details). The overarching goal of the family-based components of Fast Track is to help parents assist their children in succeeding in school. This goal is defined quite broadly to include not only academic success but also success in personal and social contexts as well.

The parent group focuses on development in four areas: a positive family–school relationship; parental self-control; reasonable and developmentally appropriate expectations for the child's behavior; and parenting skills to increase positive parent–child interaction and to decrease the occurrence of conduct problem behaviors. Because of the importance of children getting off to a good start in school, much of the material concerning the development of a positive family–school relationship is covered during the first half of the first grade academic year. Topics addressed in these sessions include how to talk with children about school, the importance of engaging in regular parent–child reading sessions, setting up a system of regular communication between the teacher and parent concerning the child's performance in school, encouraging learning-related behaviors at home, and learning appropriate ways to assist children with homework assignments.

Prior to focusing on parenting skills related to discipline, parents learn how to maintain their self-control when faced with frustrating child behavior and to develop expectations for their children's behavior that are reasonable and appropriate for their children's developmental level. Parents learn to identify the behavioral, cognitive, and affective cues that indicate that they are becoming angry and to use an anger management strategy (adapted from Hawkins et al., 1988). With respect to developmentally appropriate parental expectations, separate sessions in first and second grade are devoted to a discussion of the physical, social, behavioral, and cognitive capabilities of children in that age range and the importance of recognizing individual differences in these capabilities as well.

The majority of parent group sessions in grades 1 and 2 are concerned with teaching parenting skills to enhance positive parent–child interaction and to decrease the occurrence of conduct-problem behaviors. Many of the skills that are taught are most closely derived from the HNC parent training program, with some additional material from the group-based program (BASIC) developed by Webster-Stratton (2000) (see Chapter 2). The skills taught include ways to spend positive time with children, praise, differential attention, when–then rules, clear instructions, TO, privilege removal, and the use of house rules. By the end of grade 1, parents have been exposed to almost all of these strategies. A major focus of the parent group in grade 2 is teaching the parents a problem-solving protocol that they can use to select the most appropriate strategies for dealing with a particular situation. This protocol, which is referred to as the Problem-Solving Approach, consists of implementation of a parental self-control strategy, defining the problem in terms of a preferred positive child behavior, making sure that the expectation is developmentally appropriate and realistic, and then selecting a parenting skill.

A typical parent group is composed of five to seven parents. The primary parenting figures in the children's lives are targeted for participation in the parent group. In most cases that is the biological mother, with or without participation by her male partner and other significant family members. The parent groups are conducted by a family coordinator and, in most cases, a coleader. Parent group sessions run concurrently with children's social skills group sessions. There are 22 weekly group sessions (each lasting 60 minutes) during grade 1 and 14 biweekly sessions (each lasting 90 minutes) during grade 2. Family coordinators employ a wide variety of teaching methods during the parent group, including some didactic presentation of material, group discussion and exercises, posters and handouts, demonstration of various skills, and parental role play exercises.

At the conclusion of each parent group and children's social skills group, the parents and children meet together for "parent–child sharing time." Each session lasts 30 minutes and is led by the family coordinator with assistance from a coleader. There are two goals for this component of Fast Track. The primary goal is to foster positive parent–child relationships through the promotion of positive, cooperative verbal behavior and nonverbal interchanges between parents and children. Families participate in a variety of cooperative activities, games, and crafts; they also participate in joint reading activities. The activities that occur during parent–child sharing time often have direct tie-ins to social skills that the children have been learning in the classroom-based curriculum and the social skills group. The second goal of parent–child sharing time is to provide an opportunity for parents to practice the new skills that they learned in the parent group with their children, with appropriate support and supervision from Fast Track staff members. It also provides the children with the opportunity to learn the new strategies that their parents will be using with them at home.

The home-visiting component of Fast Track is intended to serve a variety of functions. These include (1) providing an opportunity for the family coordinator to become familiar with the entire family system; (2) providing an opportunity to promote the generalization of newly acquired parenting skills to the natural environment; (3) promoting effective parental support for the child's school adjustment; and (4) promoting parental problem-solving and coping skills.

Early results of the Fast Track intervention have indicated significant positive effects for the high-risk children and their families (Conduct Problems Prevention Research Group, 1999, 2002). At the end of first grade, compared to children in the control condition, there were consistent, moderate effects for children in the intervention condition in the following areas: social, emotional, and academic skills; peer interactions and social status; conduct problems; and special education resource use. Parents in the intervention condition reported less use of physical discipline and greater parenting satisfaction/ease of parenting, and they engaged in more appropriate/consistent discipline and warmth/positive involvement when interacting with their children. Teachers reported that the parents had more positive involvement with their children's school. Intervention effects for parenting and child behavior were generally maintained at the end of third grade.

Fast Track serves as a model comprehensive program for families with at-risk children. The inclusion of components of the HNC parenting training program as core ingredients in this efficacious multi-faceted intervention suggests that the HNC parenting program can be readily adapted for culturally diverse at-risk groups and integrated into large-scale community prevention programs. Although programs such as Fast Track are expensive in terms of resources and time, they are warranted, given the frequency, severity, and consequences of serious conduct problems in society.

CONCLUSIONS

Our research program has been a programmatic effort to design and evaluate the HNC parent training program over a 30-year period. The research efforts have progressed through various stages of evaluation, with the primary foci being the following: (1) laboratory investigations of components of the parenting program; (2) treatment effectiveness of the program; (3) treatment generalization, social validity, and positive side effects; (4) enhancement of treatment and generalization through the use of adjunctive procedures; (5) self-administered interventions; (6) comparisons to other methods of intervention; and, currently, (7) use of the parenting program for prevention of problem behavior in at-risk children. Strengths of the research include the collection of observational data in natural settings (i.e., home and school); collection of observational data on both parent and child behavior; multiple sources of data; collection of long-term follow-up data; and, perhaps of most importance, consistent findings across studies. As with any research effort, our program of research does have limitations. These include small sample sizes; failure to find generalization of treatment effects to the school setting; a neglect of fathers; and, with the exception of our prevention efforts, inclusion of predominantly middle- to lower-middle-class European American samples. Clearly, there is much work still to be done. However, we believe that our investigations have contributed to the alleviation of parenting skill difficulties and child conduct problems, particularly noncompliance. More importantly, we sincerely hope that we have been able to enrich the lives of parents and children in a meaningful way.

Parent's Consumer Satisfaction Questionnaire

Parent's Name _____   Date _____

The following questionnaire is part of our evaluation of the treatment program that you have received. It is important that you answer as honestly as possible. The information obtained will help us to evaluate and continually improve the program we offer. Your cooperation is greatly appreciated.

A. THE OVERALL PROGRAM

Please circle the response that best expresses how you honestly feel.

1. The major problem(s) that originally prompted me to begin treatment for my child is (are) at this point

| considerably worse | worse | slightly worse | the same | slightly improved | improved | greatly improved |

2. My child's problems that have been treated at the clinic are at this point

| considerably worse | worse | slightly worse | the same | slightly improved | improved | greatly improved |

3. My child's problems that have *not* been treated at the clinic are

| considerably worse | worse | slightly worse | the same | slightly improved | improved | greatly improved |

(continued)

4. My feelings at this point about my child's progress are that I am

very dissatisfied	dissatisfied	slightly dissatisfied	neutral	slightly satisfied	satisfied	very satisfied

5. To what degree has the treatment program helped with other general personal or family problems not directly related to your child?

hindered much more than helped	hindered	hindered slightly	neither helped nor hindered	helped slightly	helped	helped very much

6. At this point, my expectation for a satisfactory outcome of the treatment is

very pessimistic	pessimistic	slightly pessimistic	neutral	slightly optimistic	optimistic	very optimistic

7. I feel the approach to treating my child's behavior problems in the home by using this type of parent training program is

very inappro- priate	inappro- priate	slightly inappro- priate	neutral	slightly appro- priate	appro- priate	very appro- priate

8. Would you recommend the program to a friend or relative?

strongly recom- mend	recom- mend	slightly recom- mend	neutral	slightly not recom- mend	not recom- mend	strongly not recom- mend

9. How confident are you in managing *current* behavior problems in the home on your own?

very confident	confident	somewhat confident	neutral	somewhat uncon- fident	uncon- fident	very uncon- fident

10. How confident are you in your ability to manage *future* behavior problems in the home using what you learned from this program?

very uncon- fident	uncon- fident	somewhat uncon- fident	neutral	somewhat confident	confident	very confident

11. My overall feeling about the treatment program for my child and family is

very negative	negative	somewhat negative	neutral	slightly positive	positive	very positive

(continued)

B. TEACHING FORMAT

Difficulty

In this section, we'd like to get your ideas of how difficult each of the following types of teaching has been for you to follow. Please circle the response that most closely describes your opinion.

1. Lecture information

| extremely easy | easy | somewhat easy | neutral | somewhat difficult | difficult | extremely difficult |

2. Demonstration of skills by the therapist

| extremely easy | easy | somewhat easy | neutral | somewhat difficult | difficult | extremely difficult |

3. Practice of skills in the clinic with the therapist

| extremely easy | easy | somewhat easy | neutral | somewhat difficult | difficult | extremely difficult |

4. Practice of skills in the clinic with your child

| extremely easy | easy | somewhat easy | neutral | somewhat difficult | difficult | extremely difficult |

5. Practicing the Child's Game at home

| extremely easy | easy | somewhat easy | neutral | somewhat difficult | difficult | extremely difficult |

6. Other homework assignments

| extremely easy | easy | somewhat easy | neutral | somewhat difficult | difficult | extremely difficult |

7. The written materials you were asked to read

| extremely easy | easy | somewhat easy | neutral | somewhat difficult | difficult | extremely difficult |

(continued)

Usefulness

In this section, we'd like to get your ideas of how useful each of the following types of teaching is for you *now*. Please circle the response that most clearly describes your opinion.

1. Lecture information

   extremely not useful   not useful   somewhat not useful   neutral   somewhat useful   useful   extremely useful

2. Demonstration of skills by the therapist

   extremely not useful   not useful   somewhat not useful   neutral   somewhat useful   useful   extremely useful

3. Practice of skills in the clinic with the therapist

   extremely not useful   not useful   somewhat not useful   neutral   somewhat useful   useful   extremely useful

4. Practice of skills in the clinic with your child

   extremely not useful   not useful   somewhat not useful   neutral   somewhat useful   useful   extremely useful

5. Practicing the Child's Game at home

   extremely not useful   not useful   somewhat not useful   neutral   somewhat useful   useful   extremely useful

6. Other homework assignments

   extremely not useful   not useful   somewhat not useful   neutral   somewhat useful   useful   extremely useful

7. The written materials you were asked to read

   extremely not useful   not useful   somewhat not useful   neutral   somewhat useful   useful   extremely useful

(continued)

C. SPECIFIC PARENTING TECHNIQUES

Difficulty

In this section we'd like to get your idea of how difficult it usually is to do each of the following techniques *now*. Please circle the response that most closely describes how difficult the technique is to do.

1. Attends

| extremely easy | easy | somewhat easy | neutral | somewhat difficult | difficult | extremely difficult |

2. Rewards

| extremely easy | easy | somewhat easy | neutral | somewhat difficult | difficult | extremely difficult |

3. Ignoring

| extremely easy | easy | somewhat easy | neutral | somewhat difficult | difficult | extremely difficult |

4. Clear instructions

| extremely easy | easy | somewhat easy | neutral | somewhat difficult | difficult | extremely difficult |

5. Time out

| extremely easy | easy | somewhat easy | neutral | somewhat difficult | difficult | extremely difficult |

6. The overall group of techniques

| extremely easy | easy | somewhat easy | neutral | somewhat difficult | difficult | extremely difficult |

Usefulness

In this section, we'd like to have your opinion of how useful each of the following techniques is to you in improving your interaction with your child and decreasing his or her "not OK" behavior *now*. Please circle the response that most closely describes the usefulness of the technique.

1. Attends

| extremely not useful | not useful | somewhat not useful | neutral | somewhat useful | useful | extremely useful |

(continued)

2. Rewards

extremely not useful	not useful	somewhat not useful	neutral	somewhat useful	useful	extremely useful

3. Ignoring

extremely not useful	not useful	somewhat not useful	neutral	somewhat useful	useful	extremely useful

4. Clear instructions

extremely not useful	not useful	somewhat not useful	neutral	somewhat useful	useful	extremely useful

5. Time out

extremely not useful	not useful	somewhat not useful	neutral	somewhat useful	useful	extremely useful

6. The overall group of techniques

extremely not useful	not useful	somewhat not useful	neutral	somewhat useful	useful	extremely useful

D. THERAPIST(S)

In this section we'd like to get your ideas about your therapist(s). Please circle the response to each question that best expresses how you feel.

1. I feel that the therapist's teaching was

poor	fair	slightly below average	average	slightly above average	high	superior

2. The therapist's preparation was

poor	fair	slightly below average	average	slightly above average	high	superior

3. Concerning the therapist's interest and concern in me and my problems with my child, I was

extremely dissatisfied	dissatisfied	slightly dissatisfied	neutral	slightly satisfied	satisfied	extremely satisfied

4. At this point, I feel that the therapist in the treatment program was

extremely not helpful	not helpful	slightly not helpful	neutral	slightly helpful	helpful	extremely helpful

(continued)

5. Concerning my personal feelings toward the therapist

I dislike him/her very much	I dislike him/her	I dislike him/her slightly	I have a neutral attitude toward him/her	I like him/her slightly	I like him/her	I like him/her very much

E. YOUR OPINION PLEASE

1. What part of the program was most helpful to you?

2. What did you like most about the program?

3. What did you like least about the program?

(continued)

4. What part of the program was least helpful to you?

5. How could the program have been improved to help you more?

Thank you. Now please enclose this questionnaire in the attached envelope and drop it in the mail.

SCORING INSTRUCTIONS

Score all items on a 7-point scale.

A. Overall Program

Items 1, 2, 3, 4, 5, 6, 7, 10, and 11 are scored on a 1- to 7-point scale (i.e., if first answer is circled, the item is assigned a point value of 1, if second answer is circled, the item is assigned a point value of 2, etc.), while items 8 and 9 are scored on a 7- to 1-point scale.

B. Teaching Format

Difficulty: Score all items on a 1- to 7-point scale.
Usefulness: Score all items on a 1- to 7-point scale.

C. Specific Parenting Techniques

Difficulty: Score all items on a 1- to 7-point scale.
Usefulness: Score all items on a 1- to 7-point scale.

D. Therapist(s)

Score all items on a 1- to 7-point scale.

Parent Handouts and Record Sheets

Parent Handout 1: Introduction to Phase I

In this program, you will learn to:
- Increase your child's desirable or "OK" behavior.
- Decrease your child's undesirable or "not OK" behavior.

The goals of Phase I are to help you:
- Reestablish more positive patterns of interactions between you and your child.
- Become skilled in the use of your attention to your child as a way of increasing your child's "OK" behavior and decreasing your child's "not OK" behavior.

"OK" and "Not OK" Behaviors
- An "OK" behavior is any behavior that you would like to see your child continue to do or do more often.
- A "not OK" behavior is any behavior that you would like to see your child do less often or not at all.

Phase I is based on two assumptions:

Positive Reinforcement Rule. When a behavior is followed by a positive consequence, the behavior is more likely to occur in the future.

Attention Rule. Attention, especially from parents, is a very powerful reinforcer for children aged 3 to 8 years.
- Children will work for attention, whether it is positive (such as praise) or negative (such as criticism, scolding).
- Therefore, you can use your attention to change your child's behavior.

The major focus of Phase I is to:
- Use positive parental attention to increase positive "OK" behaviors. "Catch your child being good!"
- Decrease many "not OK" behaviors by withholding your attention from your child (ignoring).

Two situations to avoid:
- The "criticism trap" is when you provide *negative* attention (such as nagging, scolding, or yelling) after your child does a "not OK" behavior. It is a trap because the negative attention stops the "not OK" behavior, but only for a while. In the long run, it actually *increases* the "not OK" behavior!
- Ignoring your child when he or she is doing an "OK" behavior will lead to that behavior occurring less often. "Leave well enough alone" is *not* the approach to take when you want to make sure that your child is doing an "OK" behavior!

(continued)

The Skills That You Will Learn in Phase I

- How to use your attention following "OK" behavior. You will specifically learn two types of positive attention:
  Attends (describe your child's behavior)
  Rewards (praise)
- How to withhold your attention to your child (ignoring) after "not OK" behavior. Note that ignoring is used only when the behavior is not harmful or destructive. Harmful behaviors will be addressed in Phase II.
- How to use the combination of positive attention and ignoring (differential attention).

What Phase I Skills Can Do

- You can teach your child which behaviors you like ("OK" behaviors), so that he or she can do them more often. Punishing "not OK" behavior only gives your child information about what not to do.
- You can learn to observe your child's behavior closely and to notice good things that he or she does. You will find your child does many "OK" behaviors, not just "not OK" ones.
- These skills can help you to relax and have fun playing with your child. This will help to make time you spend playing with your child "quality" time.
- As your child begins to enjoy being with you more, he or she will try harder to please you by doing the things you like.
- You can be a model of good behavior for your child.
- By increasing your child's "OK" behaviors, you give him or her less time for "not OK" ones.

Parent Handout 2: Attends and the Child's Game

ATTENDS

- High-rate form of positive attention in which you provide an ongoing verbal description of your child's activity.
- Follow, rather than lead, your child's activity (by providing a running verbal commentary).
  Watch closely, and with interest, what your child is doing. A good way to describe this is "tailgating" your child.
  Describe enthusiastically what your child is doing. Pretend that you are a radio announcer—give a play-by-play account or a running commentary on your child's activity.
- Attend only to "OK" behavior.
  If your child does a "not OK" behavior, *do not attend to it!*
- Two basic types:
  Describe your child's activity (*"You just put the red block on top of the green block"*).
  Emphasize a desired "OK" behavior (*"You're talking in a regular voice"*).
- "Volume control" allows you to raise or lower the intensity and frequency of the positive attention that you give to your child. A major advantage of attending is that it can be used continuously.
- When using attends:
  Do not ask any *questions* (*"What's this you're building?" "This is a tower, isn't it?"*).
  Do not give any *commands* (*"Make the car go this way" "Hand me the block"*).
  Do not try to *teach* (*"Now, Julie, how many colors are there in a rainbow?"*).
  Questions, commands, and teaching interrupt and structure your child's play.
      REMEMBER: Your child is supposed to lead the play!

RULES FOR THE CHILD'S GAME

The Child's Game is the context for practicing all of the skills in Phase I, both in the clinic and at home. It is an excellent opportunity for establishing a positive relationship with your child. Because your child will see that you are interested in what he or she is doing, your child will want to be more cooperative with you.

- Play the Child's Game with your child for one 10- to 15-minute period each day.
  (It is helpful to schedule a time so that it becomes a regular part of your day.) Make a record of each Child's Game on Parent Handout 3: Parent Record Sheet: Child's Game.
- Allow your child to choose the activity.
  Toys that facilitate less structured activities include blocks and other building materials, drawing supplies, people and animal figures, puzzles, and cars and trucks. Board

(continued)

games and reading materials are not well suited for the Child's Game activities. Do not introduce anything new into his or her play. If your child changes activities, follow along, but do not change the activity yourself.

- *Participate* in your child's play by handing him or her materials or taking a turn.
  Be careful not to begin structuring the activity yourself. You also may participate by *imitating* his or her play. Remember that your child's activity should be the center of your attention, so continue to describe his or her activity while working on your own.
- If your child does a minor "not OK" behavior during the Child's Game, ignore it.
  However, if your child repeatedly does this, or does a "not OK" behavior that is destructive, then matter-of-factly tell your child that the Child's Game has ended for the day.

The Child's Game is a chance for you to practice your attending skills and to enrich the quality of your relationship with your child. It also will be "quality" time for your child, since he or she will have your complete attention. Your child will enjoy the Child's Game because it is a safe and positive way for him or her to be "in charge" for a little while. Relax and have fun!

REMEMBER: Attending is a skill that you can use throughout the day with your child. You want to make this (and the other kinds of positive attention that you will learn) a regular part of your daily interactions with your child.

Parent Handout 3: Parent Record Sheet: Child's Game

Date	Time spent	Activity	Child's response

Date	Time spent	Activity	Child's response

Parent Handout 4: Rewards

Rewards, like attends, are types of positive attention. Rewards and attends should be used following "OK" behaviors to help increase those behaviors.

TYPES OF REWARDS

- *Physical rewards* include various forms of physical affection such as hugs, kisses, pats, and so forth.
- *Unlabeled verbal rewards* are nonspecific praise statements that do not tell your child exactly which behavior is being rewarded.
  Examples include:
  "That's great!"
  "Wow!"
  "That's really good, I wish I could do that."
  "See what nice things you do."
  "This is such fun."
  One word "quickies":*"Beautiful!" "Fine!" "Great!" Gorgeous!" "Tremendous!"*

- *Labeled verbal rewards* are praise statements that are paired with telling your child exactly what he or she did that you liked. This helps your child to learn what is "OK" behavior. Therefore, *labeled verbal rewards should be used much more often than unlabeled verbal rewards.*
  Examples include:
  "I like it when you . . . "
  "I really appreciate it when you do what I tell you to do."
  "That's a beautiful . . . " [whatever your child makes]
  "Thank you for . . . " [whatever your child has done]
  "Good boy for . . . "
  "Hey, you're really sharp, you . . . "
  "You're doing just what Mommy wants you to do."
  "My! You're minding Daddy so well."
  "You do a good job at . . . "
  "That's a very nice [or good]." (pointing)
  "You're such a big girl for . . . "
  "Mommy's very proud of you for . . . "
  "Those . . . [pictures, towers] *are real pretty."*
  "I like playing this with you."

(continued)

GUIDELINES FOR USING REWARDS

- *Be specific*
  Use a labeled verbal reward.
- *Give immediately*
  This helps your child make the connection between the "OK" behavior and your positive
  attention.
- *Focus on improvement*
  Give rewards for steps along the way to completing a task.
- *Use consistently*
  When your child is first learning an "OK" behavior, reward the behavior *every* time that
  it occurs.
  Once the "OK" behavior is established, you can reward the behavior less frequently.
  However, never stop rewarding an "OK" behavior—it will go away!

HOMEWORK

Continue to play the Child's Game with your child for one 10- to 15-minute period each
day. Record each Child's Game session on Parent Handout 3: Parent Record Sheet: Child's
Game. Practice using both rewards and attends. *As a rough rule of thumb, try to provide
at least three to four attends for every reward.* REMEMBER: Your child chooses the activity; you are to reward and attend to "OK" behavior; there should be some imitation and
participation on your part; no questions, commands, or teaching should take place.

Parent Handout 5: Parent Record Sheet: Identifying "OK" Behaviors to Increase

On the right-hand side of the page, please list three "OK" behaviors that you would like your child to do more often. Sometimes it may be easier to first identify a "not OK" behavior that your child is doing. Then identify the "OK" positive behavior that you would like to see instead of the "not OK" behavior. If that is the case, list three "not OK" behaviors on the left-hand side of the page first. (Be sure that the "not OK" behaviors that you list are *not* ones that involve risk to people or property. We will deal with those types of problems later in the program.)

"Not OK" Behaviors I Want to See Less Of

"OK" Behaviors I Want to See More Of Instead (There can be more than one "OK" behavior for each "not OK" behavior that is listed.)

1. _____

1. _____

_____

_____

2. _____

2. _____

_____

_____

3. _____

3. _____

_____

_____

REMEMBER: THE FOCUS IS ON "OK" BEHAVIORS THAT YOU WANT TO SEE HAPPEN MORE OFTEN!

Parent Handout 6: Ignoring

Ignoring is a major way to decrease your child's "not OK" behavior. However, it is very important that you use ignoring *every* time a particular "not OK" behavior occurs and continue ignoring until the "not OK" behavior stops. Otherwise, the behavior will become worse instead of better.

HOW TO IGNORE

The ignoring procedure is very *active*.
- Decide ahead of time which "not OK" behaviors to ignore.
  Attention-seeking behaviors such as whining, nagging, and temper tantrums are "not OK" behaviors that are best ignored.
  You should *not* ignore behaviors where there is a chance of harm to your child, to someone else, or to property. We will address those situations later in the program.
- When ignoring, you actively avoid giving any attention to your child.

IGNORING STEPS

There are three things you should do when you ignore your child's behavior.
- *No eye contact or nonverbal cues.* Turn your back (or at least turn 90°) so that your child cannot get any attention (even a frown or a glance) from you.
- *No verbal contact (don't talk!).* Once you have started ignoring, do not say anything to your child. If you do, you are no longer ignoring him or her; instead, you are rewarding your child for "not OK" behavior.
- *No physical contact.* You may have to stand up or even leave the room to avoid giving physical attention to your child.
  However, do not leave the room unless necessary. If you are not in the same room, it is more difficult to determine when your child stops the "not OK" behavior. It is also more difficult to know what else your child may be up to!

WHEN TO IGNORE

- *Start* ignoring as soon as the "not OK" behavior begins.
- *Stop* ignoring soon after (10–15 seconds) the "not OK" behavior has stopped. Then give positive attention (rewards and attends) for your child's "OK" behavior.

IMPORTANT: Expect that your child's attention-seeking behavior will get worse when you first start ignoring it. This happens because children sometimes think that if they just do more of the "not OK" behavior, then you will pay attention to them.
- If you do give your child attention at this point, then the behavior will get even worse!
- The good news is that your child's attention-seeking behavior will decrease dramatically when he or she realizes that you are going to keep ignoring it. So hang in there!

Parent Handout 7: Combining Positive Attention and Ignoring (Differential Attention)

WHAT IS DIFFERENTIAL ATTENTION?

- Differential attention is using positive attention (attends and rewards) *in combination with* ignoring to increase child "OK" behaviors.
- You use attends and rewards when you see an "OK" behavior that you want to see more often.
- You use ignoring when you see a "not OK" behavior you want to decrease.
- Ignoring should *always* be used in combination with the positive attention skills of attends and rewards.
- Ignoring should never be used alone, because while it provides your child with feedback about what not to do, it does not provide your child with information about an alternative "OK" behavior.
- This combination of ignoring a "not OK" behavior while giving positive attention (attends, rewards) to an alternative "OK" behavior can be a very powerful procedure for changing your child's behavior.

STEPS IN USING DIFFERENTIAL ATTENTION

There are four steps in developing a plan for using differential attention. Use Parent Handout 5: Parent Record Sheet: Identifying "OK" Behaviors to Increase for the first two steps.

- Identify a "not OK" behavior to ignore.
  REMEMBER: Because differential attention employs ignoring, it is not to be used for "not OK" behaviors that are risky to your child, other people, or property.
- Identify at least one "OK" behavior that you would like to see instead of the "not OK" behavior.
  There may be a number of "OK" behaviors that you can identify.
- Explain and demonstrate the differential attention plan to your child.
  Do this at a time when your child is not engaging in the "not OK" behavior.
  Make sure that your child understands the plan.
- Implement the plan at home.
  Ignore the "not OK" behavior whenever it occurs and provide positive attention (attends, rewards) whenever your child engages in the "OK" behavior. It is the pairing of ignoring and positive attention that makes differential attention effective.

Parent Handout 8: Introduction to Phase II

In Phase I, you learned the skills of rewards, attends, and ignoring to:
- Increase your child's "OK" behavior.
- Decrease your child's "not OK" behavior.

In Phase II, you will learn new skills to use along with the skills you learned in Phase I.

The goal of Phase II is to learn ways to:
- Increase your child's *compliance* to your instructions.
- Decrease your child's *noncompliance* to your instructions.

THE PARENT'S GAME

Phase II skills are taught in the clinic in the context of the Parent's Game. In the Parent's Game, unlike the Child's Game, you will structure the activity and have your child follow your instructions. In other words, you are to be in control. The Parent's Game is a way to practice using the new skills with your child. You will master the skills first in the clinic in the Parent's Game and then you can use them at home.

In the Parent's Game, you will use attends, rewards, and ignoring, plus learn new skills that are part of the "clear instructions sequence." The clear instructions sequence is:
- You give clear instructions to your child.
- Your child does or does not comply.
- You provide consequences depending on whether or not your child complies.

The first new skill in the clear instructions sequence is how to give clear instructions. Other skills concern what to do depending on how your child responds. The consequences you provide can take three different paths—A, B, or C—depending on your child's response. In Phase II you will learn about each path.

Finally, you will also learn how to establish standing rules with your child.

Phase II skills do *not* replace the skills you have already mastered.
- Be sure to continue to praise and attend to your child's "OK" behavior.
- Also continue to ignore minor problem behaviors. Be consistent with the behaviors you decide to ignore.
- Continue with Child's Game sessions at home. It is a great way to structure some extended positive time with your child.
- Review the Parent Handouts from Phase I as needed.

REMEMBER: PHASE II SKILLS ARE EFFECTIVE ONLY WHEN USED IN COMBINATION WITH PHASE I SKILLS!

Parent Handout 9: The Clear Instructions Sequence: Path A

The primary Phase II skills are taught as part of the clear instructions sequence. The clear instructions sequence always begins with giving your child a clear instruction. It then follows one of three different paths. You will first learn Path A, followed by Paths B and C. Path A is summarized below. A detailed description of each step follows.

PATH A SUMMARY

Clear Instruction	$\rightarrow$	Child Complies	$\rightarrow$	Reward/ Attend

- Give your child a single clear instruction. (For example, *"Please pick up your toys now"*)
- Your child begins to comply to the clear instruction within 5 seconds.
- Provide positive attention (that is, rewards, attends). (For example, *"Thank you so much for playing quietly. I really appreciate it when you do what I ask"*)

GIVE A CLEAR INSTRUCTION

What Are Clear Instructions?

Clear instructions employ three steps that help your child understand what you want him or her to do. These make it more likely that your child will comply.
- Get your child's attention.
  Move close (to within a few feet of your child).
  Say your child's name (a maximum of two times).
  Establish eye contact.

- State the instruction clearly.
  Give one instruction at a time.
  Use a firm (but not angry) voice, a little louder than usual.
  Give the instruction as a "do" command (not a "don't" command).
      (For example, *"Please put your coloring book and crayons in the cabinet"* instead of *"Please don't color"*)
  Use simple language.
  Use gestures as appropriate.
      (For example, point to the bathroom if you are telling your child to wash his face.)
  Give any explanations or rationales *before* the clear instruction.
      (For example, *"We are having visitors tonight and I want the house to look nice. Please help me pick up the newspapers lying on the floor"*)

(continued)

- Wait 5 seconds to see if your child will *begin* to comply.
  Count silently to yourself.
  Do not say anything to your child during this time.

Types of Unclear Instructions—AVOID THESE!!

Giving the following types of unclear instructions will make it less likely that your child will comply.

Chain Commands. This is a series of commands that are strung together. This may result in information overload for your child. Chain commands also make it difficult for you to determine whether your child has complied because there are so many different instructions.
- Example: *"Put your plate in the sink, rinse it off, put it in the dishwasher, and bring me the napkins."*

Vague Commands. These commands are ambiguous because they do not specify the exact behavior expected of your child. The problem is that your child may not know what you mean. What you mean and what your child *thinks* you mean might be very different!
- Examples: *"Be careful!" "Watch out!" "Act your age!" "Be a good boy (girl)!"*

Question Commands. These are commands that are stated in the form of questions. It is important to distinguish between a clear instruction (compliance is expected) and a request (your child has the option of whether or not to do what you have asked), which is phrased as a question.
- The problem arises when you expect compliance, but have phrased what you want your child to do as a request instead of a clear instruction.
- Example: *"Would you like to take out the trash?"*

"Let's . . . " Commands. These commands are phrased so that it sounds like you will be involved in the activity. If you intend to assist your child, then this is fine. However, if you expect your child to complete the task without your assistance, then your child may feel tricked and therefore less likely to follow through on your instruction.
- Example: *"Let's go clean up your room."*

Commands Followed *by a Reason or Other Verbalization.* Rationales or explanations to your child about why you are giving a particular instruction can be very helpful. However, if the explanation or rationale *follows* your command, then it may distract your child from the command and make it less likely that your child will comply.
- A related situation is when children play the "Why Game" after a command in an attempt to avoid having to follow through on the command (*"Why do I have to pick up my toys, Mommy? . . . But* why*?"* and so on).
- Example: *"Please pick up the toys in here."* (Child: *"Why?"*) *"Because your mother's boss is coming for dinner tonight and we want the house to look nice."* (Child: *"But she won't come up here"*) And so on.

(continued)

When to Give a Clear Instruction

Indications that a clear instruction is appropriate include situations when:
- It is important to you that your child do what you tell him or her to do right away.
- You are not willing to give your child a choice as to whether to do the behavior or not.
- Your child is doing something that might harm people or property.

Consider whether differential attention skills from Phase I might be useful here instead, especially if your child's behavior is minor and is annoying, irritating, or attention seeking.

IMPORTANT: You will need to decide ahead of time when to use the clear instructions sequence. Do not give a clear instruction unless you are prepared to follow through with Paths B or C of the sequence, if necessary, as well as Path A. You will learn all the paths before using the clear instructions sequence at home.

YOUR CHILD COMPLIES

Your child's response to your clear instruction determines which path you should now follow. Compliance to your instruction (that is, your child begins to comply to your clear instruction within 5 seconds) means that you follow Path A.

REWARD/ATTEND FOR COMPLIANCE

If your child *begins* to follow your instruction (within the 5 seconds), *immediately*:
- Praise and attend to him or her. Compliance is "OK" behavior! By giving your child positive attention as soon as he or she begins to comply, then you increase the likelihood that the task will be completed, as well.
- Use *labeled verbal rewards*, so that your child makes the connection between following the clear instruction and your positive attention. (For example, *"Thanks very much for picking up the toys like I said"*)

  If the task takes some time to complete (for example, your child is picking up a number of different toys):

  Give a labeled verbal reward as soon as your child begins to comply.

  Use attends and rewards as your child continues to comply.

  Use another labeled verbal reward when your child completes the task.

  For example: *"Thank you for doing what I said! You're picking up the blocks and putting them into the box. . . . Now you've picked up some more blocks and there they go into the box. You're really working hard! . . . Thank you so much for picking up all of those blocks—you did a wonderful job!"*

Parent Handout 10: Parent Record Sheet: Clear Instructions and Child Compliance

For the next week, give your child at least *two clear instructions* each day. Record each clear instruction below, whether or not your child complied, and the rewards and attends you gave for compliance.

Remember to make these easy instructions that you are reasonably sure that your child will comply to.

Date	Clear instruction	Did child comply?		Reward/attend for compliance
____ 1. _____		Yes	No	1. _____
____ 2. _____		Yes	No	2. _____
____ 1. _____		Yes	No	1. _____
____ 2. _____		Yes	No	2. _____
____ 1. _____		Yes	No	1. _____
____ 2. _____		Yes	No	2. _____
____ 1. _____		Yes	No	1. _____
____ 2. _____		Yes	No	2. _____
____ 1. _____		Yes	No	1. _____
____ 2. _____		Yes	No	2. _____
____ 1. _____		Yes	No	1. _____
____ 2. _____		Yes	No	2. _____
____ 1. _____		Yes	No	1. _____
____ 2. _____		Yes	No	2. _____

List any unclear instructions you notice yourself giving during the week. Then change each unclear instruction to a clear instruction.

Unclear instructions	change to	*Clear instructions*
1. _____		1. _____
2. _____		2. _____
3. _____		3. _____
4. _____		4. _____
5. _____		5. _____

Parent Handout 11: The Clear Instructions Sequence: Path B

Path B of the clear instructions sequence begins the same way as Path A—with a clear instruction. But it then tells you what to do if your child does not comply. Path B is summarized below. A detailed description of each of its steps follows.

PATH B SUMMARY

Clear Instruction	→	Child Does Not Comply	→	Warning	→	Child Complies	→	Reward/ Attend

- Give your child a clear instruction.
- Your child does *not* begin to comply to the clear instruction within 5 seconds.
- Give a warning to your child: *"If you do not* [repeat the clear instruction], *you will have to go to time out."*
- Your child begins to comply to the warning within 5 seconds.
- Provide positive attention (that is, rewards, attends), especially labeled verbal rewards. (For example, *"Great job! I like it when you help Daddy clean up"*)

CLEAR INSTRUCTION

Get your child's attention.
State the instruction clearly.
Wait 5 seconds.

YOUR CHILD DOES *NOT* COMPLY

If your child does *not* begin to comply to your instruction within 5 seconds, give a warning.

GIVE A WARNING

What Are Warnings?

Warnings are "if . . . then" statements. (For example, *"If you don't pick up the toys, then you will have to go to time out"*)
- The "If" part of the warning restates the child behavior specified in the clear instruction.
- The "then" part of the warning specifies the consequence that will follow if your child does not comply to the warning.
- Do not repeat your instruction again. This will prevent you from becoming angry because you won't have to repeatedly ask your child to do something.

(continued)

How to Give a Warning

- Give the "if . . . then" warning statement.
- Wait 5 seconds to see if your child will begin to comply.
- Count silently to yourself.
- Do not say anything to your child during this time.

YOUR CHILD COMPLIES TO THE WARNING

Reward/Attend for Compliance

- If your child *begins* to comply to the warning (within 5 seconds), *immediately* praise and attend to him or her, using labeled verbal rewards. (For example, *"Thanks very much for picking up the toys like I said"*)
- Resist the urge to criticize your child for not complying to the initial clear instruction.

Parent Handout 12: The Clear Instructions Sequence: Path C

Path C of the clear instructions sequence tells you what to do when your child does not comply with the warning. It is summarized below. A detailed description of each of its steps follows.

PATH C SUMMARY

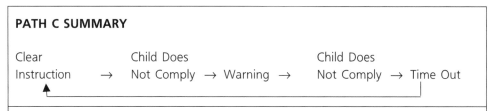

Give your child a clear instruction.
- Your child does *not* begin to comply within 5 seconds.
- Give your child a warning.
- Your child does *not* begin to comply to the warning within 5 seconds.
- Lead your child to the time-out chair without lecturing, scolding, or arguing.
- Tell your child: *"Because you did not* [the behavior in the clear instruction], *you have to sit in the chair until I say you can get up."*
- Ignore your child's shouting, protesting, and promises to comply.
- Leave your child in time out for 3 minutes (including being quiet for the last 15 seconds).
- When the time is completed, remove your child from the chair and return to the situation that elicited noncompliance.
- Restate the original clear instruction.
- Follow the clear instructions sequence (positive attention for complying to your instruction, warning and time out as necessary).

CLEAR INSTRUCTION

Get your child's attention.
State the instruction clearly.
Wait 5 seconds.

YOUR CHILD DOES *NOT* COMPLY

Your child does *not* begin to comply to the clear instruction within 5 seconds.

(continued)

GIVE A WARNING

Give your child an "If . . . then" statement describing the consequences for not complying. Wait 5 seconds to see if your child begins to comply

YOUR CHILD DOES *NOT* COMPLY

If your child does *not* begin to comply to the warning within 5 seconds, begin time out.

TIME OUT

What Is Time Out?

"Time out" means "time out from positive reinforcement." It is a punishment procedure in which you remove your child from all sources of positive reinforcement (especially your attention) for a brief period of time. In a sense, time out is a more extreme form of ignoring in which you remove *all* forms of attention to your child.

The time-out procedure that you will use requires your child to sit on a chair facing a wall for 3 minutes. If possible, the chair should be far enough away from the wall so that your child cannot kick the wall. The best location for the time-out chair is somewhere in your home that is *boring*! It should be away from toys, windows, people, TVs, radios, and the like.
- Good locations: hallway, dining room
- Poor locations: bathroom, closet
- You should decide on the best location in your home *before* you have to use time out.

How to Use Time Out

Stay calm. Do not lecture, scold, or argue with your child while you are taking him or her to time out or while your child is in time out.
- Lead your child to the time-out chair.
- Tell your child: *"Because you did not* [the behavior in the clear instruction]*, you have to sit in the chair until I say you can get up."*
- Use a matter-of-fact voice that shows that you are not pleased with your child's behavior.
- If a timer is used, set it for 3 minutes. The timer should be visible to your child, but out of reach.
- Ignore your child's shouting, protesting, and promises to comply.
- Leave your child in time out for 3 minutes.

(continued)

- Your child should be sitting quietly for the last 15 seconds. If your child is being disruptive or noisy at the end of 3 minutes, then continue with time out. You do not want your child to think that whining or crying is the reason for being released from time out. (If you use a timer, tell your child, *"You will have to stay in time out until you are quiet"*)
- After your child has been quiet for at least 15 seconds, take him or her out of the time-out chair.

IMPORTANT: RETURN TO THE START OF THE CLEAR INSTRUCTIONS SEQUENCE

Return your child to the location and activity that resulted in time out.

Restate the original clear instruction.

Follow the clear instructions sequence (positive attention for complying to your instruction, warning and time out as necessary).

When your child has finished complying to the instruction, resist the urge to criticize him or her for not complying to the first clear instruction or warning. The situation will improve over time.

These steps are critical, because they prevent your child from using time out as a way to avoid having to follow your instructions. Your child will learn that once you give a clear instruction, he or she must follow through, whether it is before or after being placed in time out.

To summarize, this flowchart shows the entire clear instructions sequence.

FLOWCHART OF THE CLEAR INSTRUCTIONS SEQUENCE

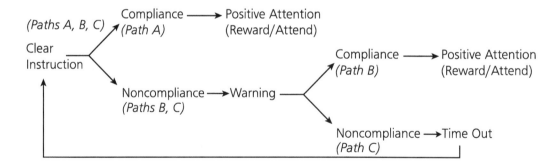

REMEMBER: *Never give your child a clear instruction unless you are prepared to follow the above procedure.* If you really don't think that it is important, don't make it a clear instruction.

Parent Handout 13: Challenges in the Use of the Clear Instructions Sequence

The following information summarizes various challenging situations that may arise as you use the clear instructions sequence with your child, and the solutions for dealing with them.

TARDY COMPLIANCE

Your child says *"I will do it now"* when you begin to take him or her to time out.

THE SOLUTION: It is critical that you *follow through with time out* at this point. If you do not, your child will learn that he or she does not have to obey the clear instruction until time out is actually initiated rather than complying to the initial clear instruction or warning.

VERBAL DISRUPTIONS IN TIME OUT

When your child is in time out, he or she may whine, yell, or cry, or say things such as *"I am going to run away," "I hate you," "You are mean," "You don't love me," "I don't care,"* or *"I don't like time out."*

THE SOLUTION: It is important to *ignore* these comments, as they are an attempt to control the situation by the child. If you do not respond, they will quickly stop.

OTHER MISBEHAVIOR IN TIME OUT

Some children "push the limits" in time out by moving the chair backward away from the corner or kicking the wall. These behaviors also are usually attempts to get parental attention and to control the situation.

THE SOLUTION: Whenever possible, *ignore* these behaviors. However, if there is a risk of harm to your child or property, then give your child a *single* warning, such as *"If you* [state the behavior] *again, then I will* [state one of the backups described below]." Only major behaviors that cannot be ignored should be treated in this manner.

REFUSAL TO *STAY IN* TIME OUT

We define "leaving time out" as when your child's buttocks leave the time-out chair, even for a second. By adopting this definition, you can avoid the situation where your child

(continued)

gradually eases more and more of his or her body off of the time-out chair, all the while maintaining that he or she is still in the chair.

THE SOLUTION: If your child leaves the chair, he or she should be immediately returned to the chair.

- The first time this occurs, give your child a warning: *"If you get off the chair again, then [specify the backup]."* This warning is only presented once *ever.*
- If your child gets off the chair again, return your child to the time-out chair and administer the backup procedure(s) described below.
- There are three different sets of backup consequences that can be used if your child refuses to stay in time out: (1) adding more time, (2) taking away a privilege, and (3) using a room time out.

Additional time. One backup involves adding an extra 3 minutes of time out.
- Tell your child, *"[Name], because you didn't stay in the chair, you have to stay in time out for an extra 3 minutes."*
- If you use a timer, add 3 minutes to the remaining time when you return your child to the chair.
- This backup procedure is used only once (that is, one additional 3-minute time out, for 6 minutes total).

Taking away a privilege. Removal of a privilege that is to occur at a slightly later time can be very effective, especially with older children. For example, you might say, *"If you get out of the chair again, you may not watch television tonight."* The consequence should:
- Occur immediately or within a few hours.
- Be moderate (no TV tonight, rather than no TV for the next two days).
- Be a logical consequence, if possible. For example, you might suspend television privileges because the reason that your child disobeyed your initial clear instruction was because he or she did not want to miss any of a favorite cartoon show on TV.

Using a room time out. A time-out *room* can be an effective backup. If your child leaves the time-out chair, then say, *"Because you left the chair, you will have to stay by yourself for a while."* Take your child to a room that is closed either by a partition or a door. Hold the door shut as necessary. The room should be well-lit, relatively spacious (*not* a closet), and free of entertaining (e.g., radio, toys) or potentially dangerous (for example, razors, medications) items. After *1* minute, take your child back to the time-out chair. Repeat this procedure as needed.

In general, we recommend the following sequence of backup procedures:
- Adding minutes to the original time out.
- For younger children (5 years and younger), next use the time-out room.
- For older children (6 to 8 years), next use the privilege removal procedure, with the time-out room as a third backup.

(continued)

REFUSAL TO *GO TO* TIME OUT

Occasionally, your child may refuse to go to the time-out chair.

THE SOLUTION: Use the same *backup procedures* described above.

REFUSAL TO *LEAVE* TIME OUT

A related situation is if your child refuses to come out of time out when the time-out period is over. This is another attempt to control the situation.

THE SOLUTION: *Either repeat the original clear instruction or give your child a clear instruction to leave the time-out chair.* In either case, if your child does not comply, then continue with the clear instructions sequence, including another 3-minute time out if necessary.

COMPLIANCE ONLY TO THE WARNING

Over time, your child may decide to wait to comply only to the warning rather than to the initial clear instruction. In this situation, your child realizes that your clear instruction is always followed by a warning, and that time out will occur only after noncompliance to the warning. (NOTE: When children are first learning about the clear instructions sequence, this is also a typical pattern, and is usually temporary.)

THE SOLUTION: In this situation, it may be necessary to employ *time out immediately following noncompliance to the clear instruction*. This strategy should be used only after several weeks of using time out, and after consulting with your therapist.

Parent Handout 14: Parent Record Sheet:
Clear Instructions Sequence

Date	Time	Clear instruction/ warning	Child's response	Reward/ attend for compliance	Time-out duration	Back-up?

Parent Handout 15: Standing Rules

WHAT ARE STANDING RULES?

- Standing rules are *"If . . . then"* statements that specify:
  A particular behavior that you do *not* want your child to do (*"If you . . . "*).
  The consequence for breaking the standing rule, which is time out (*"then you will have to go to time out"*).

Examples:
  "If you hit your sister, then *you have to go to time out."*
  "If you play with matches, then *you have to go to time out."*

- Once the standing rule is established, it is always in effect.
- If your child breaks the standing rule, the consequence (time out) is implemented immediately. There is no warning.

WHEN TO USE STANDING RULES

- Standing rules are especially useful for situations when there is a potential harm to your child, to others, or to property.

ADVANTAGES AND DISADVANTAGES

- Two *advantages* are:
  The consequence can be administered immediately.
  Standing rules represent a more developmentally advanced form of discipline. They usually cover broad classes of behavior (such as hitting or jumping on furniture), and the rule is not stated every time.
- A potential *disadvantage* to standing rules: there is no built-in reminder to provide positive attention to your child for *following* the rule.
  So, there should only be one or two standing rules in effect at any given time.
  Post the rule(s) in a prominent place (such as the refrigerator) to be a reminder.
  IMPORTANT: Be sure to provide positive attention to your child regularly for following the rule, especially when it is first established. (For example, *"You are doing such a good job of playing nicely with your sister!"*)
  Use Parent Handout 16: Parent Record Sheet: Standing Rules to list positive statements about rule following and to help you remember the steps to follow when your child *follows* the rule and when your child *breaks* the rule.
  You also may want to put a sign next to the posted rule to remind you to praise your child for following the rule.

(continued)

Partially adapted with permission from Mark W. Roberts, Idaho State University (1995). From *Helping the Noncompliant Child* (2nd ed.) by Robert J. McMahon and Rex L. Forehand. Copyright 2003 by The Guilford Press. Permission to photocopy this form is granted to purchasers of this book for personal use only (see copyright page for details).

TEACH YOUR CHILD ABOUT STANDING RULES

Once you have decided to set up a standing rule:
- Tell your child about the new rule *in advance*, when he or she is behaving appropriately.
- Provide a rationale for the rule.
- Rehearse the rule with your child. Ask your child:
  "What is it that you are not to do?"
  "What will happen if you [the "not OK" behavior]*?"*
  "What could you do instead?"
- Demonstrate the rule and practice the enforcement of the rule with your child.
- Remind your child occasionally about the rule.
- Remember to provide positive attention for following the rule.

IF YOUR CHILD BREAKS THE STANDING RULE

- Tell your child, *"Since you* [state the rule violation]*, you must go to time out."*
- Use the standard time-out procedure.
- At the end of time out, rehearse the standing rule with your child. Ask your child:
  "Why did you have to go to time out?"
  "What's wrong with [state the "not OK" behavior]*?"*
  "What will happen if you forget again?"
  "What could you have done instead?"
- If your child answers incorrectly or refuses to answer, then calmly provide the correct responses.
- Get your child involved in an activity so that you can provide positive attention for "OK" behavior.

Parent Handout 16: Parent Record Sheet: Standing Rules

The standing rule that I will work on with my child is:

_____

_____

Positive statements that I can make for following the standing rule are:

1. _____

2. _____

Date	Did my child follow the rule?	Number of times I praised my child for *following* the rule	Time out for *breaking* the rule?	Rehearse the rule after time out?
	Yes No		Yes No	Yes No
	Yes No		Yes No	Yes No
	Yes No		Yes No	Yes No
	Yes No		Yes No	Yes No
	Yes No		Yes No	Yes No
	Yes No		Yes No	Yes No
	Yes No		Yes No	Yes No

Partially adapted by permission of the authors from McMahon, Slough, and the Conduct Problems Prevention Research Group (1994). From *Helping the Noncompliant Child* (2nd ed.) by Robert J. McMahon and Rex L. Forehand. Copyright 2003 by The Guilford Press. Permission to photocopy this form is granted to purchasers of this book for personal use only (see copyright page for details).

Parent Handout 17: Dealing with Situations Outside the Home

- Plan ahead to increase the likelihood of success.
  Decide ahead of time how you want to handle the situation.
  Explain the consequences for "OK" and "not OK" behavior to your child.
- Set up brief "practice" sessions to guarantee that your child will be successful.
- In the public setting:
  Look for opportunities to "catch your child being good." Give positive attention for "OK" behaviors.

Stores
  - Let your child help with shopping (push cart, put items in cart, etc.).
  - Give your child information about shopping tasks.
  - Give your child choices about purchases when possible.
  - Keep the length of the trip reasonable.

Restaurants
  - Invite conversation (about the meal, activities, etc.).
  - Bring a coloring book or game book and pencil.

Home of Others
  - Take a set of toys from home (perhaps ones that your child only plays with on visits so that they remain novel and more interesting).
  - Help your child find good places to play and things that he or she can use before you settle down to visiting.

Car
  - Bring a set of "car toys."
  - Sing songs or play car games (alphabet, license plate counting, etc.).
  - Describe things seen from the window.
  - Stop often for treats and bathroom breaks.

- Use ignoring (as part of differential attention), the clear instructions sequence, and standing rules as needed.
- You may need to modify use of time out slightly.
  Decrease the time from 3 minutes to 1 minute.
  Possible locations for time out:
    - *Stores*
      quiet area of store
      backseat of car
      just outside the entrance

(continued)

- *Restaurants and Theaters*
  lobby
  just outside the entrance
  backseat of car
- *Parks*
  picnic table
  any specific spot (by a tree, on a rock, etc.)
  backseat of car
- *Backyard*
  steps of house
  any specific spot
- *Home of Others*
  same as at home or back bedroom away from visitors
- *Car*
  pull over to side of road

- *Never* leave your child alone. Sit or stand next to your child.

Social Learning Criterion Tests and Scoring Keys

SOCIAL LEARNING CRITERION, RATIONALE

Name _____

Date _____

Fill in the blanks in the following statements. In some cases there are several correct responses possible.

1. Behavior can be ch_____.
2. The social learning approach assumes that you are responsible for your own _____.

Circle the best answer.

3. A critical factor for achieving success in this program is
   a. authority
   b. insight
   c. consistency
   d. all of the above
4. Which of the following is a negative effect of punishment?
   a. It may be emotionally upsetting for you and your child.
   b. It has no effect on compliance per se.
   c. Your child may avoid you.
   d. All of the above are true.

Circle **T** if the statement is true; circle **F** if the statement is false.

5. Often when children behave in disturbing ways, their parents have unknowingly taught them to do so. **T F**

(continued)

6. A social learning approach to child behavior is designed primarily to teach children to be popular. **T F**
7. A problem child acts the way he or she does because he or she was born that way. **T F**
8. You can teach your child both positive and problem behaviors. **T F**
9. Punishment will permanently eliminate a problem behavior. **T F**

SOCIAL LEARNING CRITERION, PHASE I

Name _____

Date _____

Fill in the blanks in the following statements. In some cases there are several correct responses available.

1. Follow behaviors you wish to _____ with reinforcing events.
2. Behaviors can be weakened by no longer _____ them.
3. A delay in reinforcement can be bridged by t_____ your child what you are praising him or her for.
4. When teaching something new, _____ each new behavior right away.
5. It is possible to accidentally train your child to engage in inappropriate ("not OK") behavior by occasionally "giving in" and _____ _____ to the bad behavior.
6. A major assumption is that a child will work for adults' _____, which may be positive or negative.
7. To change an undesirable behavior, parents must be very _____ in not rewarding that behavior.
8. To get a new behavior going, reinforce it _____ _____ it occurs.
9. To keep the behavior going, reward _____.
10. Reinforcing small steps on the way to the desired behavior is called s_____.
11–12. The task in teaching new behavior is to find ways to _____ the undesirable behavior and to strengthen the _____ behaviors, and to pair these two events so that the child learns what is expected of him or her more quickly.
13. The parent who tries to teach children mainly by scolding instead of praising may be caught in the _____ trap.
14–15. To get out of the criticism trap, you need to _____ more and _____ less.
16. The person in the family who gives the most punishment receives the most _____.
17–18. Two general types of reinforcers are _____ reinforcers, such as "thank you" or a smile, and _____ reinforcers, such as money or candy.

Circle **T** if the statement is true; circle **F** if the statement is false.
19. If the reward is a large one, you only need to reward the child once to get his or her behavior to change. **T F**
20. You can cause your child's good behavior to occur less often or even to disappear by ignoring it. **T F**
21. An advantage of social reinforcers over material reinforcers is that they are more realistic in terms of what the child can expect to find as an adult in the real world as reinforcement for his or her behavior. **T F**

(continued)

SOCIAL LEARNING CRITERION, PHASE II

Name _____

Date _____

Fill in the blanks in the following statements. In some cases there are several correct responses possible.

1. An event that occurs following behavior and weakens the future rate of such behavior is called a _____.

2. Most of the rules about reinforcers apply to punishment, except that we are talking about _____ rather than strengthening behavior.

3–4. In itself, use of punishment is not immoral or moral. Punishment should be used when the long-term effects from the use of punishment lead to more _____ than harm. Punishment should not be used when the long-term effects are more _____ than good.

5. Punishment is one way of _____ behavior.

6. When you do use punishment, it should be given _____ after the bad behavior.

7–8. Punishment involves presenting _____ consequences or _____ reinforcing consequences.

9. If a behavior you desire your child to engage in is relatively complex, break your commands into the _____ steps necessary to achieve that behavior.

10. When your child complies to a command, it is best to reinforce him or her frequently and _____. Your reinforcement should come as soon as he or she initiates the behavior.

11. Time out means to remove your child from all sources of _____ _____.

12. When using ignoring or time out to weaken a behavior, remember to use _____ to strengthen the positive behaviors, and to pair these two events so that the child learns what is expected of him or her more quickly.

13. If you depend upon punishment alone to train your child, you will become (*more/ less*) powerful as a reinforcing agent to your child.

14–15. To be effective, punishment must prevent avoidance and _____ from the punisher, and minimize _____ reactions.

16. To be effective, the punisher should not provide a _____ of aggressive behavior.

17. Effective punishment makes use of a _____ signal, usually in the form of words.

18. Good punishment is carried out in a _____, matter-of-fact way.

19. If you really want a behavior to stop, you should not punish it sometimes and _____ it at other times.

20. You may have to use punishment if the problem behavior causes your child to _____ himself or herself or others.

(continued)

269

KEY: SOCIAL LEARNING CRITERION, RATIONALE

1. changed
2. behavior
3. c.
4. d.
5. T
6. F
7. F
8. T
9. F

KEY: SOCIAL LEARNING CRITERION, PHASE I

1. strengthen
2. reinforcing
3. telling
4. reinforce
5. paying attention
6. attention
7. consistent
8. every time
9. once in a while, intermittently, occasionally
10. shaping
11. weaken
12. desirable
13. criticism
14. praise
15. criticize
16. punishment
17. social
18. material
19. F
20. T
21. T

KEY: SOCIAL LEARNING CRITERION, PHASE II

1. punishment, punisher
2. weakening
3. good
4. harmful

(continued)

 5. weakening
 6. immediately
 7. negative, aversive
 8. taking away
 9. small, short
10. immediately
11. positive reinforcement
12. reinforcement
13. less
14. escape
15. fearful, emotional
16. model
17. warning
18. calm
19. reinforce
20. hurt

Mealtime Brochure

PROCEDURE

The first step in the mealtime program is to have the parent complete the Mealtime Behavior Checklist (see below). This checklist includes a number of behaviors that have been identified in the literature as inappropriate mealtime behaviors (e.g., Barton, Guess, Garcia, & Baer, 1970; O'Brien & Azrin, 1972; Sanders et al., 1993). These behaviors are grouped into "Inappropriate Eating Behaviors" and "Misconduct." In addition, the parent may add other inappropriate behaviors not covered on the list. The brochure is then given to the parent, who is asked to implement the procedures in the home at mealtime. The Mealtime Behavior Checklist serves as a prompt for the parent to implement the program procedures for the noted inappropriate mealtime behaviors. The TO procedure described in the brochure is somewhat different from the one taught in the parenting program. Since the brochure is often used in a totally self-administered context, the TO procedure has been simplified so that there are fewer steps involved.

(continued)

MEALTIME BEHAVIOR CHECKLIST

I. Inappropriate Eating Behaviors

_____ 1. Spilling food onto the table and/or floor on purpose

_____ 2. Eating food spilled on the table, floor, or clothing

_____ 3. Eating food by placing mouth directly on it (without use of fingers or utensils)

_____ 4. Eating too fast (not pausing between bites)

_____ 5. Putting too much food in mouth, such that chewing cannot be done with the mouth closed

_____ 6. Playing with food (e.g., patting Jello with hands, smearing food)

_____ 7. Eating food with fingers (excepting use of fingers to hold foods properly eaten with fingers such as sandwiches, potato chips, etc.)

_____ 8. Removing food from the mouth (spitting out or using fingers)

_____ 9. Using fingers to place food on utensil

_____ 10. Others:

II. Misconduct

_____ 1. Not coming to the table when called

_____ 2. Standing up or leaving table before end of meal

_____ 3. Stealing food or other objects at the table

_____ 4. Throwing or banging utensils

_____ 5. Throwing food

_____ 6. Pushing the table

_____ 7. Rocking or moving the chair (other than to sit down or leave the table)

_____ 8. Placing a foot on the table

_____ 9. Placing head on the table

_____ 10. Placing a foot on others or their chairs, or kicking them

_____ 11. Hitting others at the table

_____ 12. Whining or crying

_____ 13. Screaming or yelling

_____ 14. Others:

(continued)

"How to Handle Your Child's Inappropriate Mealtime Behaviors"
by
Robert J. McMahon, PhD, and Rex L. Forehand, PhD

In order to correct your child's inappropriate mealtime behaviors, it is very important that you decide which specific behaviors you wish to change. The list of your child's mealtime behaviors that you decided were inappropriate is included at the end of this brochure.

As a parent, your attention to your child is very important to him or her. Children quickly learn that they receive attention for some things they do. These behaviors are the ones that your child will do again and again. Therefore, it is important that you give attention to your child only when he or she is behaving correctly at the table. There are two primary ways in which you should respond positively.

1. Praise your child for acting appropriately at the table (e.g., "You're such a good boy [*or girl*] for eating your food!"). See the attached list for some more praise statements.
2. Give physical rewards such as a hug, kiss, pat, and so forth.

These two types of positive attention from you, especially the praise, are very important in helping good behavior get started and in maintaining this good behavior once it has begun.

Initially, it is important to praise your child quite often when he or she is acting appropriately at the table. Therefore, for the first week during a meal you should praise your child at least once every minute (more frequently if you wish) that he or she has acted appropriately. During the next week, you might praise the child a little less often. Never phase out your praise statements completely—always praise your child several times during every meal when he or she is being good.

We feel that the best way to establish a good relationship with your child and to eliminate the child's bad behavior at the table is by rewarding him or her for being good. However, there are times when you may need a punishment procedure to stop this bad behavior. In order to implement the following procedure, it is necessary that you use a quiet room, such as a bedroom, where you can place your child when he or she misbehaves at the table. The room should contain as few fun things (such as magazines, toys, TV) as possible. Furthermore, there should not be dangerous items like sharp objects and medicine in the room.

Use the following procedure when your child misbehaves at the table. (Note: Please use this procedure only when your child does one of the specific behaviors you listed earlier as a behavior problem; see the attached list.)

1. Tell your child to stop misbehaving. Be sure to name the bad behavior. Tell your child only once, and make your statement as brief as possible. For example, say, "[*Child's name*], stop throwing food right now!" If he or she complies (e.g., stops throwing food), reward your child. For example, say, "That's a good boy [*or girl*] for doing what Mom asks you to do."

(continued)

2. If your child does not comply immediately or complies for a moment and then does the same behavior again (say within 5 seconds), immediately take your child firmly by the hand and lead him or her to the quiet room, and while placing him or her in the quiet room say, "You didn't do what I said, so you have to stay in here." Be sure not to say anything else to your child at any time during this procedure. You don't owe your child any additional explanations.

3. Then close the door and hold it if necessary to keep your child in the room. Leave your child in the quiet room for 3 minutes, but be sure to wait until he or she has quit crying, fussing, or yelling for 15 seconds at the end of the 3-minute period before taking him or her out. It is important that you do not respond in any way (such as talking to your child) while he or she is in the room.

4. When taking your child out, open the door and say, "Now we will finish eating."

5. As soon as your child is acting appropriately at the table, praise him or her for the good table behavior.

6. If your child begins to act inappropriately at the table again, follow the above procedure, even if you have just brought him or her back to the table.

At first, you will find this procedure difficult to implement. However, once your child realizes that you are going to be consistent and not tolerate bad behavior at the table (and that you will reward good behavior), life will be much easier at mealtime and you will enjoy your child more.

Some praise statements include:

1. "I really like it when you eat so nicely!"
2. "You are such a big boy [*or girl*] to eat your food."
3. "Thank you for behaving so well at the table."
4. "I'm so proud of you—you're acting just like a grown-up."
5. "I like it when you stay at the table for Mom."
6. "You have such good manners—that's great."
7. "Thank you." "You're so nice!" "Good!"

These are just a few examples of some praise statements you can make to reward your child for good mealtime behavior. Don't be afraid to use other statements of your own.

References

Abidin, R. R. (1995). *Parenting Stress Index—professional manual* (3rd ed.). Lutz, FL: Psychological Assessment Resources.

Abidin, R. R., Jenkins, C. L., & McGaughey, M. C. (1992). The relationship of early family variables to children's subsequent behavioral adjustment. *Journal of Clinical Child Psychology, 21,* 60–69.

Abikoff, H., & Klein, R. G. (1992). Attention-deficit hyperactivity and conduct disorder: Comorbidity and implications for treatment. *Journal of Consulting and Clinical Psychology, 60,* 881–892.

Achenbach, T. M., & Edelbrock, C. S. (1981). *Behavioral problems and competencies reported by parents of normal and disturbed children aged four through sixteen* (Monographs of the Society for Research in Child Development, No. 188). Chicago: Society for Research in Child Development.

Achenbach, T. M., Howell, C. T., Quay, H. C., & Conners, C. K. (1991). National survey of problems and competencies among four- to sixteen-year-olds: Parents' reports for normative and clinical samples. *Monographs of the Society for Research and Child Development, 56,* 1–131.

Achenbach, T. M., & Rescorla, L. A. (2000). *Manual for the ASEBA preschool forms and profiles.* Burlington, VT: University of Vermont, Department of Psychiatry.

Achenbach, T. M., & Rescorla, L. A. (2001). *Manual for the ASEBA school-age forms and profiles.* Burlington, VT: University of Vermont, Research Center for Children, Youth, & Families.

Adkins, D. A., & Johnson, S. M. (1972). *What behaviors may be called deviant for children? A comparison of two approaches to behavior classification.* Paper presented at the meeting of the Western Psychological Association, Portland, OR.

Aguilar, B., Sroufe, L. A., Egeland, B., & Carlson, E. (2000). Distinguishing the early-onset/persistent and adolescent-onset antisocial behavior types: From birth to 16 years. *Development and Psychopathology, 12,* 109–132.

Alexander, J. F., Barton, C., Schiavo, R. S., & Parsons, B. V. (1976). Systems-behavioral intervention with families of delinquents: Therapist characteristics, family behavior, and outcome. *Journal of Consulting and Clinical Psychology, 44,* 656–664.

Altepeter, T. S., & Breen, M. J. (1992). Situational variation in problem behavior at home and school in attention-deficit disorder with hyperactivity: A factor analytic study. *Journal of Child Psychology and Psychiatry and Allied Disciplines, 33,* 741–748.

Alvarado, R., Kendall, K., Beesley, S., & Lee-Cavaness, C. (2000). *Strengthening America's Families: Model family programs for substance abuse and delinquency prevention.* Salt Lake City: University of Utah.

Amato, P. R., & Keith, B. (1991). Parental divorce and the well-being of children: A meta-analysis. *Psychological Bulletin, 110,* 26–46.

American Psychiatric Association. (2000). *Diagnostic and statistical manual of mental disorders* (4th ed., text rev.). Washington, DC: Author.

Ammerman, R. T., & Galvin, M. R. (1998). Child maltreatment. In R. T. Ammerman & J. V. Campo (Eds.), *Handbook of pediatric psychology and psychiatry: Vol. II. Disease, injury, and illness* (pp. 31–69). Needham Heights, MA: Allyn & Bacon.

Anastopoulos, A. D., Shelton, T. L., DuPaul, G. J., & Guevremont, D. C. (1993). Parent training for attention-deficit hyperactivity disorder: Its impact on parent functioning. *Journal of Abnormal Child Psychology, 21,* 581–596.

Anastopoulos, A. D., Smith, J. M., & Wien, E. E. (1998). Counseling and training parents. In R. A. Barkley, *Attention-deficit hyperactivity disorder: A handbook for diagnosis and treatment* (2nd ed., pp. 373–393). New York: Guilford Press.

Angold, A., Costello, E. J., & Erkanli, A. (1999). Comorbidity. *Journal of Child Psychology and Psychiatry and Allied Disciplines, 40,* 57–87.

Arnold, L. E., Abikoff, H. B., Cantwell, D. P., Conners, C. K., Elliott, G., Greenhill, L. L., Hechtman, L., Hinshaw, S. P., Hoza, B., Jensen, P. S., Kraemer, H. C., March, J. S., Newcorn, J. H., Pelham, W. E., Richters, J. E., Schiller, E., Severe, J. B., Swanson, J. M., Vereen, D., & Wells, K. C. (1997). National Institute of Mental Health collaborative multimodal treatment study of children with ADHD (the MTA). *Archives of General Psychiatry, 54,* 865–870.

Azar, S. T., & Wolfe, D. A. (1998). Child physical abuse and neglect. In E. J. Mash & R. A. Barkley (Eds.), *Treatment of childhood disorders* (2nd ed., pp. 501–544). New York: Guilford Press.

Baden, A. D., & Howe, G. W. (1992). Mothers' attributions and expectancies regarding their conduct-disordered children. *Journal of Abnormal Child Psychology, 20,* 467–485.

Barkley, R. A. (1981). *Hyperactive children: A handbook for diagnosis and treatment.* New York: Guilford Press.

Barkley, R. A. (1987). *Defiant children: A clinician's manual for parent training.* New York: Guilford Press.

Barkley, R. A. (1997). *Defiant children: A clinician's manual for assessment and parent training* (2nd ed.). New York: Guilford Press.

Barkley, R. A. (1998a). Attention-deficit/hyperactivity disorder. In E. J. Mash & R. A. Barkley (Eds.), *Treatment of childhood disorders* (2nd ed., pp. 55–110). New York: Guilford Press.

Barkley, R. A. (1998b). *Attention-deficit hyperactivity disorder: A handbook for diagnosis and treatment* (2nd ed.). New York: Guilford Press.

Barkley, R. A., & Benton, C. M. (1998). *Your defiant child: 8 steps to better behavior.* New York: Guilford Press.

Barkley, R. A., & Edelbrock, C. S. (1987). Assessing situational variation in children's behavior problems: The Home and School Situations Questionnaires. In R. Prinz (Ed.),

Advances in behavioral assessment of children and families (Vol. 3, pp. 157–176). Greenwich, CT: JAI Press.

Barkley, R. A., Guevremont, D. C., Anastopoulos, A. D., & Fletcher, K. E. (1992). A comparison of three family therapy programs for treating family conflicts in adolescents with attention-deficit hyperactivity disorder. *Journal of Consulting and Clinical Psychology, 60*, 450–462.

Barkley, R. A., Karlsson, J., & Pollard, S. (1985). Effects of age on the mother–child interactions of hyperactive children. *Journal of Abnormal Child Psychology, 13*, 631–638.

Barkley, R. A., Shelton, T. L., Crosswait, C., Moorehouse, M., Fletcher, K., Barrett, S., Jenkins, L., & Metevia, L. (2000). Multi-method psycho-educational intervention for preschool children with disruptive behavior: Preliminary results at post-treatment. *Journal of Child Psychology and Psychiatry and Allied Disciplines, 41*, 319–332.

Barton, E. S., Guess, D., Garcia, E., & Baer, D. M. (1970). Improvement of retardates' mealtime behaviors by timeout procedures using multiple baseline techniques. *Journal of Applied Behavior Analysis, 3*, 77–84.

Bates, J. E., Bayles, K., Bennett, D. S., Ridge, B., & Brown, M. M. (1991). Origins of externalizing behavior problems at eight years of age. In D. J. Pepler & K. H. Rubin (Eds.), *The development and treatment of childhood aggression* (pp. 93–120). Hillsdale, NJ: Erlbaum.

Baum, C. G., & Forehand, R. (1981). Long-term follow-up assessment of parent training by use of multiple-outcome measures. *Behavior Therapy, 12*, 643–652.

Baum, C. G., Reyna McGlone, C. L., & Ollendick, T. H. (1986, November). *The efficacy of behavioral parent training: Behavioral parent training plus clinical self-control training, and a modified STEP program with children referred for noncompliance*. Paper presented at the meeting of the Association for Advancement of Behavior Therapy, Chicago.

Beach, S. R. H., & Jones, D. J. (2002). Marital and family therapy for depression in adults. In I. H. Gotlib & C. L. Hammen (Eds.), *Handbook of depression* (pp. 422–440). New York: Guilford Press.

Beach, S. R. H., Sandeen, E. E., & O'Leary, K. D. (1990). *Depression in marriage: A model for etiology and treatment*. New York: Guilford Press.

Bean, A. W., & Roberts, M. W. (1981). The effect of time-out release contingencies on changes in child noncompliance. *Journal of Abnormal Child Psychology, 9*, 95–105.

Beautrais, A. L., Fergusson, D. M., & Shannon, F. T. (1982). Family life events and behavioral problems in preschool-aged children. *Pediatrics, 70*, 774–779.

Beck, A. T., Rush, A. J., Shaw, B. F., & Emery, G. (1979). *Cognitive therapy of depression*. New York: Guilford Press.

Beck, A. T., Steer, R. A., & Garbin, M. G. (1988). Psychometric properties of the Beck Depression Inventory: Twenty-five years of evaluation. *Clinical Psychology Review, 8*, 77–100.

Becker, W. C. (1971). *Parents are teachers: A child management program*. Champaign, IL: Research Press.

Becker, W. C. (1975). *Review tests for "Parents Are Teachers."* Champaign, IL: Research Press.

Befera, M., & Barkley, R. A. (1985). Hyperactive and normal girls and boys: Mother–child interactions, parent psychiatric status, and child psychopathology. *Journal of Child Psychology and Psychiatry and Allied Disciplines, 26*, 439–452.

Berkowitz, B. P., & Graziano, A. M. (1972). Training parents as behavior therapists: A review. *Behaviour Research and Therapy, 10*, 297–317.

Bernhardt, A. J., & Forehand, R. (1975). The effects of labeled and unlabeled praise upon lower and middle class children. *Journal of Experimental Child Psychology, 19*, 536–543.

Bierman, K. L. (1983). Cognitive development and clinical interviews with children. In B. B. Lahey & A. E. Kazdin (Eds.), *Advances in clinical child psychology* (Vol. 6, pp. 217–250). New York: Plenum Press.

Bierman, K. L., Greenberg, M. T., & the Conduct Problems Prevention Research Group. (1996). Social skills training in the Fast Track Program. In R. DeV. Peters & R. J. McMahon (Eds.), *Preventing childhood disorders, substance abuse, and delinquency* (pp. 65–89). Thousand Oaks, CA: Sage.

Blechman, E. A. (1981). Toward comprehensive behavioral family intervention: An algorithm for matching families and interventions. *Behavior Modification, 5*, 221–236.

Block, J. H., Block, J., & Morrison, A. (1981). Parental agreement-disagreement on child-rearing orientations and gender-related personality correlates in children. *Child Development, 52*, 965–974.

Bond, C. R., & McMahon, R. J. (1984). Relationships between marital distress and child behavioral problems, maternal personal adjustment, maternal personality, and maternal parenting behavior. *Journal of Abnormal Psychology, 93*, 348–351.

Braukmann, C. J., Ramp, K. K., Tigner, D. M., & Wolf, M. M. (1984). The Teaching-Family approach to training group-home parents: Training procedures, validation research, and outcome findings. In R. F. Dangel & R. A. Polster (Eds.), *Parent training: Foundations of research and practice* (pp. 144–161). New York: Guilford Press.

Breen, M. J., & Altepeter, T. S. (1990). *Disruptive behavior disorders in children: Treatment-focused assessment*. New York: Guilford Press.

Breiner, J. (1989). Training parents as change agents for their developmentally disabled children. In C. E. Schaefer & J. M. Briesmeister (Eds.), *Handbook of parent training: Parents as co-therapists for children's behavior problems* (pp 269–304). New York: Wiley.

Breiner, J., & Beck, S. (1984). Parents as change agents in the management of their developmentally delayed children's noncompliant behaviors: A critical review. *Applied Research in Mental Retardation, 5*, 259–278.

Breiner, J., & Forehand, R. (1981). An assessment of the effects of parent training on clinic-referred children's school behavior. *Behavioral Assessment, 3*, 31–42.

Breiner, J., & Forehand, R. (1982, November). *Training groups of parents in the management of their developmentally and language delayed children*. Paper presented at the meeting of the Association for Advancement of Behavior Therapy, Los Angeles.

Brestan, E. V., & Eyberg, S. M. (1998). Effective psychosocial treatments of conduct-disordered children and adolescents: 29 years, 82 studies, and 5,272 kids. *Journal of Clinical Child Psychology, 27*, 180–189.

Briesmeister, J. M., & Schaefer, C. E. (Eds.). (1998). *Handbook of parent training: Parents as co-therapists for children's behavior problems* (2nd ed.). New York: Wiley.

Brody, G., & Forehand, R. (1985). The efficacy of parent training with maritally distressed and non-distressed mothers: A multimethod assessment. *Behaviour Research and Therapy, 23*, 291–296.

Brumfield, B. D., & Roberts, M. W. (1998). A comparison of two measurements of child compliance with normal preschool children. *Journal of Clinical Child Psychology, 27*, 109–116.

Butcher, J. N., Dahlstrom, W. G., Graham, J. R., Tellegen, A., & Kaemmer, B. (1989). *Minnesota Multiphasic Personality Inventory-2 (MMPI-2): Manual for administration and scoring*. Minneapolis: University of Minnesota Press.

Campbell, S. B. (1995). Behavior problems in preschool children: A review of recent research. *Journal of Child Psychology and Psychiatry and Allied Disciplines, 36,* 113–149.

Campbell, S. B., Shaw, D. S., & Gilliom, M. (2000). Early externalizing behavior problems: Toddlers and preschoolers at risk for later maladjustment. *Development and Psychopathology, 12,* 467–488.

Campbell, R. V., O'Brien, S., Bickett, A. D., & Lutzker, J. R. (1983). In-home parent training, treatment of migraine headaches, and marital counseling as an ecobehavioral approach to prevent child abuse. *Journal of Behavior Therapy and Experimental Psychiatry, 14,* 147–154.

Capage, L. C., Bennett, G. M., & McNeil, C. B. (2001). A comparison between African American and Caucasian children referred for treatment of disruptive behavior disorders. *Child & Family Behavior Therapy, 23*(1), 1–13.

Capaldi, D. M. (1991). Co-occurrence of conduct problems and depressive symptoms in early adolescent boys: I. Familial factors and general adjustment at age 6. *Development and Psychopathology, 3,* 277–300.

Capaldi, D. M. (1992). Co-occurrence of conduct problems and depressive symptoms in early adolescent boys: II. A 2–year follow-up at grade 8. *Development and Psychopathology, 4,* 125–144.

Capaldi, D. M., Degarmo, D., Patterson, G. R., & Forgatch, M. (2002). Contextual risk across the early life span and association with antisocial behavior. In J. B. Reid, G. R. Patterson, & J. Snyder (Eds.), *Antisocial behavior in children and adolescents: A developmental analysis and model for intervention* (pp. 123–145). Washington, DC: American Psychological Association.

Cavell, T. A. (2000). *Working with parents of aggressive children: A practitioner's guide.* Washington, DC: American Psychological Association.

Cerezo, M. A. (1988). Community Interaction Checklist. In M. Hersen & A. S. Bellack (Eds.), *Dictionary of behavioral assessment techniques* (pp. 135–138). New York: Pergamon Press.

Chamberlain, P., & Patterson, G. R. (1995). Discipline and child compliance in parenting. In M. H. Bornstein (Ed.), *Handbook of parenting: Vol. 4. Applied and practical parenting* (pp. 205–225). Hillsdale, NJ: Erlbaum.

Chamberlain, P., Patterson, G., Reid, J., Kavanagh, K., & Forgatch, M. (1984). Observation of client resistance. *Behavior Therapy, 15,* 144–155.

Chamberlain, P., Reid, J. B., Ray, J., Capaldi, D. M., & Fisher, P. (1997). Parent Inadequate Discipline (PID). In T. A. Widiger, A. J. Frances, H. A. Pincus, R. Ross, M. B. First, & W. Davis (Eds.), *DSM-IV sourcebook* (Vol. 3, pp. 569–629). Washington, DC: American Psychiatric Association.

Charlop, M. H., Parrish, J. M., Fenton, L., R., & Cataldo, M. F. (1987). Evaluation of hospital-based outpatient pediatric psychology services. *Journal of Pediatric Psychology, 12,* 485–503.

Chen, W. J., Faraone, S. V., Biederman, J., & Tsuang, M. T. (1994). Diagnostic accuracy of the Child Behavior Checklist scales for attention-deficit hyperactivity disorder: A receiver-operating characteristic analysis. *Journal of Consulting and Clinical Psychology, 62,* 1017–1025.

Coie, J. D., & Dodge, K. A. (1998). Aggression and antisocial behavior. In W. Damon (Series Ed.) & N. Eisenberg (Vol. Ed.), *Handbook of child psychology: Vol. 3. Social, emotional, and personality development* (5th ed., pp. 779–862). New York: Wiley.

Coie, J. D., Lochman, J. E., Terry, R., & Hyman, C. (1992). Predicting early adolescent disorder from childhood aggression and peer rejection. *Journal of Consulting and Clinical Psychology, 60,* 783–792.

Coleman, M., Ganong, L., & Fine, M. (2000). Reinvestigating remarriage: Another decade of progress. *Journal of Marriage and the Family, 62,* 1288–1307.

Conduct Problems Prevention Research Group. (1992). A developmental and clinical model for the prevention of conduct disorders: The FAST Track Program. *Development and Psychopathology, 4,* 509–527.

Conduct Problems Prevention Research Group. (1999). Initial impact of the Fast Track prevention trial for conduct problems: I. The high-risk sample. *Journal of Consulting and Clinical Psychology, 67,* 631–647.

Conduct Problems Prevention Research Group. (2000). Merging universal and indicated prevention programs: The Fast Track model. *Addictive Behaviors, 25,* 913–927.

Conduct Problems Prevention Research Group. (2002). Evaluation of the first three years of the Fast Track prevention trial with children at high risk for adolescent conduct problems. *Journal of Abnormal Child Psychology, 30,* 19–35.

Conners, C. K. (2001). Multimodal treatment of ADHD in the MTA: An alternative outcome analysis. *Journal of the American Academy of Child and Adolescent Psychiatry, 40,* 159–167.

Conners, C. K., & Erhardt, D. (1998). Attention-deficit hyperactivity disorder in children and adolescents. In M. Hersen & A. Bellack (Eds.), *Comprehensive clinical psychology* (pp. 487–525). New York: Pergamon Press.

Conway, J. G., & Bucher, B. D. (1976). Transfer and maintenance of behavior change in children: A review and suggestions. In E. J. Mash, L. A. Hamerlynck, & L. C. Handy (Eds.), *Behavior modification and families* (pp. 119–159). New York: Brunner/Mazel.

Cowen, E. L., Huser, J., Beach, D. R., & Rappaport, J. (1970). Parental perceptions of young children and their relation to indexes of adjustment. *Journal of Consulting and Clinical Psychology, 34,* 97–103.

Crick, N. R., & Dodge, K. A. (1994). A review and reformulation of social information-processing mechanisms in children's social adjustment. *Psychological Bulletin, 115,* 74–101.

Crittenden, P. M., & DiLalla, D. L. (1988). Compulsive compliance: The development of an inhibitory coping strategy in infancy. *Journal of Abnormal Child Psychology, 16,* 585–599.

Crnic, K. A., & Greenberg, M. T. (1990). Minor parenting stresses with young children. *Child Development, 61,* 1628–1637.

Cross Calvert, S., & McMahon, R. J. (1987). The treatment acceptability of a behavioral parent training program and its components. *Behavior Therapy, 18,* 165–179.

Cummings, E. M., & Davies, P. T. (1994). Maternal depression in child development. *Journal of Child Psychology and Psychiatry and Allied Disciplines, 35,* 73–112.

Cunningham, C. E. (1989). A family systems-oriented training program for parents of language-delayed children with behavior problems. In C. E. Schaefer & J. M. Briesmeister (Eds.), *Handbook of parent training: Parents as co-therapists for children's behavior problems* (pp. 133–175). New York: Wiley.

Cunningham, C. E., & Barkley, R. A. (1979). The interactions of normal and hyperactive children with their mothers in free play and structured tasks. *Child Development, 50,* 217–224.

Cushing, P., Adams, A., & Rincover, A. (1983). Research on the education of autistic children. In M. Hersen, R. M. Eisler, & P. M. Miller (Eds.), *Progress in behavior modification* (Vol. 14, pp. 1–48). New York: Academic Press.

Dachman, R. S., Halasz, M. M., Bickett, A. D., & Lutzker, J. R. (1984). A home-based ecobehavioral parent-training and generalization package with a neglectful mother. *Education and Treatment of Children, 7*, 183–202.

Dangel, R. F., & Polster, R. A. (Eds.). (1984). *Parent training: Foundations of research and practice.* New York: Guilford Press.

Darling, N., & Steinberg, L. (1993). Parenting style as context: An integrative model. *Psychological Bulletin, 113*, 487–496.

Davies, G. R., McMahon, R. J., Flessati, E., & Tiedemann, G. L. (1984). Verbal rationales and modeling as adjuncts to a parenting technique for child compliance. *Child Development, 55*, 1290–1298.

Davies, P. T., & Cummings, E. M. (1994). Marital conflict and child adjustment: An emotional security hypothesis. *Psychological Bulletin, 116*, 387–411.

Day, D. E., & Roberts, M. W. (1983). An analysis of the physical punishment component of a parent training program. *Journal of Abnormal Child Psychology, 11*, 141–152.

Deater-Deckard, K. (1998). Parenting stress and child adjustment: Some old hypotheses and new questions. *Clinical Psychology: Science and Practice, 5*, 314–332.

Demo, D. H., & Cox, M. J. (2000). Families with young children: A review of research in the 1990s. *Journal of Marriage and the Family, 62*, 876–895.

Dinkmeyer, D., & McKay, G. D. (1976). *Systematic training for effective parenting.* Circle Pines, MN: American Guidance Services.

Dische, S., Yule, W., Corbett, J., & Hand, D. (1983). Childhood nocturnal enuresis: Factors associated with outcome of treatment with an enuresis alarm. *Developmental Medicine and Child Neurology, 25*, 67–80.

Dishion, T. J., Patterson, G. R., Stoolmiller, M., & Skinner, M. L. (1991). Family, school, and behavioral antecedents to early adolescent involvement with antisocial peers. *Developmental Psychology, 27*, 172–180.

Dishion, T. J., & Patterson, S. G. (1996). *Preventive parenting with love, encouragement, and limits: The preschool years.* Eugene, OR: Castalia.

Dreikurs, R. (1964). *Children: The challenge.* New York: Hawthorn Books.

Dreyer, C. A., & Dreyer, A. S. (1973). Family dinner time as a unique behavior habitat. *Family Process, 12*, 291–301.

Dubey, D. R., O'Leary, S. G., & Kaufman, K. F. (1983). Training parents of hyperactive children in child management: A comparative outcome study. *Journal of Abnormal Child Psychology, 11*, 229–246.

Ducharme, J. M. (1996). Errorless compliance training: Optimizing clinical efficacy. *Behavior Modification, 20*, 259–280.

Ducharme, J. M., Popynick, M., Pontes, E., & Steele, S. (1996). Errorless compliance to parental requests: III. Group parent training with parent observation data and long-term follow-up. *Behavior Therapy, 27*, 353–372.

Dumas, J. E. (1984a). Child, adult-interactional, and socioeconomic setting events as predictors of parent training outcome. *Education and Treatment of Children, 7*, 351–364.

Dumas, J. E. (1984b). Indiscriminate mothering: Empirical findings and theoretical speculations. *Advances in Behaviour Research and Therapy, 7*, 13–27.

Dumas, J. E. (1989). Treating antisocial behavior in children: Child and family approaches. *Clinical Psychology Review, 9*, 197–222.

Dumas, J. E. (1996). Why was this child referred? Interactional correlates of referral status in families of children with disruptive behavior problems. *Journal of Clinical Child Psychology, 25*, 106–115.

Dumas, J. E., & LaFreniere, P. J. (1993). Mother–child relationships as sources of support or stress: A comparison of competent, average, aggressive, and anxious dyads. *Child Development, 64*, 1732–1754.

Dumas, J. E., & Lechowicz, J. G. (1989). When do noncompliant children noncomply? Implications for family behavior therapy. *Child & Family Behavior Therapy, 11*(3–4), 21–38.

Dumas, J. E., & Serketich, W. J. (1994). Maternal depressive symptomatology and child maladjustment: A comparison of three process models. *Behavior Therapy, 25*, 161–181.

Dumas, J. E., & Wahler, R. G. (1983). Predictors of treatment outcome in parent training: Mother insularity and socioeconomic disadvantage. *Behavioral Assessment, 5*, 301–313.

Dumas, J. E., & Wahler, R. G. (1985). Indiscriminate mothering as a contextual factor in aggressive-oppositional child behavior: "Damned if you do and damned if you don't." *Journal of Abnormal Child Psychology, 13*, 1–17.

Edelbrock, C. (1985). *Conduct problems in childhood and adolescence: Developmental patterns and progressions.* Unpublished manuscript.

Edelbrock, C., Costello, A. J., Dulcan, M. K., Kalas, R., & Conover, N. C. (1985). Age differences in the reliability of the psychiatric interview of the child. *Child Development, 56*, 265–275.

Egeland, B., Sroufe, L. A., & Erickson, M. (1983). The developmental consequences of different patterns of maltreatment. *Child Abuse and Neglect, 7*, 459–469.

El-Sheikh, M., & Flanagan, E. (2001). Parental problem drinking and children's adjustment: Family conflict and parental depression as mediators and moderators of risk. *Journal of Abnormal Child Psychology, 29*, 417–432.

Embry, L. H. (1984). What to do? Matching client characteristics and intervention techniques through a prescriptive taxonomic key. In R. F. Dangel & R. A. Polster (Eds.), *Parent training: Foundations of research and practice* (pp. 443–473). New York: Guilford Press.

Emery, R. E. (1999). *Marriage, divorce, and children's adjustment* (2nd ed.). Thousand Oaks, CA: Sage.

Emery, R. E., & Forehand, R. (1994). Parental divorce and children's well-being: A focus on resilience. In R. J. Haggerty, N. Garmezy, M. Rutter, & L. Sherrod (Eds.), *Risk and resilience in children* (pp. 64–99). London: Cambridge University Press.

Epstein, N., & Baucom, D. H. (2002). *Enhanced cognitive-behavioral therapy for couples: A contextual approach.* Washington, DC: American Psychological Association.

Erhardt, D., & Baker, B. L. (1990). The effects of behavioral parent training on families with young hyperactive children. *Journal of Behavior Therapy and Experimental Psychiatry, 21*, 121–132.

Estrada, A. V., & Pinsof, W. M. (1995). The effectiveness of family therapies for selected behavioral disorders of childhood. *Journal of Marital and Family Therapy, 21*, 403–440.

Evans, I. M., & Nelson, R. O. (1986). Assessment of children. In A. R. Ciminero, K. S. Calhoun, & H. E. Adams (Eds.), *Handbook of behavioral assessment* (2nd ed., pp. 601–630). New York: Wiley.

Eyberg, S. (1993). Consumer satisfaction measures for assessing parent training programs. In L. VandeCreek, S. Knapp, & T. L. Jackson (Eds.), *Innovations in clinical practice: A source book* (Vol. 12, pp. 377–382). Sarasota, FL: Professional Resource Press.

Eyberg, S., Bessmer, J., Newcomb, K., Edwards, D., & Robinson, E. (1994). *Dyadic Parent–Child Interaction Coding System II: A manual.* Unpublished manuscript, University of Florida, Gainesville.

Eyberg, S. M., & Boggs, S. R. (1998). Parent–child interaction therapy: A psychosocial intervention for the treatment of young conduct-disordered children. In J. M. Briesmeister & C. S. Schaefer (Eds.), *Handbook of parent training: Parents as co-therapists for children's behavior problems* (2nd ed., pp. 61–97). New York: Wiley.

Eyberg, S. M., & Matarazzo, R. G. (1980). Training parents as therapists: A comparison between individual parent–child interaction training and parent group didactic training. *Journal of Clinical Psychology, 36,* 492–499.

Eyberg, S. M., & Pincus, D. (1999). *The Eyberg Child Behavior Inventory and Sutter-Eyberg Student Behavior Inventory: Professional manual.* Lutz, FL: Psychological Assessment Resources.

Eyberg, S. M., Schuhmann, E. M., & Rey, J. (1998). Child and adolescent psychotherapy research: Developmental issues. *Journal of Abnormal Child Psychology, 26,* 71–82.

Farrington, D. P. (2003). Key results from the first forty years of the Cambridge Study in Delinquent Development. In T. P. Thornberry & M. D. Krohn (Eds.), *Taking stock of delinquency: An overview of findings from contemporary longitudinal studies* (pp. 137–183). New York: Kluwer Academic/Plenum Press.

Fauber, R., Forehand, R., Thomas, A. M., & Wierson, M. (1990). A mediational model of the impact of marital conflict on adolescent adjustment in intact and divorced families: The role of disrupted parenting. *Child Development, 61,* 1112–1123.

Fincham, F. D. (1998). Child development and marital relations. *Child Development, 69,* 543–574.

Fincham, F. D., Grych, J. H., & Osborne, L. N. (1994). Does marital conflict cause child maladjustment? Directions and challenges for longitudinal research. *Journal of Family Psychology, 8,* 128–140.

Finney, J. W. (1986). Preventing common feeding problems in infants and young children. *Pediatric Clinics of North America, 33,* 775–788.

Fischer, M. (1990). Parenting stress and the child with attention deficit hyperactivity disorder. *Journal of Clinical Child Psychology, 19,* 337–346.

Fischer, M., Barkley, R. A., Fletcher, K., & Smallish, L. (1993). The adolescent outcome of hyperactive children diagnosed by research criteria: V. Predictors of outcome. *Journal of the American Academy of Child and Adolescent Psychiatry, 32,* 324–332.

Fleischman, M. J. (1979). Using parenting salaries to control attrition and cooperation in therapy. *Behavior Therapy, 10,* 111–116.

Forehand, R. (1977). Child noncompliance to parental requests: Behavioral analysis and treatment. In M. Hersen, R. M. Eisler, & P. M. Miller (Eds.), *Progress in behavior modification* (Vol. 5, pp. 111–147). New York: Academic Press.

Forehand, R. (1986). Parental positive reinforcement with deviant children: Does it make a difference? *Child & Family Behavior Therapy, 8*(3), 19–25.

Forehand, R. (1993). Family psychopathology and child functioning. *Journal of Child and Family Studies, 2,* 81–86.

Forehand, R., Armistead, L., Neighbors, B., & Klein, K. (1994). *Parent training for the noncompliant child: A guide for training therapists* [Videotape]. South Burlington, VT: Child Focus.

Forehand, R., & Atkeson, B. M. (1977). Generality of treatment effects with parents as therapists: A review of assessment and implementation procedures. *Behavior Therapy, 8,* 575–593.

Forehand, R., Breiner, J., McMahon, R. J., & Davies, G. (1981). Predictors of cross setting behavior change in the treatment of child problems. *Journal of Behavior Therapy and Experimental Psychiatry, 12,* 311–313.

Forehand, R., & Brody, G. (1985). The association between parental personal adjustment and parent–child interactions in a clinic sample. *Behaviour Research and Therapy, 23,* 211–212.

Forehand, R., Cheney, T., & Yoder, P. (1974). Parent behavior training: Effects on the noncompliance of a deaf child. *Journal of Behavior Therapy and Experimental Psychiatry, 5,* 281–183.

Forehand, R., Furey, W., & McMahon, R. J. (1984). The role of maternal distress in a parent training program to modify child noncompliance. *Behavioural Psychotherapy, 12,* 93–108.

Forehand, R., Griest, D., & Wells, K. C. (1979). Parent behavioral training: An analysis of the relationship among multiple outcome measures. *Journal of Abnormal Child Psychology, 7,* 229–242.

Forehand, R., Griest, D. L., Wells, K., & McMahon, R. J. (1982). Side effects of parent counseling on marital satisfaction. *Journal of Counseling Psychology, 29,* 104–107.

Forehand, R., & King, H. E. (1974). Pre-school children's non-compliance: Effects of short-term behavior therapy. *Journal of Community Psychology, 2,* 42–44.

Forehand, R., & King, H. E. (1977). Noncompliant children: Effects of parent training on behavior and attitude change. *Behavior Modification, 1,* 93–108.

Forehand, R., King, H. E., Peed, S., & Yoder, P. (1975). Mother–child interactions: Comparisons of a non-compliant clinic group and a non-clinic group. *Behaviour Research and Therapy, 13,* 79–84.

Forehand, R., & Kotchick, B. A. (1996). Cultural diversity: A wake-up call for parent training. *Behavior Therapy, 27,* 187–206.

Forehand, R., Lautenschlager, G. J., Faust, J., & Graziano, W. G. (1986). Parent perceptions and parent–child interactions in clinic referred children: A preliminary investigation of the effects of maternal depressive moods. *Behaviour Research and Therapy, 24,* 73–75.

Forehand, R., & Long, N. (1988). Outpatient treatment of the acting out child: Procedures, long term follow-up data, and clinical problems. *Advances in Behaviour Research and Therapy, 10,* 129–177.

Forehand, R., & Long, N. (1996). *Parenting the strong-willed child: The clinically-proven five-week program for parents of two- to six-year-olds.* Chicago: McGraw-Hill.

Forehand, R., & Long, N. (2002). *Parenting the strong-willed child: The clinically-proven five-week program for parents of two- to six-year-olds* (2nd ed.). New York: McGraw-Hill.

Forehand, R., McCombs, A., & Brody, G. H. (1987). The relationship between parental depressive mood states and child functioning. *Advances in Behaviour Research and Therapy, 9,* 1–20.

Forehand, R., McCombs, A., Long, N., Brody, G., & Fauber, R. (1988). Early adolescent adjustment to recent parental divorce: The role of interparental conflict and adolescent sex as mediating variables. *Journal of Consulting and Clinical Psychology, 56,* 624–627.

Forehand, R. L., & McMahon, R. J. (1981). *Helping the noncompliant child: A clinician's guide to parent training.* New York: Guilford Press.

Forehand, R., Middlebrook, J., Rogers, T. R., & Steffe, M. (1983). Dropping out of parent training. *Behaviour Research and Therapy, 21,* 663–668.

Forehand, R., Rogers, T., McMahon, R. J., Wells, K. C., & Griest, D. L. (1981). Teaching parents to modify child behavior problems: An examination of some follow-up data. *Journal of Pediatric Psychology, 6,* 313–322.

Forehand, R., & Scarboro, M. E. (1975). An analysis of children's oppositional behavior. *Journal of Abnormal Child Psychology, 3,* 27–31.

Forehand, R., Steffe, M., Furey, W. M., & Walley, P. M. (1983). Mothers' evaluation of a parent training program completed three and one-half years earlier. *Journal of Behavior Therapy and Experimental Psychiatry, 14,* 339–342.

Forehand, R., Sturgis, E. T., McMahon, R. J., Aguar, D., Green, K., Wells, K., & Breiner, J. (1979). Parent behavioral training to modify child noncompliance: Treatment generalization across time and from home to school. *Behavior Modification, 3,* 3–25.

Forehand, R., Wells, K. C., & Griest, D. L. (1980). An examination of the social validity of a parent training program. *Behavior Therapy, 11,* 488–502.

Forehand, R., Wells, K. C., McMahon, R. J., Griest, D. L., & Rogers, T. (1982). Maternal perceptions of maladjustment in clinic-referred children: An extension of earlier research. *Journal of Behavioral Assessment, 4,* 145–151.

Forehand, R., Wells, K. C., & Sturgis, E. T. (1978). Predictors of child noncompliant behavior in the home. *Journal of Consulting and Clinical Psychology, 46,* 179.

Forehand, R., & Wierson, M. (1993). The role of developmental factors in planning behavioral interventions for children: Disruptive behavior as an example. *Behavior Therapy, 24,* 117–141.

Forgatch, M. S. (1994). *Parenting through change: A training manual.* Eugene: Oregon Social Learning Center.

Forgatch, M. S., Patterson, G. R., & Skinner, M. L. (1988). A mediational model for the effect of divorce on antisocial behavior in boys. In E. M. Hetherington & J. D. Arasteh (Eds.), *Impact of divorce, single parenting, and stepparenting on children* (pp. 135–154). Hillsdale, NJ: Erlbaum.

Frick, P. J. (1994). Family dysfunction and the disruptive behavior disorders: A review of recent empirical findings. In T. H. Ollendick & R. J. Prinz (Eds.), *Advances in clinical child psychology* (Vol. 16, pp. 203–226). New York: Plenum Press.

Frick, P. J., Lahey, B. B., Loeber, R., Stouthamer-Loeber, M., Christ, M. A. G., & Hanson, K. (1992). Familial risk factors to oppositional defiant disorder and conduct disorder: Parental psychopathology and maternal parenting. *Journal of Consulting and Clinical Psychology, 60,* 49–55.

Frick, P. J., & Loney, B. R. (2002). Understanding the association between parent and child antisocial behavior. In R. J. McMahon & R. DeV. Peters (Eds.), *The effects of parental dysfunction on children* (pp. 105–126). New York: Kluwer Academic/Plenum Press.

Furey, W. M., & Basili, L. A. (1988). Predicting consumer satisfaction in parent training for noncompliant children. *Behavior Therapy, 19,* 555–564.

Furtkamp, E., Giffort, D., & Schiers, W. (1982). In-class evaluation of behavior modification knowledge: Parallel tests for use in applied settings. *Journal of Behavior Therapy and Experimental Psychiatry, 13,* 131–134.

Garcia, M. M., Shaw, D. S., Winslow, E. B., & Yaggi, K. E. (2000). Destructive sibling conflict and the development of conduct problems in young boys. *Developmental Psychology, 36,* 44–53.

Gardner, F. E. M. (1987). Positive interaction between mothers and conduct-problem children: Is there training for harmony as well as fighting? *Journal of Abnormal Child Psychology, 15,* 283–293.

Gardner, F. (2000). Methodological issues and the direct observation of parent–child interactions: Do observational findings reflect the natural behavior of participants? *Clinical Child and Family Psychology Review, 3,* 185–198.

Gardner, H. L., Forehand, R., & Roberts, M. (1976). Time-out with children: Effects of an explanation and brief parent training on child and parent behaviors. *Journal of Abnormal Child Psychology, 4,* 277–288.

Glogower, F., & Sloop, E. W. (1976). Two strategies of group training of parents as effective behavior modifiers. *Behavior Therapy, 7,* 177–184.

Gmeinder, K. L., & Kratochwill, T. R. (1998). Short-term, home-based intervention for child noncompliance using behavioral consultation and a self-help manual. *Journal of Educational and Psychological Consultation, 9,* 91–117.

Goodman, S. H., & Gotlib, I. (1999). Risk for psychopathology in children of depressed mothers: A developmental model for understanding mechanisms of transmission. *Psychological Review, 106,* 458–490.

Greenberg, M. T. (1999). Attachment and psychopathology in childhood. In J. Cassidy & P. R. Shaver (Eds.), *Handbook of attachment: Theory, research, and clinical applications* (pp. 469–496). New York: Guilford Press.

Greenberg, M. T., Domitrovich, C., & Bumbarger, B. (2001, March 30). The prevention of mental disorders in school-age children: Current state of the field. *Prevention & Treatment, 4,* Article 1 [Online]. Available: *http://journals.apa.org/prevention/volume4/pre004000a.html*

Greene, R. W., & Doyle, A. E. (1999). Toward a transactional conceptualization of oppositional defiant disorder: Implications for assessment and treatment. *Clinical Child and Family Psychology Review, 2,* 129–148.

Greenspan, S. (1991). *The clinical interview of the child* (2nd ed.). Washington: American Psychiatric Press.

Griest, D. L., Forehand, R., Rogers, T., Breiner, J., Fury, W., & Williams, C. A. (1982). The effects of parent enhancement therapy on treatment outcome and generalization of a parent training program. *Behaviour Research and Therapy, 20,* 429–436.

Griest, D. L., Forehand, R., & Wells, K. C. (1981). The follow-up assessment of parent behavioral training: An analysis of who will participate. *Child Study Journal, 11,* 221–229.

Griest, D. L., Forehand, R., Wells, K. C., & McMahon, R. J. (1980). An examination of differences between nonclinic and behavior problem clinic-referred children and their mothers. *Journal of Abnormal Psychology, 89,* 497–500.

Griest, D. L., & Wells, K. C. (1983). Behavioral family therapy with conduct disorders in children. *Behavior Therapy, 14,* 37–53.

Griest, D., Wells, K. C., & Forehand, R. (1979). An examination of predictors of maternal perceptions of maladjustment in clinic-referred children. *Journal of Abnormal Psychology, 88,* 277–281.

Grusec, J. E., & Kuczynski, L. (Eds.). (1997). *Parenting and children's internalization of values: A handbook of contemporary theory.* New York: Wiley.

Haley, J. (1976). *Problem-solving therapy: New strategies for effective family therapy.* San Francisco: Jossey-Bass.

Handen, B. L. (1998). Mental retardation. In E. J. Mash & R. A. Barkley (Eds.), *Treatment of childhood disorders* (2nd ed., pp. 369–415). New York: Guilford Press.

Hanf, C. (1969). *A two-stage program for modifying maternal controlling during mother–child (M-C) interaction.* Paper presented at the meeting of the Western Psychological Association, Vancouver, BC, Canada.

Hanf, C. (1970). *Shaping mothers to shape their children's behavior.* Unpublished manuscript, University of Oregon Medical School.

Hanf, C., & Kling, J. (1973). *Facilitating parent–child interaction: A two-stage training model.* Unpublished manuscript, University of Oregon Medical School.

Hawkins, J. D., Catalano, R. F., Brown, E. O., Vadasy, P. F., Roberts, C., Fitzmahan, D., Starkman, N., & Ransdell, M. (1988). *Preparing for the drug (free) years: A family activity book*. Seattle, WA: Comprehensive Health Education Foundation.

Haynes, S. N. (1991). Behavioral assessment. In M. Hersen, A. E. Kazdin, & A. S. Bellack (Eds.), *The clinical psychology handbook* (pp. 430–464). New York: Pergamon Press.

Hembree-Kigin, T. L., & McNeil, C. B. (1995). *Parent–child interaction therapy*. New York: Plenum Press.

Hetherington, E. M., Cox. M., & Cox, R. (1982). The effects of divorce on parents and children. In M. E. Lamb (Ed.), *Nontraditional families* (pp. 233–288). Hillsdale, NJ: Erlbaum.

Hinshaw, S. P., Lahey, B. B., & Hart, E. L. (1993). Issues of taxonomy and comorbidity in the development of conduct disorder. *Development and Psychopathology, 5*, 31–49.

Hobbs, S. A., & Forehand, R. (1975). Effects of differential release from time-out on children's deviant behavior. *Journal of Behavior Therapy and Experimental Psychiatry, 6*, 256–257.

Hobbs, S. A., Forehand, R., & Murray, R. G. (1978). Effects of various durations of timeout on the noncompliant behavior of children. *Behavior Therapy, 9*, 652–656.

Holleran, P. A., Littman, D. C., Freund, R. D., & Schmaling, K. B. (1982). A signal detection approach to social perception: Identification of negative and positive behaviors by parents of normal and problem children. *Journal of Abnormal Child Psychology, 10*, 547–557.

Horn, W. F., Ialongo, N., Greenberg, G., Packard, T., & Smith-Winberry, C. (1990). Additive effects of behavioral parent training and self-control therapy with attention deficit hyperactivity disordered children. *Journal of Clinical Child Psychology, 19*, 98–110.

Horn, W. F., Ialongo, N. S., Pascoe, J. M., Greenberg, G., Packard, T., Lopez, M., Wagner, A., & Puttler, L. (1991). Additive effects of psychostimulants, parent training, and self-control therapy with ADHD children. *Journal of the American Academy of Child and Adolescent Psychiatry, 30*, 233–240.

Houlihan, D., Sloan, H. N., Jones, R. N., & Patten, C. (1992). A review of behavioral conceptualizations in treatment of child noncompliance. *Education and Treatment of Children, 15*, 56–77.

Houseknecht, S. K. (1979). Childlessness and marital adjustment. *Journal of Marriage and the Family, 41*, 259–265.

Hudson, A., & Blane, M. (1985). The importance of non verbal behavior in giving instructions to children. *Child & Family Behavior Therapy, 7*(2), 1–10.

Hughes, H. M., & Haynes, S. M. (1978). Structured laboratory observation in the behavioral assessment of parent–child interactions: A methodological critique. *Behavior Therapy, 9*, 428–447.

Humphreys, L., Forehand, R., McMahon, R., & Roberts, M. (1978). Parent behavioral training to modify child noncompliance: Effects on untreated siblings. *Journal of Behavior Therapy and Experimental Psychiatry, 9*, 235–238.

Huszti, H., & Olson, R. (1999). Noncompliance. In S. D. Netherton, D. Holmes, & C. E. Walker (Eds.), *Child and adolescent psychological disorders: A comprehensive textbook* (pp. 567–581). New York: Oxford University Press.

Ialongo, N. S., Horn, W. F., Pascoe, J. M., Greenberg, G., Packard, T., Lopez, M., Wagner, A., & Puttler, L. (1993). The effects of a multimodal intervention with attention-deficit hyperactivity disorder children: A 9–month follow-up. *Journal of the American Academy of Child and Adolescent Psychiatry, 32*, 182–189.

Jacobs, J. R., Boggs, S. R., Eyberg, S. M., Edwards, D., Durning, P., Querido, J. G., McNeil, C. B., & Funderburk, B. W. (2000). Psychometric properties and reference point data for the Revised Edition of the School Observation Coding System. *Behavior Therapy, 31*, 695–712.

Jacobson, N. S., & Anderson, E. A. (1980). The effects of behavior rehearsal and feedback on the acquisition of problem-solving skills in distressed and non-distressed couples. *Behaviour Research and Therapy, 18*, 25–36.

Jacobson, N. S., & Christensen, A. (1996). *Integrative couples therapy.* New York: Norton.

Jensen, B. J., & Haynes, S. N. (1986). Self-report questionnaires and inventories. In A. R. Ciminero, K. S. Calhoun, & H. E. Adams (Eds.), *Handbook of behavioral assessment* (2nd ed., pp. 150–175). New York: Wiley.

Johnson, S. M. (1996). *Creating connections.* New York: Brunner/Mazel.

Johnson, S. M., Bolstad, O. D., & Lobitz, G. K. (1976). Generalization and contrast phenomena in behavior modification with children. In E. J. Mash, L. A. Hamerlynck, & L. C. Handy (Eds.), *Behavior modification and families* (pp. 160–188). New York: Brunner/Mazel.

Johnson, S. M., & Lobitz, G. K. (1974). Parental manipulation of child behavior in home observations. *Journal of Applied Behavior Analysis, 7*, 23–31.

Johnston, C. (1996a). Addressing parent cognitions in interventions with families of disruptive children. In K. S. Dobson & K. D. Craig (Eds.), *Advances in cognitive-behavioral therapy* (pp. 193–209). Thousand Oaks, CA: Sage.

Johnston, C. (1996b). Parent characteristics and parent–child interactions in families of nonproblem children and ADHD children with higher and lower levels of oppositional-defiant behavior. *Journal of Abnormal Child Psychology, 24*, 85–104.

Jones, R. N., Sloane, H. N., & Roberts, M. W. (1992). Limitations of "don't" instructional control. *Behavior Therapy, 23*, 131–140.

Kazdin, A. E. (1977). Assessing the clinical or applied importance of behavior change through social validation. *Behavior Modification, 1*, 427–252.

Kazdin, A. E. (1985). *Treatment of antisocial behavior in children and adolescents.* Homewood, IL: Dorsey Press.

Kazdin, A. E. (1990). Premature termination from treatment among children referred for antisocial behavior. *Journal of Child Psychology and Psychiatry and Allied Disciplines, 31*, 415–425.

Kazdin, A. E. (1995). *Conduct disorders in childhood and adolescence* (2nd ed.). Thousand Oaks, CA: Sage.

Kazdin, A. E. (2002). *Research design in clinical psychology* (4th ed.). Boston: Allyn & Bacon.

Kazdin, A. E., Holland, L., & Crowley, M. (1997). Family experience of barriers to treatment and premature termination from child therapy. *Journal of Consulting and Clinical Psychology, 65*, 453–463.

Kelley, M. L. (1990). *School–home notes: Promoting children's classroom success.* New York: Guilford Press.

Kendall, P. C., Hollon, S. D., Beck, A. T., Hammen, C. L., & Ingram, R. E. (1987). Issues and recommendations regarding use of the Beck Depression Inventory. *Cognitive Therapy and Research, 11*, 289–299.

Kimmel, D., & van der Veen, F. (1974). Factors of marital adjustment in Locke's Marital Adjustment Test. *Journal of Marriage and the Family, 36*, 57–63.

Klein, R. G., & Mannuzza, S. (1991). Long-term outcome of hyperactive children: A review. *Journal of the American Academy of Child and Adolescent Psychiatry, 30*, 383–387.

Knapp, P. A., & Deluty, R. H. (1989). Relative effectiveness of two behavioral parent training programs. *Journal of Clinical Child Psychology, 18,* 314–322.

Kochanska, G., & Aksan, N. (1995). Mother–child mutually positive affect, the quality of child compliance to requests and prohibitions, and maternal control as correlates of early internalization. *Child Development, 68,* 94–112.

Kochanska, G., Coy, K. C., & Murray, K. T. (2001). The development of self-regulation in the first four years of life. *Child Development, 72,* 1091–1111.

Kochanska, G., & Thompson, R. A. (1997). The emergence and development of conscience in toddlerhood and early childhood. In J. E. Grusec & L. Kuczynski (Eds.), *Parenting and children's internalization of values: A handbook of contemporary theory* (pp. 53–77). New York: Wiley.

Kochanska, G., Tjebkes, T. L., & Forman, D. R. (1998). Children's emerging regulation of conduct: Restraint, compliance, and internalization from infancy to the second year. *Child Development, 69,* 1378–1389.

Koegel, R. L., Rincover, A., & Egel, A. L. (Eds.) (1982). *Educating and understanding autistic children.* San Diego, CA: College-Hill Press.

Koegel, R. L., Russo, D. C., & Rincover, A. (1977). Assessing and training teachers in the generalized use of behavior modification with autistic children. *Journal of Applied Behavior Analysis, 10,* 197–205.

Koenig, A. L., Cicchetti, D., & Rogosch, F. A. (2000). Child compliance/noncompliance and maternal contributors to internalization in maltreating and nonmaltreating dyads. *Child Development, 71,* 1018–1032.

Kopp, C. B. (1982). Antecedents of self-regulation: A developmental prospective. *Developmental Psychology, 18,* 199–214.

Kotchick, B. A., & Forehand, R. (2002). Putting parenting in perspective: A discussion of the social-contextual factors that shape parenting practices. *Journal of Child and Family Studies, 11,* 255–269.

Kotchick, B. A., Shaffer, A., Dorsey, S., & Forehand, R. (in press). Parenting antisocial children and adolescents. In M. Hoghughi & N. Long (Eds.), *Handbook of parenting.* London: Sage.

Kotler, J. S., & McMahon, R. J. (2003). *Compliance and noncompliance in anxious, aggressive, and socially competent children: The impact of the Child's Game.* Manuscript submitted for publication.

Kratzer, L., & Hodgins, S. (1997). Adult outcomes of child conduct problems: A cohort study. *Journal of Abnormal Child Psychology, 25,* 65–81.

Krumboltz, J. D., & Krumboltz, H. B. (1972). *Changing children's behavior.* Englewood Cliffs, NJ: Prentice-Hall.

Kuczynski, L., & Hildebrandt, N. (1997). Models of conformity and resistance in socialization theory. In J. Grusec & L. Kuczynski (Eds.), *Parenting and the socialization of values: A handbook of contemporary theory* (pp. 227–256). New York: Wiley.

Kuczynski, L., & Kochanska, G. (1990). Development of children's noncompliance strategies from toddlerhood to age 5. *Developmental Psychology, 26,* 398–408.

Kuczynski, L., Kochanska, G., Radke-Yarrow, M., & Girnius-Brown, O. (1987). A developmental interpretation of young children's noncompliance. *Developmental Psychology, 23,* 799–806.

Lahey, B. B., Loeber, R., Hart, E. L., Frick, P. J., Applegate, B., Zhang, Q., Green, S. M., & Russo, M. F. (1995). Four-year longitudinal study of conduct disorder in boys: Patterns and predictors of persistence. *Journal of Abnormal Psychology, 104,* 83–93.

Landauer, T. K., Carlsmith, J. M., & Lepper, M. (1970). Experimental analysis of the factors determing obedience of four-year-old children to adult females. *Child Development, 41,* 601–611.

Lang, A. R., Pelham, W. E., Atkeson, B. M., & Murphy, D. A. (1999). Effects of alcohol intoxication on parenting behavior and interactions with child confederates exhibiting normal or deviant behavior. *Journal of Abnormal Child Psychology, 27,* 177–189.

Lawton, J. M., & Sanders, M. R. (1994). Designing effective behavioral family interventions for stepfamilies. *Clinical Psychology Review, 14,* 463–496.

Lay, K., Waters, E., & Park, K. A. (1989). Maternal responsiveness and child compliance: The role of mood as a mediator. *Child Development, 60,* 1405–1411.

Lloyd, B. M., Case, L., Ducharme, J., & Feldman, M. A. (1988, May). *Teaching child behavior management skills to developmentally handicapped persons.* Paper presented at the meeting of the Association of Applied Behavior Analysis, Philadelphia.

Loeber, R., & Keenan, K. (1994). Interaction between conduct disorder and its comorbid conditions: Effects of age and gender. *Clinical Psychology Review, 14,* 497–523.

Long, N., & Forehand R. (2000a). Modifications of a parental training program for implementation beyond the clinical setting. In N. N. Singh, J. P. Leung, & A. N. Singh (Eds.), *International perspectives on child and adolescent mental health* (pp. 293–310). New York: Elsevier.

Long, N., & Forehand, R. (2000b). *Parenting the strong-willed child: Leader's guide for the 6–week parenting class.* (Available from Nicholas Long, Department of Pediatrics, University of Arkansas School for Medical Sciences, 1612 Marily St., Little Rock, AR 72202.)

Long, N., & Forehand, R. (2002a, June). *Evaluation of a parenting class for parents of young strong-willed children.* Paper presented at the Third International Conference on Child and Adolescent Mental Health, Brisbane, Australia.

Long, N., & Forehand, R. (2002b). *Making divorce easier on your child: 50 effective ways to help children adjust.* New York: McGraw-Hill.

Long, N., Rickert, V. I., & Ashcraft, E. W. (1993). Bibliotherapy as an adjunct to stimulant medication in the treatment of attention deficit hyperactivity disorder. *Journal of Pediatric Health Care, 7,* 82–88.

Long, P., Forehand, R., Wierson, M., & Morgan, A. (1994). Moving into adulthood: Does parent training with young noncompliant children have long term effects? *Behaviour Research and Therapy, 32,* 101–107.

Lovaas, O. I., & Newsom, C. D. (1976). Behavior modification with psychotic children. In H. Leitenberg (Ed.), *Handbook of behavior modification and behavior therapy* (pp. 303–360). Englewood Cliffs, NJ: Prentice-Hall.

Lutzker, J. R. (1984). Project 12–Ways: Treating child abuse and neglect from an ecobehavioral perspective. In R. F. Dangel & R. A. Polster (Eds.), *Parent training: Foundations of research and practice* (pp. 260–297). New York: Guilford Press.

Lutzker, J. R., Campbell, R. V., Newman, M. R., & Harrold, M. (1989). Ecobehavioral interventions for abusive, neglectful, and high-risk families. In G. H. S. Singer & L. K. Irvin (Eds.), *Support for caregiving families: Enabling positive adaptation to disability* (pp. 313–326). Baltimore: Paul H. Brookes.

Lyon, G. R. (Ed.). (1994). *Frames of reference for the assessment of learning disabilities: New views on measurement issues.* Baltimore: Paul H. Brookes.

Lyons-Ruth, K. (1996). Attachment relationships among children with aggressive behavior problems: The role of disorganized early attachment patterns. *Journal of Consulting and Clinical Psychology, 64,* 64–73.

Maccoby, E. A., & Martin, J. A. (1983). Socialization in the context of the family: Parent–child interaction. In P. H. Mussen (Ed.), *Handbook of child psychology* (4th ed., Vol. 4, pp. 1–101). New York: Wiley.

MacKenzie, E. P., & Hilgedick, J. M. (1999). The computer-assisted parenting program (CAPP): The use of a computerized behavioral parent training program as an educational tool. *Child & Family Behavior Therapy, 21*(4), 23–43.

Manne, S. L. (1998). Treatment adherence and compliance. In R. T. Ammerman & J. V. Campo (Eds.), *Handbook of pediatric psychology and psychiatry: Vol. II. Disease, injury, and illness* (pp. 103–132). Needham Heights, MA: Allyn & Bacon.

March, J. S., Wells, K. C., & Conners, C. K. (1995). Attention-deficit/hyperactivity disorder: Part I. Assessment and diagnosis. *Journal of Practical Psychiatry and Behavioral Health, 1*, 219–228.

Margolin, G. (1990). Marital conflict. In G. H. Brody & I. E. Sigel (Eds.), *Methods of family research: Bibliographies and research projects: Vol. 2. Clinical populations* (pp. 191–225). Hillsdale, NJ: Erlbaum.

Margolin, G., Oliver, P. H., Gordis, E. B., O'Hearn, H. G., Medina, A. M., Ghosh, C. M., & Morland, L. (1998). The nuts and bolts of behavioral observation of marital and family interaction. *Clinical Child and Family Psychology Review, 1*, 195–213.

Marholin, D., Siegel, L. J., & Phillips, D. (1976). Treatment and transfer: A search for empirical procedures. In M. Hersen, R. M. Eisler, & P. M. Miller (Eds.), *Progress in behavior modification* (Vol. 3, pp. 293–342). New York: Academic Press.

Marsiglio, W., Amato, P., Day, R. D., & Lamb, M. E. (2000). Scholarship on fatherhood in the 1990s and beyond. *Journal of Marriage and the Family, 62*, 1173–1191.

Mash, E. J., & Johnston, C. (1982). A comparison of the mother–child interactions of younger and older hyperactive and normal children. *Child Development, 53*, 1371–1381.

Mash, E. J., & Johnston, C. (1990). Determinants of parenting stress: Illustrations from families of hyperactive children and families of physically abused children. *Journal of Clinical Child Psychology, 19*, 313–328.

Mash, E. J., Lazere, R., Terdal, L., & Garner, A. (1973). Modification of mother–child interactions: A modeling approach for groups. *Child Study Journal, 3*, 131–143.

Mash, E. J., & Terdal, L. (1973). Modification of mother–child interactions: Playing with children. *Mental Retardation, 11*, 44–49.

Mash, E. J., & Terdal, L. G. (1997). Assessment of child and family disturbance: A behavioral-systems approach. In E. J. Mash & L. G. Terdal (Eds.), *Assessment of childhood disorders* (3rd ed., pp. 3–68). New York: Guilford Press.

McElreath, L. H., & Eisenstadt, T. H. (1994). Child directed interaction: Family play therapy for developmentally delayed preschoolers. In C. E. Schaefer & L. Carey (Eds.), *Family play therapy* (pp. 271–292). Northvale, NJ: Aronson.

McKee, W. T. (1984). *Acceptability of alternative classroom treatment strategies and factors affecting teachers' ratings.* Unpublished master's thesis, University of British Columbia, Vancouver.

McMahon, R. J. (1987). Some current issues in the behavioral assessment of conduct disordered children and their families. *Behavioral Assessment, 9*, 235–252.

McMahon, R. J. (1991). Parent management training. In V. E. Caballo (Ed.), *Manual de técnicas de terapia y modificacion de conducta [Handbook of behavior therapy methods and techniques]* (pp. 445–471). Madrid, Spain: Siglo XXI de España Editores, S.A.

McMahon, R. J. (1999). Parent training. In S. W. Russ & T. H. Ollendick (Eds.), *Handbook of psychotherapies with children and adolescents* (pp. 153–180). New York: Kluwer Academic/Plenum Press.

McMahon, R. J., & Davies, G. R. (1980). A behavioral parent training program and its side effects on classroom behavior. *B. C. Journal of Special Education, 4,* 165–174.

McMahon, R. J., Davies, G. R., & Tiedemann, G. L. (1983, December). *Developmental considerations in using time out: Adjunctive procedures and age effects.* Paper presented at the meeting of the World Congress on Behavior Therapy, Washington, DC.

McMahon, R. J., & Estes, A. (1994). *Fast Track parent–child interaction task: Observational data collection manuals.* Unpublished manuscript, University of Washington.

McMahon, R. J., & Estes, A. M. (1997). Conduct problems. In E. J. Mash & L. G. Terdal (Eds.), *Assessment of childhood disorders* (3rd ed., pp. 130–193). New York: Guilford Press.

McMahon, R. J., & Forehand, R. (1978). Nonprescription behavior therapy: Effectiveness of a brochure in teaching mothers to correct their children's inappropriate mealtime behavior. *Behavior Therapy, 9,* 814–820.

McMahon, R. J., & Forehand, R. (1980). Self-help behavior therapies in parent training. In B. B. Lahey & A. E. Kazdin (Eds.), *Advances in clinical child psychology* (Vol. 3, pp. 149–176). New York: Plenum Press.

McMahon, R. J., & Forehand, R. (1981). Suggestions for evaluating self-administered materials in parent training. *Child Behavior Therapy, 3*(1), 38–39.

McMahon, R. J., & Forehand, R. L. (1983). Consumer satisfaction in behavioral treatment of children: Types, issues, and recommendations. *Behavior Therapy, 14,* 209–225.

McMahon, R. J., & Forehand, R. L. (1988). Conduct disorders. In E. J. Mash & L. G. Terdal (Eds.), *Behavioral assessment of childhood disorders* (2nd ed., pp. 105–157). New York: Guilford Press.

McMahon, R. J., Forehand, R., & Griest, D. L. (1981). Effects of knowledge of social learning principles on enhancing treatment outcome and generalization in a parent training program. *Journal of Consulting and Clinical Psychology, 49,* 526–532.

McMahon, R. J., Forehand, R., Griest, D. L., & Wells, K. C. (1981). Who drops out of treatment during parent behavioral training? *Behavioral Counseling Quarterly, 1,* 79–85.

McMahon, R. J., Forehand, R., & Tiedemann, G. (1985, November). *Relative effectiveness of a parent training program with children of different ages.* Paper presented at the meeting of the Association for Advancement of Behavior Therapy, Houston.

McMahon, R. J., Johnson, K. K., & Robbins, K. H. (2003). *Acceptability of written instructions versus therapist administration of a parent training program.* Manuscript submitted for publication.

McMahon, R. J., & Lehman, K. (2003). *Effectiveness of written instructions in teaching mothers to give clear instructions to their children.* Manuscript submitted for publication.

McMahon, R. J., Slough, N. M., & the Conduct Problems Prevention Research Group. (1994). *Fast Track Parent Group Curriculum.* Unpublished manuals, University of Washington.

McMahon, R. J., Slough, N. M., & the Conduct Problems Prevention Research Group. (1996). Family-based intervention in the Fast Track Program. In R. DeV. Peters & R. J. McMahon (Eds.), *Preventing childhood disorders, substance abuse, and delinquency* (pp. 90–110). Thousand Oaks, CA: Sage.

McMahon, R. J., Tiedemann, G. L., & Davies, G. R. (1987, June). *Contingent parental attention: Enhancing its effects with verbal rationales and modeling.* Paper presented at the meeting of the Canadian Psychological Association, Vancouver, BC.

McMahon, R. J., Tiedemann, G., Forehand, R., & Griest, D. L. (1984). Parental satisfaction with parent training to modify child noncompliance. *Behavior Therapy, 15*, 295–303.

McMahon, R. J., & Wells, K. C. (1998). Conduct problems. In E. J. Mash & R. A. Barkley (Eds.), *Treatment of childhood disorders* (pp. 111–207). New York: Guilford Press.

McNeil, C. B., Eyberg, S., Eisenstadt, T. H., Newcomb, K., & Funderburk, B. (1991). Parent–child interaction therapy with behavior problem children: Generalization of treatment effects to the school setting. *Journal of Clinical Child Psychology, 20*, 140–151.

Mellon, M. W., & Houts, A. C. (1998). Home-based treatment for primary enuresis. In J. M. Briesmeister & C. E. Schaefer (Eds.), *Handbook of parent training: Parents as co-therapists for children's behavior problems* (2nd ed., pp. 384–417). New York: Wiley.

Mellon, M. W., & Stern, H. P. (1998). Elimination disorders. In R. T. Ammerman & J. V. Campo (Eds.), *Handbook of pediatric psychology and psychiatry: Vol. 1. Psychological and psychiatric issues in pediatric settings* (pp. 182–198). Needham Heights, MA: Allyn & Bacon.

Metzler, C., Eddy, M., & Taylor, T. K. (2002, May). The evidence standards of ten "best practices" lists and the evidence base of the top family-focused programs. In C. Metzler (Chair), *Finding common ground among "best practices" lists: The evidence base and program elements of top family-focused and school-based programs.* Symposium conducted at the meeting of the Society for Prevention Research, Seattle, WA.

Miller, G. E., & Prinz, R. J. (1990). Enhancement of social learning family interventions for childhood conduct disorder. *Psychological Bulletin, 108*, 291–307.

Miller, W. H. (1975). A systematic comparison of instructional techniques for parents. *Behavior Therapy, 6*, 14–21.

Minuchin, S. (1974). *Families and family therapy.* Cambridge, MA: Harvard University Press.

Moffitt, T. E. (1993). "Adolescence-limited" and "life-course-persistent" antisocial behavior: A developmental taxonomy. *Psychological Review, 100*, 674–701.

Monti, P. M., Kadden, R. M., Rohsenow, D. J., Cooney, N. L., & Abrams, D. B. (2002). *Treating alcohol dependence: A coping skills training guide* (2nd ed.). New York: Guilford Press.

Newsom, C. (1998). Autistic disorder. In E. J. Mash & R. A. Barkley (Eds.), *Treatment of childhood disorders* (2nd ed., pp. 416–467). New York: Guilford Press.

Nicholson, J. M., & Sanders, M. R. (1999). Randomized control trial of behavioral family intervention for the treatment of child behavior problems in stepfamilies. *Journal of Marriage & Remarriage, 30*, 1–23.

O'Brien, F., & Azrin, N. H. (1972). Developing proper mealtime behaviors of the institutionalized retarded. *Journal of Applied Behavior Analysis, 5*, 389–399.

O'Dell, S. L (1974). Training parents in behavior modification: A review. *Psychological Bulletin, 81*, 418–433.

O'Dell, S. L. (1985). Progress in parent training. In M. Hersen, R. M. Eisler, & P. M. Miller (Eds.), *Progress in behavior modification* (Vol. 9, pp. 57–108). New York: Academic Press.

O'Dell, S. L., Flynn, J. M., & Benlolo, L. A. (1977). A comparison of parent training techniques in child behavior modification. *Journal of Behavior Therapy and Experimental Psychiatry, 8*, 261–268.

O'Dell, S. L., Tarler-Benlolo, L. A., & Flynn, J. M. (1979). An instrument to measure knowledge of behavioral principles as applied to children. *Journal of Behavior Therapy and Experimental Psychiatry, 10*, 29–34.

O'Farrell, T. J. (1993). *Treating alcohol problems: Marital and family interventions.* New York: Guilford Press.

Oldershaw, L., Walters, G. C., & Hall, D. K. (1986). Control strategies and noncompliance: An observational study. *Child Development, 57,* 722–732.

O'Leary, K. D., & Emery, R. E. (1984). Marital discord and child problems. In M. D. Levine & P. Satz (Eds.), *Developmental variation in dysfunction* (pp. 345–364). New York: Academic Press.

Ollendick, T. H., & King, N. J. (1994). Diagnosis, assessment, and treatment of internalizing problems in children: The role of longitudinal data. *Journal of Consulting and Clinical Psychology, 62,* 918–927.

Parpal, M., & Maccoby, E. E. (1985). Maternal responsiveness and subsequent child compliance. *Child Development, 56,* 1326–1334.

Parrish, J. M., Cataldo, M. F., Kolko, D. J., Neef, N. A., & Egel, A. L. (1986). Experimental analysis of response covariation among compliant and inappropriate behaviors. *Journal of Applied Behavior Analysis, 19,* 241–254.

Patterson, G. R. (1974). Interventions for boys with conduct problems: Multiple settings, treatments and criteria. *Journal of Consulting and Clinical Psychology, 42,* 471–481.

Patterson, G. R. (1975). *Families: Applications of social learning to family life* (rev. ed.). Champaign, IL: Research Press.

Patterson, G. R. (1976). *Living with children: New methods for parents and teachers* (rev. ed.). Champaign, IL: Research Press.

Patterson, G. R. (1982). *Coercive family process.* Eugene, OR: Castalia.

Patterson, G. R. (1997). Performance models for parenting: A social interactional perspective. In J. E. Grusec & L. Kuczynski (Eds.), *Parenting and children's internalization of values: A handbook of contemporary theory* (pp. 193–226). New York: Wiley.

Patterson, G. R. (2002). The early development of coercive family process. In J. B. Reid, G. R. Patterson, & J. Snyder (Eds.), *Antisocial behavior in children and adolescents: A developmental analysis and model for intervention* (pp. 25–44). Washington, DC: American Psychological Association.

Patterson, G. R., Capaldi, D., & Bank, L. (1991). An early starter model for predicting delinquency. In D. J. Pepler & K. H. Rubin (Eds.), *The development and treatment of childhood aggression* (pp. 139–168). Hillsdale, NJ: Erlbaum.

Patterson, G. R., & Chamberlain, P. (1988). Treatment process: A problem at three levels. In L. C. Wynne (Ed.), *The state of the art in family therapy research: Controversies and recommendations* (pp. 189–223). New York: Family Process Press.

Patterson, G. R., & Chamberlain, P. (1994). A functional analysis of resistance during parent training therapy. *Clinical Psychology: Science and Practice, 1,* 53–70.

Patterson, G. R., Cobb, J. A., & Ray, R. S. (1973). A social engineering technology for retraining the families of aggressive boys. In H. E. Adams & I. P. Unikel (Eds.), *Issues and trends in behavior therapy* (pp. 139–210). Springfield, IL: Charles C Thomas.

Patterson, G. R., & Forgatch, M. S. (1985). Therapist behavior as a determinant for client noncompliance: A paradox for the behavior modifier. *Journal of Consulting and Clinical Psychology, 53,* 846–851.

Patterson, G. R., Reid, J. B., & Dishion, T. J. (1992). *Antisocial boys.* Eugene, OR: Castalia.

Patterson, G. R., Reid, J. B., Jones, R. R., & Conger, R. E. (1975). *A social learning approach to family intervention: Vol. 1. Families with aggressive children.* Eugene, OR: Castalia.

Patterson, G. R., & Yoerger, K. (2002). A developmental model for early and late-onset delinquency. In J. B. Reid, G. R. Patterson, & J. Snyder (Eds.), *Antisocial behavior in children and adolescents: A developmental analysis and model for intervention* (pp. 147–172). Washington, DC: American Psychological Association.

Peed, S., Roberts, M., & Forehand, R. (1977). Evaluation of the effectiveness of a standardized parent training program in altering the interactions of mothers and their noncompliant children. *Behavior Modification, 1,* 323–350.

Pelham, W. E., & Lang, A. R. (1993). Parental alcohol consumption and deviant child behavior: Laboratory studies and reciprocal effects. *Clinical Psychology Review, 13,* 763–784.

Pelham, W. E., Schnedler, R. W., Bender, M. E., Nilsson, D. E., Miller, J., Budrow, M. S., Ronnei, M., Paluchowski, C., & Marks, D. A. (1988). The combination of behavior therapy and methylphenidate in the treatment of attention deficit disorders: A therapy outcome study. In L. Bloomingdale (Ed.), *Attention deficit disorders* (Vol. 3, pp. 29–48). London: Pergamon Press.

Pelham, W. E., Wheeler, T., & Chronis, A. (1998). Empirically supported psychosocial treatments for attention deficit hyperactivity disorder. *Journal of Clinical Child Psychology, 27,* 190–205.

Peterson, S. L., Robinson, E. A., & Littman, I. (1983). Parent–child interaction training for parents with a history of mental retardation. *Applied Research in Mental Retardation, 4,* 329–342.

Phares, V., & Compas, B. E. (1992). The role of fathers in child and adolescent psychopathology: Make room for daddy. *Psychological Bulletin, 111,* 387–412.

Pisterman, S., Firestone, P., McGrath, P., Goodman, J. T., Webster, I., Mallory, R., & Goffin, B. (1992a). The effects of parent training on parenting stress and sense of competence. *Canadian Journal of Behavioural Science, 24,* 41–58.

Pisterman, S., Firestone, P., McGrath, P., Goodman, J. T., Webster, I., Mallory, R., & Goffin, B. (1992b). The role of parent training in treatment of preschoolers with ADDH. *American Journal of Orthopsychiatry, 62,* 397–408.

Pisterman, S., McGrath, P., Firestone, P., Goodman, J. T., Webster, I., & Mallory, R. (1989). Outcome of parent-mediated treatment of preschoolers with attention deficit disorder with hyperactivity. *Journal of Consulting and Clinical Psychology, 57,* 628–635.

Pollard, S., Ward, E. M., & Barkley, R. A. (1983). The effects of parent training and Ritalin on the parent–child interactions of hyperactive boys. *Child & Family Behavior Therapy, 5*(4), 51–69.

Porter, B., & O'Leary, K. D. (1980). Marital discord and childhood behavior problems. *Journal of Abnormal Child Psychology, 8,* 287–295.

Prinz, R. J., & Miller, G. E. (1994). Family-based treatment for childhood antisocial behavior: Experimental influences on dropout and engagement. *Journal of Consulting and Clinical Psychology, 62,* 645–650.

Prinz, R. J., & Miller, G. E. (1996). Parental engagement in interventions for children at risk for conduct disorder. In R. Dev. Peters & R. J. McMahon (Eds.), *Preventing childhood disorders, substance abuse, and delinquency* (pp. 161–183). Thousand Oaks, CA: Sage.

Ramsey, E., Patterson, G. R., & Walker, H. M. (1990). Generalization of the antisocial trait from home to school settings. *Journal of Applied Developmental Psychology, 11,* 209–223.

Rayfied, A., Monaco, L., & Eyberg, S. M. (1999). Parent–child interaction therapy with oppositional children: Review and clinical strategies. In S. W. Russ & T. H. Ollendick (Eds.), *Handbook of psychotherapies with children and families* (pp. 327–343). New York: Kluwer Academic/Plenum Press.

Richters, J. E., Arnold, L. E., Jensen, P. S., Abikoff, H., Conners, C. K., Greenhill, L. L., Hechtman, L., Hinshaw, S. P., Pelham, W. E., & Swanson, J. M. (1995). NIMH collaborative multisite multimodal treatment study of children with ADHD: I. Background and rationale. *Journal of the American Academy of Child and Adolescent Psychiatry, 34,* 987–1000.

Rickard, K. M., Forehand, R., Atkeson, B. M., & Lopez, C. (1982). An examination of the effects of marital satisfaction and divorce on parent–child interactions. *Journal of Clinical Child Psychology, 11,* 61–65.

Rickard, K. M., Forehand, R., Wells, K. C., Griest, D. L., & McMahon, R. J. (1981). Factors in the referral of children for behavioral treatment: A comparison of mothers of clinic-referred deviant, clinic-referred non-deviant, and non-clinic children. *Behaviour Research and Therapy, 19,* 201–205.

Risley, T. R., Clark, H. B., & Cataldo, M. F. (1976). Behavioral technology for the normal middle-class family. In E. J. Mash, L. A. Hamerlynck, & L. C. Handy (Eds.), *Behavior modification and families* (pp. 34–60). New York: Brunner/Mazel.

Robbins, M. S., Alexander, J. F., Newell, R. M., & Turner, C. W. (1996). The immediate effect of reframing on client attitude in family therapy. *Journal of Family Psychology, 10,* 28–34.

Robbins, M. S., Alexander, J. F., & Turner, C. W. (2000). Disrupting defensive family interactions in family therapy with delinquent adolescents. *Journal of Family Psychology, 14,* 688–701.

Roberts, M. W. (1982). The effects of warned versus unwarned time-out procedures on child noncompliance. *Child & Family Behavior Therapy, 4*(1), 37–53.

Roberts, M. W. (1988). Enforcing chair timeouts with room timeouts. *Behavior Modification, 12,* 353–370.

Roberts, M. W. (1995). *Parent handouts.* Unpublished material, Idaho State University.

Roberts, M. W. (2001). Clinic observations of structured parent–child interaction designed to evaluate externalizing problems. *Psychological Assessment, 13,* 46–58.

Roberts, M. W., Hatzenbuehler, L. C., & Bean, A. W. (1981). The effects of differential attention and time out on child noncompliance. *Behavior Therapy, 12,* 93–99.

Roberts, M. W., Joe, V. C., & Rowe-Hallbert, A. L. (1992). Oppositional child behavior and parental locus of control. *Journal of Clinical Child Psychology, 21,* 170–177.

Roberts, M. W., McMahon, R. J., Forehand, R., & Humphreys, L. (1978). The effect of parental instruction-giving on child compliance. *Behavior Therapy, 9,* 793–798.

Roberts, M. W., & Powers, S. W. (1988). The Compliance Test. *Behavioral Assessment, 10,* 375–398.

Roberts, M. W., & Powers, S. W. (1990). Adjusting chair timeout enforcement procedures for oppositional children. *Behavior Therapy, 21,* 257–271.

Rogers, T. R., Forehand, R., Griest, D. L., Wells, K. C., & McMahon, R. J. (1981). Socioeconomic status: Effects on parent and child behaviors and treatment outcome of parent training. *Journal of Clinical Child Psychology, 10,* 98–101.

Ross, C. N., Blanc, H. M., McNeil, C. B., Eyberg, S. M., & Hembree-Kigin, T. L. (1998). Parenting stress in mothers of young children with oppositional defiant disorder and other severe behavior problems. *Child Study Journal, 28,* 93–110.

Rothbart, M. K., & Bates, J. E. (1998). Temperament. In W. Damon (Series Ed.) & N. Eisenberg (Vol. Ed.), *Handbook of child psychology: Vol. 3. Social, emotional and personality development* (5th ed., pp. 105–176). New York: Wiley.

Russo, D. C., Cataldo, M. F., & Cushing, P. J. (1981). Compliance training and behavioral covariation in the treatment of multiple behavior problems. *Journal of Applied Behavior Analysis, 14,* 209–222.

Rutter, M. (1994). Family discord and conduct disorder: Cause, consequence, or correlate? *Journal of Family Psychology, 8,* 170–186.

Sajwaj, T., & Dillon, A. (1977). Complexities of an "elementary" behavior modification procedure: Differential adult attention used for children's behavior disorders. In B. C. Etzel, J. M. LeBlanc, & D. M. Baer (Eds.), *New developments in behavioral research: Theory, method, and application* (pp. 303–315). Hillsdale, NJ: Erlbaum.

Salzinger, K., Feldman, R. S., & Portnoy, S. (1970). Training parents of brain-injured children in the use of operant conditioning procedures. *Behavior Therapy, 1,* 4–32.

Sanders, M. R., & Dadds, M. R. (1992). Children's and parents' cognitions about family interaction: An evaluation of video-mediated recall and thought listing procedures in the assessment of conduct-disordered children. *Journal of Clinical Child Psychology, 21,* 371–379.

Sanders, M. R., & Dadds, M. R. (1993). *Behavioral family intervention.* Boston: Allyn & Bacon.

Sanders, M. R., & Lawton, J. M. (1993). Discussing assessment findings with families: A guided participation model of information transfer. *Child & Family Behavior Therapy, 15*(2), 5–35.

Sanders, M. R., & Markie-Dadds, C. (1992). Toward a technology of prevention of disruptive behaviour disorders: The role of behavioural family intervention. *Behaviour Change, 9,* 186–200.

Sanders, M. R., Markie-Dadds, C., Tully, L. A., & Bor, W. (2000). The Triple P-Positive Parenting Program: A comparison of enhanced, standard, and self-directed behavioral family intervention for parents of child with early onset conduct problems. *Journal of Consulting and Clinical Psychology, 68,* 624–640.

Sanders, M. R., Patel, R. K., Le Grice, B., & Shepherd, R. W. (1993). Children with persistent feeding difficulties: An observational analysis of the feeding interactions of problem and non-problem eaters. *Health Psychology, 12,* 64–73.

Sanders, M. R., & Plant, K. (1989). Programming for generalization to high and low risk parenting situations in families with oppositional developmentally disabled preschoolers. *Behavior Modification, 13,* 283–305.

Sanson, A., Oberklaid, F., Pedlow, R., & Prior, M. (1991). Risk indicators: Assessment of infancy predictors of pre-school behavioural maladjustment. *Journal of Child Psychology and Psychiatry, 32,* 609–626.

Sarason, I. G., Johnson, J. H., & Siegel, J. M. (1978). Assessing the impact of life changes: Development of the Life Experiences Survey. *Journal of Consulting and Clinical Psychology, 46,* 932–946.

Saunders, B. E., Berliner, L., & Hanson, R. F. (2001). *Guidelines for the psychosocial treatment of intrafamilial child physical and sexual abuse (Final draft report: July 30, 2001)* [Online]. Charleston, SC: Authors. Available: *http://www.musc.edu/cvc/*

Saunders, J. D., Aasland, O. G., Babor, T. F., de la Fuente, J. R., & Grant, M. (1993). Development of the Alcohol Use Disorders Identification Test (AUDIT): WHO collaborative project on early detection of persons with harmful alcohol consumption—II. *Addiction, 88,* 791–804.

Scarboro, M. E., & Forehand, R. (1975). Effects of response-contingent isolation and ignoring on compliance and oppositional behavior of children. *Journal of Experimental Child Psychology, 19,* 252–264.

Schaefer, C. E., & Briesmeister, J. M. (Eds.). (1989). *Handbook of parent training: Parents as co-therapists for children's behavior problems.* New York: Wiley.

Schindler, F., & Arkowitz, H. (1986). The assessment of mother–child interactions in physically abusive and nonabusive families. *Journal of Family Violence, 1,* 247–257.

Schoen, S. F. (1983). The status of compliance technology: Implications for programming. *Journal of Special Education, 17,* 483–496.

Schroeder, C. S., & Gordon, B. N. (2002). *Assessment and treatment of childhood problems: A clinician's guide* (2nd ed.). New York: Guilford Press.

Selzer, M. L., Vinokur, A., & van Rooijen, L. (1975). A self-administered short Michigan Alcoholism Screening Test. *Journal of Studies on Alcohol, 36,* 117–126.

Serketich, W. J., & Dumas, J. E. (1996). The effectiveness of behavioral parent training to modify antisocial behavior in children: A meta-analysis. *Behavior Therapy, 27,* 171–186.

Shaw, D. S., Bell, R. Q., & Gilliom, M. (2000). A truly early starter model of antisocial behavior revisited. *Clinical Child and Family Psychology Review, 3,* 155–172.

Shaw, D. S., Keenan, K., & Vondra, J. I. (1994). Developmental precursors of externalizing behavior: Ages 1 to 3. *Developmental Psychology, 30,* 355–364.

Slabach, E. H., Morrow, J., & Wachs, T. D. (1991). Questionnaire measurement of infant and child temperament: Current status and future directions. In J. Strelau & A. Angleitner (Eds.), *Explorations in temperament: International perspectives on theory and measurement* (pp. 205–234). New York: Plenum Press.

Slep, A. M., & O'Leary, S. G. (1998). The effects of maternal attributions on parenting: An experimental analysis. *Journal of Family Psychology, 12,* 234–243.

Sloane, H. N., Endo, G. T., Hawkes, T. W., & Jenson, W. R., (1990). Improving child compliance through self-instructional parent training materials. *Child & Family Behavior Therapy, 12*(4), 39–64.

Snyder, J. (1991). Discipline as a mediator of the impact of maternal stress and mood on child conduct problems. *Development and Psychopathology, 3,* 263–276.

Snyder, J., & Stoolmiller, M. (2002). Reinforcement and coercion mechanisms in the development of antisocial behavior: The family. In J. B. Reid, G. R. Patterson, & J. Snyder (Eds.), *Antisocial behavior in children and adolescents: A developmental analysis and model for intervention* (pp. 65–100). Washington, DC: American Psychological Association.

Sobell, M. B., & Sobell, L. C. (1993). *Problem drinkers: Guided self-change treatment.* New York: Guilford Press.

Spanier, G. B. (1976). Measuring dyadic adjustment: New scales for assessing the quality of marriage and similar dyads. *Journal of Marriage and the Family, 38,* 15–28.

Spitzer, A., Webster-Stratton, C., & Hollinsworth, T. (1991). Coping with conduct-problem children: Parents gaining knowledge and control. *Journal of Clinical Child Psychology, 20,* 413–427.

Stolberg, A. L., Zacharias, M. A., & Camplair, C. W. (1991). *Children of divorce: Leader's guide, kids book, & parents book.* Circle Pines, MN: American Guidance Service.

Stoolmiller, M., Duncan, T., Bank, L., & Patterson, G. R. (1993). Some problems and solutions in the study of change: Significant patterns in client resistance. *Journal of Consulting and Clinical Psychology, 61,* 920–928.

Strain, P. S., Lambert, D. L., Kerr, M. M., Stagg, V., & Lenkner, D. A. (1983). Naturalistic assessment of children's compliance to teachers' requests and consequences for compliance. *Journal of Applied Behavior Analysis, 16,* 243–249.

Swanson, J. (1993). Effect of stimulant medication on hyperactive children: A review of reviews. *Exceptional Children, 60,* 154–162.

Tallmadge, J., & Barkley, R. A. (1983) The interactions of hyperactive and normal boys with their fathers and mothers. *Journal of Abnormal Child Psychology, 11,* 565–580.

Tavormina, J. B. (1975). Relative effectiveness of behavioral and reflective group counseling with parents of mentally retarded children. *Journal of Consulting and Clinical Psychology*, *43*, 22–31.

Tavormina, J. B., Henggeler, S. W., & Gayton, W. F. (1976). Age trends in parental assessments of the behavior problems of their retarded children. *Mental Retardation*, *14*, 38–39.

Taylor, T. K., & Biglan, A. (1998). Behavioral family interventions for improving child-rearing: A review of the literature for clinicians and policy makers. *Clinical Child and Family Psychology Review*, *1*, 41–60.

Taylor, E., Sandberg, S., Thorley, G., & Giles, S. (1991). *The epidemiology of childhood hyperactivity*. Oxford, UK: Oxford University Press.

Tharp, R. G., & Wetzel, R. J. (1969). *Behavior modification in the natural environment*. New York: Academic Press.

Thomas, A., Chess, S., & Birch, H. G. (1968). *Temperament and behavior*. New York: New York University Press.

Urquiza, A. J., & McNeil, C. B. (1996). Parent–child interaction therapy: An intensive dyadic intervention for physically abusive families. *Child Maltreatment*, *1*, 134–144.

Wahler, R. G. (1980). The insular mother: The problems in parent–child treatment. *Journal of Applied Behavior Analysis*, *13*, 207–219.

Wahler, R. G., & Afton, A. D. (1980). Attentional processes in insular and noninsular mothers: Some differences in their summary reports about child problem behaviors. *Child Behavior Therapy*, *2*(2), 25–41.

Wahler, R. G., & Bellamy, A. (1997). Generating reciprocity with conduct problem children and their mothers: The effectiveness of compliance teaching and responsive parenting. *Journal of Social and Personal Relationships*, *14*, 549–564.

Wahler, R. G., Cartor, P. G., Fleischman, J., & Lambert, W. (1993). The impact of synthesis teaching and parent training with mothers of conduct-disordered children. *Journal of Abnormal Child Psychology*, *21*, 425–440.

Wahler, R. G., & Cormier, W. H. (1970). The ecological interview: A first step in out-patient child behavior therapy. *Journal of Behavior Therapy and Experimental Psychiatry*, *1*, 279–289.

Wahler, R. G., & Dumas, J. E. (1984). Changing the observational coding styles of insular and noninsular mothers: A step toward maintenance of parent training effects. In R. F. Dangel & R. A. Polster (Eds.), *Parent training: Foundations of research and practice* (pp. 379–416). New York: Guilford Press.

Wahler, R. G., & Dumas, J. E. (1989). Attentional problems in dysfunctional mother–child interactions: An interbehavioral model. *Psychological Bulletin*, *105*, 116–130.

Wahler, R. G., Herring, M., & Edwards, M. (2001). Coregulation of balance between children's prosocial approaches and acts of compliance: A pathway to mother–child cooperation? *Journal of Clinical Child Psychology*, *30*, 473–478.

Wahler, R. G., Leske, G., & Rogers, E. S. (1979). The insular family: A deviance support system for oppositional children. In L. A. Hamerlynck (Ed.), *Behavioral systems for the developmentally disabled: Vol 1. School and family environments* (pp. 102–127). New York: Brunner/Mazel.

Wahler, R. G., & Sansbury, L. E. (1990). The monitoring skills of troubled mothers: Their problems in defining child deviance. *Journal of Abnormal Child Psychology*, *18*, 577–589.

Walker, H. M. (1995). *The acting-out child: Coping with classroom disruption* (2nd ed.). Longmont, CO: Sopris West.

Walker, H. M., Block-Pedego, A., Todis, B., & Severson, H. (1991). *School archival records search (SARS): User's guide and technical manual.* Longmont, CO: Sopris West.

Walker, H. M., Colvin, G., & Ramsey, E. (1995). *Antisocial behavior in school: Strategies and best practices.* Pacific Grove, CA: Brooks/Cole.

Walker, H. M., Shinn, M. R., O'Neill, R. E., & Ramsey, E. (1987). A longitudinal assessment of the development of antisocial behavior in boys: Rationale, methodology, and first-year results. *RASE: Remedial and Special Education, 8,* 7–16, 27.

Walker, H. M., & Walker, J. E. (1991). *Coping with noncompliance in the classroom: A positive approach for teachers.* Austin, TX: Pro-Ed.

Webster-Stratton, C. (1990a). Enhancing the effectiveness of self-administered videotape parent training for families with conduct-problem children. *Journal of Abnormal Child Psychology, 18,* 479–492.

Webster-Stratton, C. (1990b). Stress: A potential disruptor of parent perceptions and family interactions. *Journal of Clinical Child Psychology, 19,* 302–312.

Webster-Stratton, C. (1992). *The incredible years: A trouble-shooting guide for parents of children aged 3–8.* Toronto: Umbrella Press.

Webster-Stratton, C. (1994). Advancing videotape parent training: A comparison study. *Journal of Consulting and Clinical Psychology, 62,* 583–593.

Webster-Stratton, C. (1998). Preventing conduct problems in Head Start children: Strengthening parenting competencies. *Journal of Consulting and Clinical Psychology, 66,* 715–730.

Webster-Stratton, C. (2000). *"The Incredible Years training series" bulletin.* Washington, DC: U. S. Department of Justice, Office of Juvenile Justice and Delinquency Prevention.

Webster-Stratton, C., & Herbert, M. (1994). *Troubled families—Problem children.* Chichester, England: Wiley.

Webster-Stratton, C. Hollinsworth, T., & Kolpacoff, M. (1989). The long-term effectiveness and clinical significance of three cost-effective training programs for families with conduct-problem children. *Journal of Consulting and Clinical Psychology, 56,* 558–566.

Webster-Stratton, C., & Taylor, T. (2001). Nipping early risk factors in the bud: Preventing substance abuse, delinquency, and violence in adolescence through interventions targeted at young children (0–8 years). *Prevention Science, 2,* 165–192.

Wehman, P., & McLaughlin, P. (1979). Teachers' perceptions of behavior problems with severely and profoundly handicapped students. *Mental Retardation, 1,* 20–21.

Weiss, B., Dodge, K. A., Bates, J. E., & Pettit, G. S. (1992). Some consequences of early harsh discipline: Child aggression and a maladaptive social information processing style. *Child Development, 63,* 1321–1335.

Weiss, G., & Hechtman, L. T. (1993). *Hyperactive children grown up: ADHD in children, adolescents, and adults* (2nd ed.). New York: Guilford Press.

Wells, K. C. (1985). Behavioral family therapy. In A. S. Bellack & M. Hersen (Eds.), *Dictionary of behavior therapy techniques* (pp. 25–30). New York: Pergamon Press.

Wells, K. C. (1987). What do we know about the use and effects of behavior therapies in the treatment of ADD? In J. Loney (Ed.), *The young hyperactive child: Answers to questions about diagnosis, prognosis, and treatment* (pp. 111–122). New York: Haworth Press.

Wells, K. C., & Egan, J. (1988). Social learning and systems family therapy for childhood oppositional disorder: Comparative treatment outcome. *Comprehensive Psychiatry, 29,* 138–146.

Wells, K. C., Forehand, R., & Griest, D. L. (1980). Generality of treatment effects from treated to untreated behaviors resulting from a parent training program. *Journal of Clinical Child Psychology, 8*, 217–219.

Wells, K. C., Griest, D. L., & Forehand, R. (1980). The use of a self-control package to enhance temporal generality of a parent training program. *Behaviour Research and Therapy, 18*, 347–358.

Wells, K. C., Pelham, W., Kotkin, R., Hoza, B., Abikoff, H., Abramowitz, A., Arnold, E., Cantwell, D., Conners, C. K., Elliot, G., Greenhill, L., Hechtman, L., Hibbs, E., Hinshaw, S., Jensen, P., March, J., Swanson, J., & Schiller, E. (2000). Psychosocial treatment strategies in the MTA study: Rationale, methods, and critical issues in design and implementation. *Journal of Abnormal Child Psychology, 28*, 483–505.

Wells, K. C., Pfiffner, L. Abramowitz, A., Abikoff, H., Courtney, M., Cousins, L., Del Carmen, R., Eddy, M., Eggers, S., Fleiss, K., Heller, T., Hibbs, E., Hinshaw, S., Hoza, B., & Pelham, W. (1996). *Parent training for attention-deficit/hyperactivity disorder: The MTA study.* Unpublished manual.

Wenar, C. (1982). On negativism. *Human Development, 25*, 1–23.

West, M. O., & Prinz, R. J. (1987). Parental alcoholism and child psychopathology. *Psychological Bulletin, 102*, 204–218.

Whipple, E. E., Fitzgerald, H. E., & Zucker, R. A. (1995). Parent–child interactions in alcoholic and nonalcoholic families. *American Journal of Orthopsychiatry, 65*, 153–159.

Whiting, B. B., & Edwards, C. P. (1988). *Children of different worlds: The formation of social behavior.* Cambridge, MA: Harvard University Press.

Williams, C. A., & Forehand, R. (1984). An examination of predictor variables for child compliance and noncompliance. *Journal of Abnormal Child Psychology, 12*, 491–504.

Williams, C. D. (1959). The elimination of tantrum behaviors by extinction procedures. *Journal of Abnormal and Social Psychology, 59*, 269–270.

Willner, A. G., Braukmann, C. J., Kirigin, K. A., Fixsen, D. L., Phillips, E. L., & Wolf, M. M. (1977). The training and validation of youth-preferred social behaviors of child-care personnel. *Journal of Applied Behavior Analysis, 10*, 219–230.

Wittes, G., & Radin, N. (1968). *Parent manual on child rearing.* Unpublished manuscript. (Available from Ypsilanti Early Education Program, Ypsilanti, Michigan.)

Wolf, M. M. (1978). Social validity: The case for subjective measurement or how applied behavior analysis is finding its heart. *Journal of Applied Behavior Analysis, 11*, 203–214.

Wolfe, D. A. (1999). *Child abuse: Implications for child development and psychopathology* (2nd ed.). Thousand Oaks, CA: Sage.

Wolfe, D. A., Edwards, B., Manion, I., & Koverola, C. (1988). Early intervention for child abuse and neglect: A preliminary investigation. *Journal of Consulting and Clinical Psychology, 56*, 40–47.

Wolfe, D. A., & Sandler, J. (1981). Training abusive parents in effective child management. *Behavior Modification, 5*, 320–335.

Wruble, M. K., Sheeber, L. B., Sorensen, E. K., Boggs, S. R., & Eyberg, S. (1991). Empirical derivation of child compliance time. *Child & Family Behavior Therapy, 13*(1), 57–68.

Zucker, R. A., & Fitzgerald, H. E. (1992). *The Antisocial Behavior Checklist.* East Lansing: Michigan State University Family Study, Department of Psychology.

Index

Page numbers followed by an *f* indicate figure; *t*, table.